Contents

Section V: Methods and Effects of Training   193

Section VI: Training Plans   309

Foreword

I am pleased to be associated with this book for a number of reasons. Firstly, I have known Brent Rushall for many years, since the days when he was a coach with my own school of swimming at Ryde in Sydney in the early 1960s, progressing to his work with the famed Dr Jim Counsilman in the United States and then throughout his academic and coaching careers where he has become one of the foremost sports psychologists in the world. I have great respect both for his knowledge and for his ability to apply it in a variety of sporting situations.

I am also familiar with Frank Pyke who, as an exercise physiologist, has made a significant contribution to sport, particularly in Australia. The quality of his writing and lecturing skills in both community-based coaching and tertiary-level physical education courses is widely acknowledged.

Brent and Frank met at Indiana University and formed a bond of friendship through their common interest and expertise in sports science. This finally culminated in a book that skilfully draws upon both the biological and behavioral sciences to better explain the responses of athletes to sports training. The breadth of experience of both authors with many sports in several different countries is clearly evident throughout the book which makes a unique contribution to the literature available in this field.

The authors underline clearly the importance of being systematic and careful when prescribing effective training programs. They present a definite point of view on many of the controversial issues that surround the application of modern training practices in sport and the book will challenge the thoughtful coach and trainer to evaluate his or her methods closely. I commend it to you.

Forbes Carlile, MBE
Sydney, Australia

Preface

The principal aim of this book is to present the major issues of planning and implementing sports training programs as a means of developing the physical capacities that underlie athletes' performances. It is intended to serve as a resource handbook for coaches and athletes who are serious about their involvement in sport. It attempts to relate the latest thinking and practices of sport conditioning. The prescriptive principles that are developed are intended to allow a practitioner to understand, plan, and maximize the usefulness of physical training for sport.

To achieve this aim we have relied upon research, first-hand knowledge of the practices of world-class programs and coaches, and our own experiences as consultants, coaches, and researchers. In synthesizing the available research it was necessary to survey many more references than those included in the bibliography. The references that are cited there are, however, good examples of the type of formative research or existing expert opinion. For readers who need more background knowledge on any of the recommendations, we advise consulting the cited references, then using them as a source for more extensive knowledge by reviewing the items included in their own reference lists.

The motivation for this text was the time in the late 1960s when both authors were Australians studying at Indiana University. We decided then to focus on different areas of performance enhancement, psychology and physiology. We have always respected and recognized the importance of each other's specialization for determining the quality of an athlete's performance. The fields of psychology and physiology are linked in the implementation of coaching practices. Since we have both been involved in the development of the field of coaching science, we have collaborated in different countries on numerous occasions over the past twenty years in presenting to practitioners symposia, workshops, and institutes that have focused on communicating scientific knowledge and its implications. Our annual visits have allowed each of us to supplement the other's knowledge of advances in the fields of sport that are occurring around the world, and these implications are provided in this text.

We have recognized for some time that the coaching practices of Western coaches have been inappropriate in many cases, outmoded, and potentially harmful. This necessitated our looking at the practices of other cultures and the way that they had supplanted Western nations in sporting supremacy, particularly in Olympic sports. We have been fortunate to participate in international symposia on sports science and as participants at Olympic and other international games. Those experiences have served as the springboard for considering coaching alternatives to those which have been popular in Australia, Canada, and the USA.

Another stimulus for producing this text was the publication of Tudor Bompa's 1986 book *Theory and Methodology of Training*. He presented ideas concerning training theory that had not previously been available in English. We believe that our text extends Bompa's ideas in the way the content is presented, the research bases are referenced, and with the extra training principles that have been added to produce a complete package covering scientifically based implications for contemporary coaching. We also thought that it was necessary for the text to be produced for an international audience, although there are a number of references and examples that stamp it as being 'Australian'. We focus on the principles of sports science so that the book will be useful to interested people in any country.

This book is meant to achieve a number of objectives that involve altering commonly observed and stereotyped coaching practices. It should also make the reader aware that recovery is as important as workload. When athletes work hard, they need an appropriate amount of time to recover for the effects of the work to be beneficial — that is, for training effects to occur. The reader should understand that the physical capacities of individuals have a finite level to which they can be developed, and no amount of extra 'hard' work will improve these capacities. Usually, the prescription of extra work will cause the performance and the physical state of an athlete to deteriorate, producing the phenomenon of 'overtraining' or 'burn-out'. In subtle ways there have been attempts to debunk popular clichés such as 'miles make champions' or 'the more you work, the better the dividend'; these are neither sane nor supported by objective research. There are many common training practices and testimonies of coaches that, if followed, could not only decrease athletes' motivation for participating in sport, but actually injure them.

We have attempted to suggest the best way of achieving the highest level of fitness that can be attained by athletes without spending much time on quibbling over erroneous assumptions. *There are principles of training that need to be implemented to maximize the training responses of athletes.* These have been fully covered in the text.

Finally, the book recognizes the place of physical conditioning in relation to skill and psychology. Physical fitness is the finite energizing capacity for performance. If it is to be further maximized, advances in performance have to be achieved by improving skill and/or psychology. We believe that total coaching programs should consider the three sciences that govern sport performance and consider their balance when prescribing training programs. Modern coaches cannot justify their coaching practices by emphasizing one sport science over another. If a national coach proposes that the way for a nation to elevate its standards of sporting performance is through physical training, without equally stressing skill and psychological factors, that is a recipe for failure. We hope that this text will impress upon the reader that physical fitness is merely one of the three emphases of training that have to be provided in modern and beneficial training programs.

The book is structured according to a particular plan. Section I, Fitness and Training, describes the bases for determining the importance of physical fitness, and the factors which affect it. The macro-capacities of the body's physiology are described, so that when they are mentioned in later sections, the reader will be familiar with their meaning.

Section II, Principles of Training, is a unique presentation of the basic principles that have to be considered when prescribing training programs. For each principle, there are many sub-principles specific to directing particular changes in the physical status of athletes. It is in this section that the case is made for the importance of recovery in the conduct of training and practices.

Section III, Training Modifiers, describes those factors which will alter the training responses of athletes. In understanding these biophysical and psychosocial factors, appropriate changes to the training prescription can be made so that the training responses of athletes are maximized and their modified capabilities accommodated.

Section IV, Analysis of Training Requirements, argues for physical capacity testing. It is intended to make the reader aware of the importance of testing for gaining knowledge, allowing a coach to make better decisions. We recommend to the reader that if a feeling of inadequacy in this area of sport science exists, then expert help from local sports scientists should be sought.

Section V covers the Methods and Effects of Training. This suggests the general formats and structures of training items to improve (i) muscular and aerobic endurance, (ii) strength, (iii) power and speed, and (iv) flexibility. A section has been added on training for team sports, because they usually require consideration of most physical capacities, as well as individual and team techniques, and have restricted training times. Australian football is used for examples, with the understanding that coaches of other sports will be able to apply these to their own situation.

Section VI considers the structure of Training Plans. It is divided into three chapters. The first looks at the appropriate structuring of practice sessions, microcycles (weekly plans), and macrocycles (longer periods of training with particular objectives). The other chapters look at long-term planning. The final chapter, Coaching Implications, serves as a brief summary of the major themes of the text.

The Appendixes supplement what is presented in the text.

Although it is difficult to write a general textbook, we have attempted to concentrate on describing and relating principles that pervade a majority of sports. This text never was intended to be a book for the coaches of one sport. The examples that are provided are intended to give the reader an idea of how each principle could function, and it is the responsibility of the reader to understand the principle and then adapt it to his or her particular sporting situation. If the book motivates coaches to work together to discover and agree upon ways in which the principles can be applied to their particular situations, then we will have achieved one of the major objectives of our labours.

The material in Appendix A, *Daily Analyses of Life Demands for Athletes*, at the end of the book, is a psychological evaluation procedure that is valid for competitive athletes over the age of eleven years. Results can be used to assist a coach to make better judgments. This assessment tool is reproduced by kind permission of Sports Science Associates — Canada (4225 Orchard Drive, Spring Valley, California 92077), and cannot be reproduced in part or in total without the express permission of the copyright holder.

A text that is developed by individuals on separate sides of the world's largest ocean could not be completed without the assistance of others, and we would like to recognize the contributions of a number. The Department of Physical Education at San Diego State University made it possible for us to meet in order to formulate the structure and ideas of the book, and it would not have eventuated without that opportunity. San Diego State University, the University of Wollongong, and the University of Queensland provided resources to produce the book as part of our professional responsibilities as faculty members. Sports Science Associates — Canada provided the facilities for manuscript preparation and word-processing. To these organizations, we are extremely grateful. We also appreciate the willingness of Mr Peter Debus of Macmillan Australia to publish the text.

Brent Rushall
San Diego, California
Frank Pyke
Brisbane, Australia
January 1990

Acknowledgments

The authors and publishers are grateful to the following for permission to reproduce copyright material:

Australian Coaching Council, photos 6.1, 10.1, 10.2, 11.1, 12.1, 14.1a, 14.1b, 20.1;
Aussie Sports, Queensland, photo 9.1;
Cliff Russell, Australian Institute of Sport, photos 5.1, 8.1;
Garry Taylor, Brisbane, photo 9.2;
Herald and Weekly Times, photo 1.2;
Janet Pyke, photos 1.1, 7.1, 13.1, 15.1, 18.1;
John Fairfax and Sons, photo 4.1;
The Age, photo 1.3;
West Australian Newspapers, photo 17.1.

While every care has been taken to trace and acknowledge copyright, the publishers tender their apologies for any accidental infringement where copyright has proved untraceable. They would be pleased to come to a suitable arrangement with the rightful owner in each case.

Fitness and Training

1
The Place of Fitness in Sports

Sporting performances are governed by three general factors: skilled techniques, physiological fitness and psychological skills. For recreational activities, where participation is the main objective and training is rarely undertaken, one can perform satisfactorily with low levels of development in each factor. Competent performances can be attained by individuals who aspire to higher levels of achievement if one or more of the factors are developed through training, to a high level of inherent potential. At one time it was possible to be a world-class performer with a 'weakness' in one area, but that is no longer the case. Champions require highly skilled competencies that are energized by an appropriately developed level of fitness and which are controlled by a specific set of psychological skills and attributes. This text focuses on sporting fitness as the energizer of performance.

While each of the three general factors is important in any sport, there are differences in the degree to which optimal performance relies on any one of them. For example, a golfer depends heavily on technical skills which need to be maintained for the duration of a game. Unless a player can consistently reproduce the action of swinging a club in the appropriate manner, low scores cannot be expected. However, selecting the right club swing at the right time is another matter, as is the ability to concentrate for the full duration of the competition. Fitness plays an important role in golf. While golfers do not require the fitness of a marathon runner, they do need to have sufficient endurance capacities to prevent the erosion of skills and concentration due to physical fatigue. By contrast, a marathon runner must pay primary attention to fitness

3

and physical training, although other factors cannot be ignored. A tough-minded approach to tolerating high fatigue states must be developed. Success also depends on manufacturing a smooth and economical gait, thus maximizing efficiency.

While the golfer should concentrate more on skill and the marathon runner more on fitness, in other sports the decision as to what general factors should be emphasized is not as simple. A soccer player needs a high degree of technical skill in actions such as heading, kicking, and dribbling. Tactical skills involving a sense of anticipation or the ability to 'read the game' ensure that the player is in the right place at the right time. Players need to adopt a confident, disciplined, and enthusiastic approach to the sport. High levels of both endurance and speed are also necessary to maximize the ability to keep running throughout the duration of a game. In soccer, and sports with similar requirements, attention to the three attributes of the individual — skill, fitness, and mental control — should be given an equal weighting.

While this book is about fitness, the complex interactions between this factor and the skills and psychology of sports performance must be constantly recognized by the reader. Fitness determines the level of energy that is available for use in sporting events. Fitness is the energizer of sports performance.

Components of Fitness

Figure 1.1 illustrates the basic components of sports fitness. *Endurance fitness* plays an important role in many sports. There are two types of endurance. *Aerobic endurance* determines the ability to sustain a whole-body activity for a considerable time in sports such as running, swimming, and rowing. The transport of oxygen to the muscles by the respiratory and cardiovascular systems is critical in this type of endurance. *Muscular endurance* is more regionalized and depends on the ability of specific muscle groups to sustain an activity for a short time in the face of considerable local fatigue. It requires additional *anaerobic* energy above that provided by the oxygen transport system, which leads to the accumulation of a movement-limiting product called lactic acid. The tolerance for lactic acid ultimately determines the capability of a muscle to sustain its action. Push-ups, bar-chins, and sit-ups are examples of activities that are limited by the endurance of local muscle groups

Muscular strength is the ability to exert force in a single effort. It is required while lifting a heavy weight, resisting a static wrestling hold, or pushing an opponent aside in a football scrimmage. When force is applied quickly, the resulting product of *muscular strength*

and *muscular speed* is referred to as *muscular power*. This attribute is important in many single-effort activities such as hitting, throwing, and jumping. In explosive power movements such as pitching a baseball, throwing a javelin, and hitting a golf ball, where the resistance is light, the speed factor is dominant. In other movements such as Olympic weight-lifting, shot-putting, and high-jumping, where the resistance is heavier, the strength factor is more important in generating power. Sprints lasting less than ten seconds are other high-powered activities that require fitness that is related more to strength and power than to more obvious forms of endurance.

Figure 1.1 Basic Components of Sports Fitness

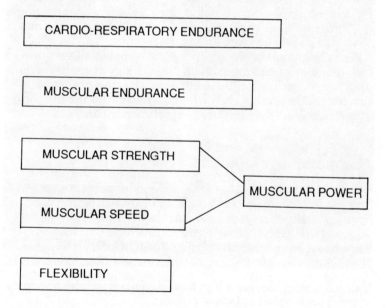

Finally, some consideration must be given to joint *flexibility* which governs the range of movement. This is vital in many sports, not only from a performance viewpoint, but also for preventing injuries in certain circumstances. Sports in which joint flexibility plays a crucial role include gymnastics, swimming, and golf.

Different sports require different fitness components. Determining the essential features of fitness that are required for a particular sport is an important coaching decision.

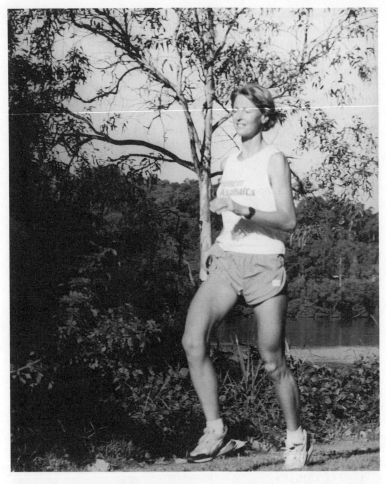

Distance running requires a high level of cardio-respiratory endurance, involving the transport and use of oxygen

Fitness for the Individual

The possession of fitness attributes varies from person to person. Some athletes have an excellent capacity for endurance but little for sprinting, while in others the qualities are reversed. Some individuals have moderate quantities of both. When sports participation becomes specialized, it is essential to make a wise choice of sport for an individual based on that person's inherited attributes.

Training programs should then be prescribed that are geared towards developing individual strengths and removing weaknesses.

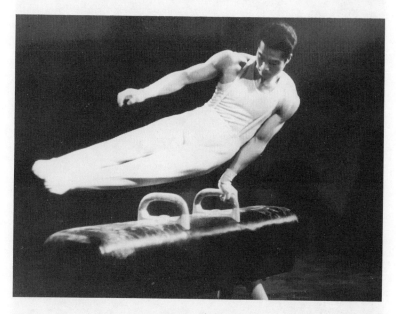

Gymnastic routines on the pommel horse require highly developed upper body muscular strength and endurance

It is important to know the caliber of the attributes of each individual athlete. Not only will such assessments permit individualized training programs to be developed, but they may dictate the strategy employed by the athlete in a particular performance. For example, a distance swimmer may well try to improve speed for a finishing effort, but may still be reluctant to employ a go-slow or negative-split strategy early in the race for fear of being beaten by opponents with superior finishing speed. A soccer player may develop endurance to keep pace with the general demand for this component of fitness in the match, but may still prefer to play in a position which does not tax this capacity to the limit. A style of play based on accurate reading of the game and quick breakaway moves may be preferred. A boxer may choose to fight over 10 or 12 rounds rather than 15 and rely more on speed and skill than endurance. He therefore avoids the risk of being worn down late in the fight.

People should be encouraged to select sports which match their physical attributes. Training programs then need to be devised by a coach to stimulate the development of these capacities.

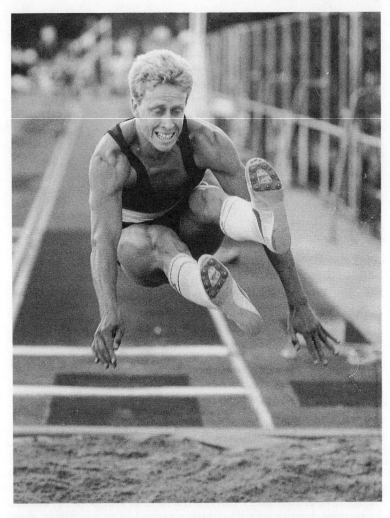

A champion long-jumper must possess explosive power during the approach and take-off phase, and flexibility during the airborne and landing phase

Variations in Attention to Fitness

As will become evident in the chapters on the principles of training, there are certain critical times during a season when the attention to fitness work should vary. As a training strategy, it is simply not wise to merely keep increasing the training load. Ultimately, an athlete will not be able to tolerate the demands of training and will break down. There are limits to which an athlete's physiological capacities can be developed. Once those have been developed fully, further improvements in performance must be sought by attending to skill and psychological factors. Montpetit, Duvallet, Serveth, and Cazorla (1981) demonstrated the ceiling effect on endurance capacity. They assessed performance and maximum oxygen uptake ($\dot{V}O_2$ max) of 16 members of the French national swimming team on four occasions over a three-month period. They found that $\dot{V}O_2$ max did not change and that performance fluctuations were independent of that measure. $\dot{V}O_2$ max did not predict performance during peak training. Dudley, Abraham, and Terjung (1982) demonstrated the ceiling effects of training in animals. What this means for the practitioner is that once the ceiling effects of fitness training are achieved, the rewards of training are few, if any, if fitness still continues to be the main focus.

The possibility exists that the lack of rewards could discourage and/or frustrate athletes. Thus training emphases and sources of reward have to change when the maximum benefits from fitness training are achieved. The concept of finite ceilings in the development of fitness capacities will be new to many coaches. It means that once peak fitness is obtained, coaching strategies will have to change to produce further performance increases.

It is important to alternate days or periods of heavy training with lighter ones in order to provide ample opportunity for recovery. It is particularly necessary to reduce the training load for a week or two before important competitions (peaking or tapering). This has been shown to assist performance considerably. However, in some sports which are played on a weekly schedule it is simply not possible to peak for each performance. If a weekly peak were attempted, it could result in no hard training ever being done. Hence physiological deterioration would occur, with an accompanying decrease in performance. Fitness is a temporary state that can be lost quickly, particularly if a sedentary life-style is adopted between periods of participation. Because of the substantial losses in fitness that usually occur during lay-offs, an athlete is presented with a time-consuming and arduous task to recover to the previous levels of fitness during the first part of the next training period. Athletes who try to accelerate this readaptation process by training too hard too early, can find themselves unduly fatigued or injured in the early stages of the season. Such a setback can seriously hamper the types and effects of training that occur in the rest of the season. If optimal adaptation is sought, there is no substitute for a gradual stepped progression in workload over an extended period.

Modern coaching theory and research evidence promote the concept that training is cyclic, consisting of judicious alternations of training loads as stimuli, and unloading periods for recovery. Training stresses which do not allow periods of recovery are no longer acceptable. Since sports fitness can reach a maximum level, a balanced approach to training emphasizing fitness maintenance alongside skill and psychological development can often offer the best alternative for preparing athletes.

Factors Which Modify Training and Performance

The ability of an athlete to train and perform effectively can be modified by the presence of a number of factors that may exist in the individual's background or environment. These are directly related to fitness and can ultimately decide the capability of an athlete to reach potential. They are mentioned briefly below but are discussed in detail in the section of the text titled Training Modifiers (see Figure 1.2).

☐ Constitutional Factors

Genetically-controlled studies have underlined the significant role of heredity in determining the success of the athlete. It has often been said that sporting achievement is dependent on the wise choice of one's parents. Certainly, the ceiling of physiological adaptation appears to be decided at birth. No matter how much training is done on a specific fitness component, it is simply not possible to outperform an individual with superior genetic endowment who has undergone a similar training program. Champion sprinters and endurance athletes are favored in that particular direction at birth and have developed their talents fully with specifically prescribed training programs.

However, this does not mean that unless the blood lines are of thoroughbred quality, all is lost in sport. Most sports involve several different components of fitness and low levels in one component may be balanced by high levels in another. Also, deficiencies in fitness may be compensated by superior skill and a resolute attitude to training and performance. Despite genetic limitations, it is still possible to coach athletes to achieve their maximum potential, even if that potential is not of world-champion caliber.

Other constitutional factors, such as age and sex, also determine performance limits. Female athletes have substantially increased their levels of sports participation in recent years and have produced some outstanding performances in a wide range of sports. However, there are fundamental biological differences between the sexes which usually manifest themselves in sports which require, for example, muscular strength and power. The average male simply develops more muscle than the average female and consistently outperforms her in strength-dominated activities.

Figure 1.2 Factors Influencing Sports Training and Performance

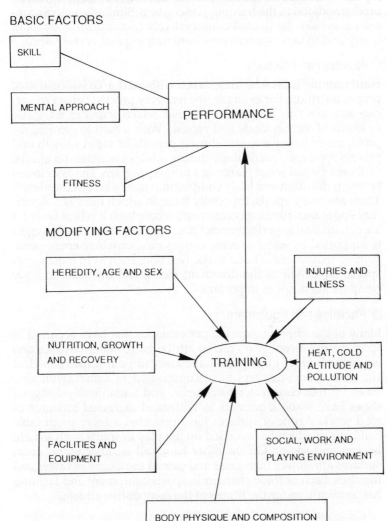

The basic factors are balanced according to each sport's requirements. The modifying factors need to be controlled as much as possible in the training and competition environment.

There are also limitations imposed by age. Younger athletes require considerable energy for growth which can substantially detract from the resources that are available for hard training. They are also more likely to experience heat-related and bone-related injuries than the average adult. Differences such as these should be accommodated in the training prescription. Similarly, veteran athletes must also be trained conservatively to minimize the risk of injury and to facilitate recovery from training and performance.

□ Nutrition and Growth

Hard training cannot be undertaken without due consideration of proper nutrition. For example, the recovery process between exercise sessions can be aided by a diet which includes adequate amounts of carbohydrate and protein. With regard to growth, the problems of heavy exercise during periods of rapid growth and protein synthesis, particularly during adolescence, should also be well understood when planning a fitness program. The association between nutrition and body composition must also be considered. There are many sports, especially those in which there is a significant endurance running component, where high levels of body fat are detrimental to performance. Other sports in which body weight is supported by water or some conveyance, or where energy-consuming movement is not a major function, such as in most target sports, have skill as the dominant factor, and attention to body composition is not as important.

□ Facilities and Equipment

Many of the improvements in performance that have occurred in sport during recent years can be attributed to better facilities and equipment. Fiber glass poles have assisted pole-vaulters to clear six metres, lane-markers have contributed to faster swimming times by reducing water turbulence, and scientifically-designed shoes have assisted runners to withstand increased amounts of road work. Artificial surfaces have provided a more predictable ball bounce which has speeded up the play in sports such as field hockey and soccer. On the other hand, all-weather tennis court surfaces are slower than grass and extend the length of rallies and matches. Each of these changes in sports equipment and facilities has implications for the fitness of the competitive athlete.

□ Injuries and Illness

As sports training and performance have taken on a higher profile in society, the Sports Medicine profession has been called upon to treat a myriad of sports injuries and illnesses, many of which result specifically from excessive or incorrect training. These problems range from sports anemia in the overtrained distance athlete, to Osgood–Schlatter's disease in the exercising adolescent, to Achilles tendinitis in the road runner. There are also many injuries that might occur in contact and collision sports such as football, hockey, boxing, and motocrosse. Disruptions to training programs through injury and illness will require coaches to reconsider the schedules of fitness development of athletes.

□ Physical Environment

It is well known that performance and training, particularly where a high endurance component is required, suffer in hot conditions. When a pollution factor is added, the situation is even worse. The same is true of endurance sports conducted at high altitude. In all cases, periods of acclimatization to unusual environmental factors are essential to allow time for beneficial physiological adjustments to occur. Cold weather sports also require special preparation. While the scope for physiological adaptation is much more limited in the cold, there are important considerations to be made when preparing for training and performance in such conditions.

□ Life-style Factors

There are influences that exist both in the sporting situation and in everyday life that can impinge on the ability of the athlete to train and perform effectively. Emotional disturbances associated with interpersonal relationships, and the lengthy periods that often must be devoted to work and study commitments, are two examples of life-style events which detract from the available energies of a hard-training athlete. Within a sport, poor relationships between players and between the players and the coaching staff can interfere with team morale, training, and performance. Travel schedules require athletes to adjust to time-zone shifts and strange conditions. Some individuals are affected more by these disruptions than others. The life-style of an athlete must be monitored if the training response is to be optimized.

Summary

One cannot train for sports by viewing fitness as a general concept. Each performance and fitness component must instead be considered. The focus of training each component appropriately will enhance the levels and precision of fitness for each sport. The components which need to be planned separately are aerobic endurance, muscular or anaerobic endurance, muscular strength, speed, and flexibility.

The individual needs and response capacities of athletes must be accommodated when developing training programs. The common approach of applying one program to a group of athletes violates this need. That approach does not maximize the development of fitness components in each athlete.

Fitness components are best developed by alternating work and rest in appropriate amounts. Continuous, highly fatiguing work without rest does not yield beneficial training effects. As a final product, fitness achieves a maximum level and will not improve through further increases in workload. Once the ceiling level of sports fitness is attained, programs of fitness maintenance should be instituted to replace programs designed to change fitness.

Training responses are modified by a number of factors which are inherent in the athlete or which occur in the athlete's sporting life and that outside sport. The impact of these factors will make the planning and implementation of training programs more complex.

2
The Physiological Capacities of the Body

The Energy Systems

A basic understanding of how energy is produced in the human body is essential before physical training can be prescribed accurately.

The energy required for short explosive activities is provided by the breakdown of high-energy phosphate compounds in the muscles. One of these, *adenosine triphosphate (ATP)*, must be present before a muscle will contract. ATP could be called the 'chemical of contraction' as the body-machine will not work if it is absent. ATP is stored in small amounts in the muscle and can only sustain activity for one to two seconds. If activity is to continue, ATP must be replenished from other energy sources in the muscle. This occurs when another high-energy phosphate compound found in the muscle, *creatine phosphate (CP)*, is degraded to produce ATP and provide the energy for continued activity for 5 to 10 seconds. Only short recovery periods (about 30 seconds) are required for these energy sources to be sufficiently replenished to provide for a repeat effort.

This facility is the main reason why high work intensities can be maintained when short work periods are employed in training. The activity of the ATP–CP energy system does not require the presence of oxygen and is considered to be part of the anaerobic (without oxygen) energy system. Since lactic acid is not produced by this system it is also called the alactacid system. It is used in speed and strength activities.

15

Other forms of fuel are also stored and made available in the muscles for more sustained bouts of work. These are stored sugar (glycogen) and fat which are degraded by different mechanisms to again produce the chemical of contraction, ATP. During a sustained high-powered sprint, when both stored ATP and CP and the delivery of oxygen are insufficient to meet the demands of the effort, the high-energy carbohydrate compound *glycogen* can be broken down by enzyme reactions, to *glucose* (glycogenolysis) and then to *lactic acid*. This latter anaerobic reaction, called *glycolysis*, produces limited quantities of ATP which, along with stored ATP and CP, can maintain muscular contractions for between 30 and 40 seconds. The system that produces energy from this source is called the *lactacid* or *glycolytic energy system*. It is used in sustained sprint or muscular endurance activities. Ultimately, the presence of large amounts of lactic acid interferes with the mechanical events associated with muscle shortening and a person is forced to cease activity. While the subsequent removal of lactic acid is facilitated by light exercise (walking or slow jogging) during recovery, it still takes a considerable time. If maximum performances are to be expected in swimming, cycling, or running events that involve a large accumulation of lactic acid, they should be spaced at least an hour apart.

If exercise is not very intense, it can be prolonged. The rate of energy release in the muscles can then be maintained by the process of *oxidation* which provides much larger quantities of ATP. For oxidation to occur, oxygen must be transported from the air to the muscles by the cardio-respiratory system and then used for the production of energy. This process is termed *aerobic metabolism*, and can occur with the oxidation of both the glycogen and fat stores contained in the body. The system that uses oxygen in energy production is called the *aerobic energy system*, and is used in activities requiring cardio-respiratory endurance. For more intensive prolonged work, such as in a squash match lasting about an hour, glycogen is preferred to fat as the fuel because it yields energy more efficiently. However, the problem with glycogen is that it is limited in supply. The heavy-legged feeling referred to by marathon runners as 'hitting-the-wall' is closely associated with severe muscle glycogen depletion. This can also occur, at the expense of skill, in many team and individual sports that last more than an hour.

Usually there is a mixture of glycogen and fat used as fuel in prolonged efforts. It has been shown that, unlike middle-distance runners, champion marathon runners use a higher proportion of fat to produce oxidative energy when their muscles work. This spares the limited resource of muscle glycogen and allows them to finish a race without 'hitting-the-wall'. Theoretically, the availability of fat is unlimited, but its energy yield is much slower.

Ultra-marathoners, iron-men, triathletes, and other individuals who exercise for extremely long periods, rely heavily on the utilization of fat as the fuel for energy. The ability to exercise for long periods at a high intensity is related to what has been termed the *anaerobic threshold*, or sometimes the 'lactate' or 'ventilatory' threshold. This is the effort level that if exceeded requires some supplementation from anaerobic energy sources, particularly the splitting of glycogen to form lactic acid. It is dependent on the aerobic qualities of the muscles and usually is high in endurance athletes involved in prolonged efforts.

In summary, the high-energy phosphates are the predominant energy source for brief efforts lasting less than 10 seconds. The splitting of glycogen into lactic acid provides the major energy resources for sustained sprints and feats of muscular endurance lasting between 10 and 60 seconds. Both these energy sources are *anaerobic* and are associated with high-power activities. The energy for lower-power efforts over longer periods of time is provided by the oxidation of glycogen and fat and requires a supply of oxygen to the working muscles via the cardio-respiratory system. This is *aerobic* energy.

Sports in which high-power efforts are made intermittently, such as many individual sports (e.g., tennis, squash, boxing) and team sports (e.g, rugby, cricket, volleyball), rely on the continual breakdown and restoration of anaerobic energy sources. The process of resynthesis during recovery periods requires the provision of aerobic energy. Hence, athletes in these sports require both aerobic and anaerobic training. Also, if these efforts are prolonged, the availability of glycogen as the preferred fuel becomes a limiting factor in performance. A summary of this energy system analysis is presented in Table 2.1 and Figure 2.1.

Muscle Characteristics

The sprint and endurance qualities of an athlete depend to a large extent on the ability of the muscles to contract with speed and force. Microscopic examination of muscle by the needle biopsy technique has made it possible to identify two different types of fibers in human muscle. These are termed *fast-twitch and slow-twitch fibers*. The nerve supply to these determines which type they are. One neuron (nerve) may supply several muscle fibers. This is called a *motor unit*. Fast-twitch motor units involve a large (thick) neuron which can serve up to several hundred muscle fibers. A slow-twitch unit has a small (thin) neuron connected to a smaller group of fibers (usually less than 100). Fast-twitch motor units develop considerably more force in a faster time than slow-twitch motor units, but they fatigue more easily (see Figure 2.2). Fast-twitch motor units are closely related to muscular strength, speed, and power and are the prized attribute of the explosive athlete. On the other hand, slow-twitch motor units are well-endowed aerobically and offer advantages to the endurance athlete.

Table 2.1 Dominant Physiological Attributes and Energy Sources for Different Activities

Activity	Duration	Dominant Physiological Attribute	Dominant Energy System
Short explosive effort: jump, hit	< 5 sec	Muscular strength, speed, power	Alactacid (ATP–CP)
Short sprint (high power)	5–10 sec	Muscular strength, speed, power	Alactacid (ATP–CP)
Sustained sprint (high power)	10–60 sec	Muscular strength, speed, power, muscular endurance	Lactacid
Middle distance (moderate power)	60 sec – 10 min	Muscular endurance, aerobic endurance, anaerobic threshold	Lactacid, aerobic
Long distance (low power)	10–60 min	Aerobic endurance anaerobic threshold	Aerobic
Marathon (low power)	60+ min	Aerobic endurance anaerobic threshold, fuel availability	Aerobic
Intermittent (high and low power)	60+ min	Muscular strength, speed, power, muscular endurance, aerobic endurance, fuel availability	Alactacid (ATP–CP), lactacid, aerobic

Figure 2.1 Contributions of the Energy Systems to Sports Performance

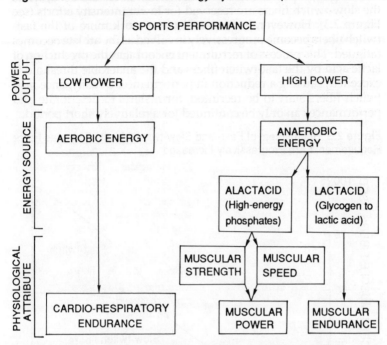

Figure 2.2 Characteristics of Fast- and Slow-twitch Motor Units

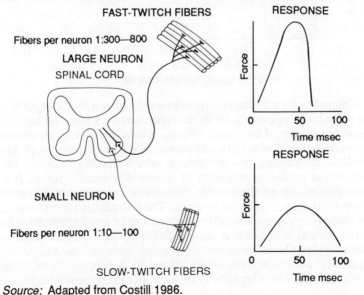

Source: Adapted from Costill 1986.

During high-power activities, fast-twitch fibers are used, while the slow-twitch fibers are reserved for lower intensity efforts (see Figure 2.3). However, in longer distance work more of the fast-twitch fibers become progressively involved as the athlete becomes fatigued. This process of recruitment encourages the production of lactic acid by the fast-twitch fibers and the anaerobic threshold is exceeded, causing a reduction in performance. Usually, once fast-twitch fibers start to be recruited, form starts to deteriorate and performance can only be continued for a relatively short period.

Figure 2.3 Recruitment of Fast- and Slow-twitch Muscle Fibers as Force Requirements Are Progressively Increased

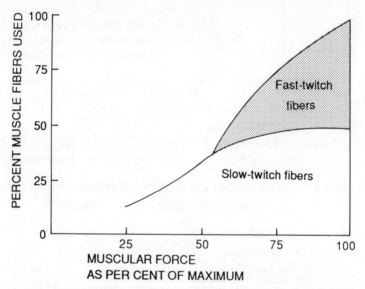

Champion long-distance runners usually have a high proportion of slow-twitch fibers (> 80%), whereas sprinters have an equally greater number of fast-twitch fibers. While these proportions are essentially decided at birth and do not change with either sprint or endurance training, the endurance athlete can significantly improve the oxidative potential of fast-twitch muscle fibers. It is possible to extend the aerobic endurance capacities of a person born with a better capacity to sprint. The trainability for endurance of these fibers is evidenced by the number of good sprinters who have been able to become quite capable distance runners later in their careers. On the other hand, it is much more difficult to develop sprinting ability in individuals with a high proportion of slow-twitch fibers. The adaptability of these fibres for generating force and power is not as high as that of the fast-twitch fibers for improving endurance.

Transport of Oxygen

The ultimate source of energy for sporting activity comes from the oxidation of fuel. In low-power efforts this may occur during the activity itself and in high-power efforts during the recovery period following it. It is important to understand the sequence of events involved in the transport of oxygen from the air to the working muscles. These are:

1. Ventilation of the lungs with air.
2. Diffusion of oxygen from the lungs into the blood.
3. Carriage of oxygen in the blood, mainly in combination with hemoglobin contained in red blood cells.
4. Pumping of blood by the heart.
5. Delivery of oxygen to the muscle fibers via a system of capillaries.
6. Delivery of oxygen from the blood permitting its diffusion into the muscle fibers.
7. Production of ATP in the mitochondria of the muscle fibers through the oxidation of glycogen and fat.

The maximum amount of oxygen that can be consumed by the body during exhausting exercise is referred to as the $\dot{V}O_2$ max. Physiologically, it is the product of the amount of blood pumped by the heart (cardiac output) and the amount of oxygen taken from the blood as it passes through the body tissues, in particular, exercising muscles. The amount of oxygen used is measured as the difference in the oxygen content of arterial and venous blood. This is known as the arterio-venous oxygen difference. Oxygen consumption can be quantified in the following manner:

$\dot{V}O_2$ max = Cardiac output
$\qquad\qquad$ × arterio-venous oxygen difference
$\qquad$ = (Stroke volume × heart rate)
$\qquad\qquad$ × arterio-venous oxygen difference

Example: The following data were obtained on a runner during a maximum effort:

Cardiac output	= 30 liters of blood per minute
Stroke volume	= 150 mL of blood per beat
Heart rate	= 200 beats per minute
Oxygen content of arterial blood	
	= 210 mL of oxygen per liter of blood

Oxygen content of venous blood
$$= 50 \text{ mL of oxygen per mL of blood}$$

$\dot{V}O_2$ max $=$ Cardiac output $\times$ arterio-venous oxygen difference
$$= (150 \text{ mL} \times 200 \text{ bpm}) \times (210 - 50) \text{ mL per liter}$$
$$= 30 \text{ liters per minute} \times 160 \text{ m}^1 \text{ per liter}$$
$$= 4800 \text{ mL } O_2 \text{ per minute}$$
$$= 4\cdot8 \text{ liters of } O_2 \text{ per minute}$$

If the athlete were an 80 kilogram man, the 4·8 figure would translate into a $\dot{V}O_2$ max of 60 (4800/80) milliliters of oxygen per kilogram of body weight per minute. Measurements of oxygen consumption are very important for determining the energy costs and capacities that are suitable for different types of sports.

It is not possible in the laboratory to take direct measurements of these particular variables on exercising athletes. However, the measurement of gases exchanged in the lungs during a maximum exercise test permits easy determination of $\dot{V}O_2$ max. It is regarded as the best single indicator of endurance potential. Figure 2.4 illustrates the major factors that determine maximum oxygen consumption.

Flexibility

Joint flexibility is dependent on the anatomical structure of the bones comprising the joint itself, the looseness and/or pliability of the ligaments which bind the joint together, and the extensibility of the muscles which cross the joint. While extreme flexibility may not be desirable in certain contact and combative sports, it certainly is important in other activities where a wide range of motion can positively benefit speed of movement at the extremities. This is the case in sports that involve throwing and striking skills. There are also several aesthetic or artistic sports which require athletes to reach difficult positions that demand good joint flexibility. For sports which require flexibility, it has to be trained as does any other performance capacity.

Physiological Capacities and Sports Performance

The energy requirements of continuous sports have been well studied and are usually depicted by the energy-contribution/performance-time relationship as exampled in Figure 2.5. Performances of short duration depend on anaerobic energy sources and as performance time is extended, so does the relative contribution from aerobic sources. However, these estimates may not be exactly

Figure 2.4 Major Factors Determining Maximum Oxygen Uptake

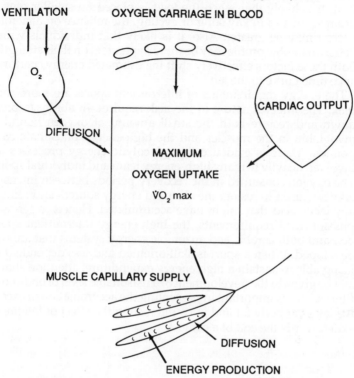

Figure 2.5 The Contribution of the Alactacid and Lactacid Anaerobic and the Aerobic Energy Systems in Performances of Different Durations

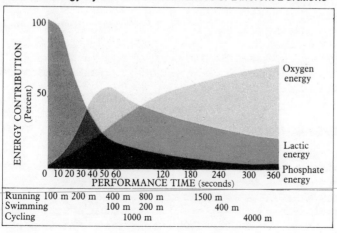

the same for each continuous sport nor for each individual engaged in it. It is likely that when the load is placed on smaller muscle groups, such as in kayaking or cycling, the reliance on anaerobic energy may be greater. Also, it is likely that individuals with a better anaerobic profile may be more dependent on their strengths. Both these factors effectively shift the estimated energy/performance time-curve to the left.

The energy requirements of intermittent sports are more complex. The interval nature of the task requires an ability to break down and restore both the small amount of oxygen bound to myoglobin in the muscles and the high-energy phosphate compounds. There is evidence that glycolytic energy processes are involved heavily in many high-energy team and individual sports. The oxygen consumed in the recovery periods between intensive efforts is used to restore the alactacid energy sources and remove any lactic acid that might have accumulated. Hence, in terms of physiological requirements, the high-energy intermittent sports demand both aerobic and anaerobic energy systems that are well developed. When a sport is skill-oriented and less dependent on being able to sustain a high energy expenditure, attention should still be given to the development of a reasonable level of endurance fitness. This is important in preventing the accumulation of excessive levels of body fat and in counteracting the effect of fatigue on skill towards the end of a contest.

🔲🔲
Principles of Training

③
Generalized Responses to Training

The structure of a training session for an athlete can vary greatly depending upon a number of factors. Table 3.1 lists the terminologies used to describe what is included in a training session. The basic unit is a *training unit*, one execution of a defined task, for example, one 200 meter swim, a discus throw, or an attempt to jump two meters. Training units are usually repeated, for the repetitions allow an athlete's ability to perform to the state of being 'overloaded'. That overloading, if done correctly, stimulates a training response in a performer. A series of repetitions of a training unit is called a *training segment*. Examples of training segments are 4 repetitions of 400 meters freestyle swimming, completing 1 every 5 minutes; 6 discus throws of slightly below maximum effort attempting to achieve a distance of 180 feet (54·8 meters); or 8 consecutive attempts to clear 2 meters while practicing for the high jump. A training session usually entails some variety in the type of tasks that are performed: that is, a number of training segments are programmed. Those tasks constitute the *training program*.

The energy cost of training items is called 'overload'. The amount of overload for a training segment is called a *training stimulus*. The total training stimuli producing the overloads in the training segments constitute a general load demand of the training session, termed the *session load* and, in some cases, the *training load*. Since each athlete has a different capacity to tolerate a session load, the impact of the same program of training on individuals will vary. This variation in reaction capacity is called the *strain* of the load on the athlete. The result of the modification of the session load by an individual's strain is the *training stress*. Individual athletes will respond differently to the same training stimuli which, when summed, produce a particularly individual reaction to the training load.

Table 3.1 Labels, Examples, and Outcomes of Training Response Features

Label	Examples	Features
1. Training unit	200 m	Single performance trials, which are the most basic units of training
2. Training segment	Total of like training units: 8 × 200 m	A segment produces an overload, the training stimulus. Fatigue and recovery needs are developed for the particular activity.
3. Training session	Total of training segments: 8 × 200 m 16 × 50 m 3,000 m	Fatigue effects of each segment accrue but are diminished by what little recovery can occur in the session. The quantifiable amount of work done is the training load.
4. Individual capacity to handle loads	Training modifiers such as age, state of training	Strain is how the athlete copes with and perceives the training load.
5. Training stress	Load × Strain	A general state of fatigue and need for recovery in the individual

Although athletes respond differently when they are subjected to the same training stimulus, the form of the response is similar. This is basic to understanding the nature of the training adaptation. The response comprises several stages, each being modified by a number of factors. A large proportion of the remainder of this text considers these modifiers, so that coaches and athletes can develop better training programs. If the form of the response and its modifiers are understood, then training prescriptions can be devised that will more closely approximate the best possible.

The Form of the Basic Training Response

Figure 3.1 illustrates the form of the basic reaction of an athlete to a training stimulus. It produces an overload with regard to the athlete's capacity to perform a particular training segment. Each stage of the response is described below.

Figure 3.1 A Stylized Curve of the Response to a Training Stimulus, Showing the Five Phases of Reaction

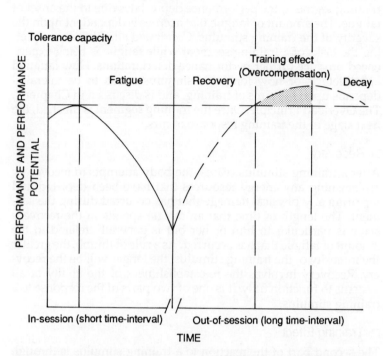

Note: The time axis is not of consistent duration, the out-of-session section being contracted purely to be accommodated more effectively in the picture.

□ Tolerance Capacity

When a training segment is attempted, generally the initial response is one of adequate performance. An athlete can normally tolerate the demand of a training stimulus that is placed on the body's resources for a period of time. At the start of the segment, there is usually some warm-up effect and performance quality improves over the standard of the initial attempt. After that occurs, the athlete tolerates the training stimulus with adequate performance. The major factors that govern the duration of the response adequacy are the state of training and the athletes's degree of fatigue. In time, an athlete's resources are taxed beyond their capacities, and performance starts to deteriorate. The onset of that deterioration marks the transition into the next stage of the overall reaction.

□ Fatigue

When an athlete can no longer adequately perform the tasks of a training segment, the performance depreciates due to the onset of fatigue. The amount of fatigue that accrues is dependent upon the severity of the training stimulus. Continued attempts at completing the tasks of a training segment while fatigue is being experienced produce further performance deteriorations. How fatigued an athlete is or how long this stimulus needs to be tolerated depends upon the aims of training, and is discussed in Chapter 4, The Overload Principle. Once the training segment is finished, the next stage of the training response occurs.

□ Recovery

After a training stimulus ceases, the body attempts to recover by replenishing any energy resources that have been depleted and repairing any physical damage that has occurred during the segment. The length of time that an athlete spends in the recovery stage is particular to him or her but is generally related to the amount of fatigue that has occurred. As a rule of thumb, the greater the intensity of the training stimulus, the longer will be the recovery. Recovery involves the re-establishment of the ability of all systems to function fully. It is one of two parts of the response to a training stimulus.

□ Training Effect

The second part of the reaction to a training stimulus is through the reorganization of the structural and functional systems of the body. This means that if the body were subjected to the same training stimulus again, after sufficient recovery and adaptation had occurred, its performance would be different: it would be improved. A common term used to describe this adaptation effect is 'overcompensation'. The improvement that results from recovery and overcompensation is called the *training effect*. It is the purpose of training to produce as many training effects as possible. Effective training allows time for recovery and overcompensation to occur. Once a training effect has been achieved, its longevity is limited. If no further training stimuli are experienced, the training response enters its final stage.

□ Decay

Due to the temporary nature of a training effect, its lack of use will result in a diminution of performance potential. There will be a return to the pre-stimulus state, that is, the performance level that is normally possible for the individual without specific training.

The specific features of each of these stages of the training response are detailed in later chapters. The curve of the response depicted in Figure 3.1 is largely hypothetical. Real performances do not produce smooth curves of tolerance and fatigue, while the stages of recovery, training effect, and decay indicate only the potential for performance, not real performance. The body's attempt to tolerate the demands of a training stimulus is quite complex, since various resources are mobilized to produce adequate responses. The nature of those, and when and how they are used, governs the response variability during the training segment.

The Microcycle of a Training Segment

In realistic circumstances, it is not possible to control an athlete's training response with sufficient precision to guarantee that an ideal training effect will occur through one experience of a training stimulus. For practical purposes, it is usually advisable to repeat the training stimulus in at least three training sessions, assuming that adequate rest between sessions is provided. As well, there is always the possibility of not gauging the recovery processes correctly. If that occurs, then an athlete may not have sufficient time to achieve a training effect and fatigue will accumulate across training sessions. Thus it is a wise procedure to be conservative in developing training plans by concluding a series of exposures to a training stimulus with a much lighter training stimulus or even a prolonged rest period. That final reduction in the intensity of the training stimulus is called the 'unloading' phase of the segment microcycle. Active unloading phases in a microcycle are preferred because recovery is accelerated through activity rather than passive rest.

To this point, the discussion has indicated that repetitions of training stimuli within a component microcycle are of the same activity. If this were followed strictly, there is a strong chance that training programs would become very boring for participants. Variety in training stimuli is a necessary feature to maintain high levels of motivation in athletes. In a practical sense, successive presentations of training stimuli within a component microcycle can be different training items, but the amount and nature of overload should be constant. For example, a swimmer may view the following training items as being equally stressful: eight 200 meters freestyle repeats on 2 minutes 45 seconds, aiming at holding 85 percent of best 200 meters time for each repeat; four 400 meters freestyle repeats on 6 minutes at 85 percent of best 400 meters time for each repeat; and sixteen 100 meters freestyle repeats on 1 minute

15 seconds, aiming at holding the split time of 85 percent of best 200 meters time for each repeat. A coach could schedule these different training items as being steps for the same fitness component since they are roughly equivalent in performance level and training load (work intensity, duration, and between repeat recovery opportunity). For some sports, particularly continuous activities such as swimming, running, and cycling, it is relatively easy to develop equivalent load activities that could be used to provide variety in training programs. However, for other activities it is not so easy. When equivalence between training items is determined, the intensity, duration, and recovery opportunities need to be equated. Some experimentation and evaluation of these determinations needs to be undertaken to validate their use. For the remainder of this text, it is assumed that training variety will be accommodated in training programs through the use of equivalent training tasks, which can be interchanged to present repeated stimulations of the same overload factor.

Because of the imprecisions which are inherent in the practical realities of training, the *segment microcycle* becomes the building block of all training programs. As a rule of thumb, a microcycle is constituted of at least three exposures to a training stimulus aimed at developing a specific fitness component (e.g, muscular power), each experience being followed by an opportunity for full recovery so that a training effect can be achieved. The segment microcycle should not be confused with the *session microcycle* which considers the *general accumulated effects* of a number of training segments which occur in a series of training sessions (see Chapter 18).

It is perhaps best to consider the response to a training segment in light of a few examples that occur in typical training situations.

□ Exact Programming

Figure 3.2 illustrates a response schema for repetitions of an exact training stimulus with sufficient recovery between each exposure. It can be seen that the onset of the second exposure to the training stimulus occurs when the maximum training effect is achieved during the first training response. On successive occasions the next exposure to the training stimulus also occurs at the time when the training effect is maximized. Thus, repeated exposures accumulate training effects and the athlete improves in the most efficient manner. Unfortunately, such a perfect program is rarely attainable. However, there are some interesting generalities that can be derived from this exact model.

Over a period of repeated exposures, as the training effects accumulate, the reorganizations that result from repeated stimulation by a segment of training are successively refined to produce more efficient forms of a particular performance. Each exposure is perceived to be easier than the previous stimulus because the training effects derived from previous experience better equip the athlete to cope with the next segment repetition's demands. Another feature that occurs is that, as repetitions occur, the size of each training effect diminishes. It becomes more difficult to produce noticeable training effects with repeated exposures to a constant training stimulus. An athlete has limited physical resources with which to respond to training and once these resources are fully used, no further improvement is possible. As a consequence of this finite limitation on adaptation resources, the performance potential of a physiological attribute levels off. Fitness levels may be maintained but not improved. Further improvements in performance will only occur if the intensity of the training stimulus is increased. Under this model of exact programming, optimum performance gains are always possible up to a ceiling limit.

Figure 3.2 A Stylized Presentation of Responses to Exact Training Stimuli when Sufficient Recovery between Exposures is Provided

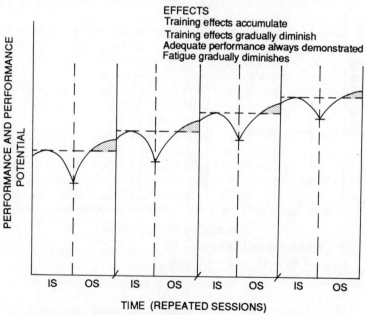

EFFECTS
Training effects accumulate
Training effects gradually diminish
Adequate performance always demonstrated
Fatigue gradually diminishes

IS = In-session (short time-interval)
OS = Out-of-session (long time-interval)

This ideal model allows one to interpret circumstances which frequently arise during attempts to increase sports fitness. Some interpretations are considered below.

□ Heavy Training Stimuli

Figure 3.3 illustrates the responses to repeated exposures of 'heavy' or 'intense' training stimuli where insufficient recovery is provided. This is a typical approach to training where there is an exaggerated emphasis on the belief: 'the more work that is done, the better will be an athlete's performance'.

Figure 3.3 Stylized Presentation of Responses to Heavy or Excessive Training Stimuli when Insufficient Recovery between Exposures is Provided

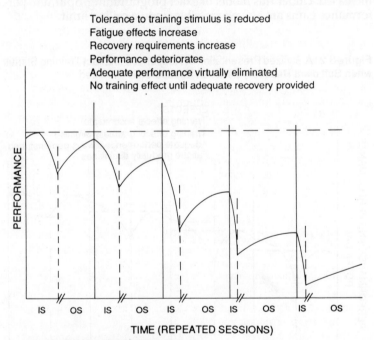

EFFECTS

Tolerance to training stimulus is reduced
Fatigue effects increase
Recovery requirements increase
Performance deteriorates
Adequate performance virtually eliminated
No training effect until adequate recovery provided

IS = In-session (short time-interval)
OS = Out-of-session (long time-interval)

When training stimuli are repeated with insufficient time to allow full recovery and overcompensation, the second training stimulus occurs before performance potential has even recovered to the pre-stimulus level of the first exposure. When this happens, the performance decrement due to fatigue accumulates. Athletes become more tired with each successive training segment when insufficient recovery is allowed. No training effects, and thus performance improvements, occur. Several features of the excessive training regime that are illustrated in Figure 3.3 should be noted.

The first segment induces a normal, untrained, and non-fatigued response to the training stimulus. With each successive exposure to the stimulus, the tolerance capacity for the stimulus is reduced. It is usually not long, even as early as the second exposure, as illustrated here, before no tolerance is exhibited, that is, adequate performances do not occur. Since the onset of the second training stimulus happens before sufficient recovery has occurred, adequate performance is not possible. The fatigue effects become more rapid and larger in magnitude with each successive exposure. The athlete's performances decline faster and faster, with each repetition of the stimulus and inadequate recovery cycle. As the athlete descends deeper into the accumulated fatigue state, recovery occurs more slowly and takes longer.

The value of this approach to training should be questioned. It does not allow the body to develop the reorganization feature of recovery that produces the overcompensated training effect. It is usually accompanied by other side-effects, particularly worsening psychological features and skill deterioration. This text strongly advises against this training philosophy. The ingredient that is missing from this continual heavy-training model is sufficient opportunity for recovery and training effects to occur. Without adequate recovery and overcompensation, the development of sports fitness cannot be realized in the most efficient manner.

□ Unprogrammed Recovery

Many coaches claim that they train their athletes 'hard' and that the athletes still improve in performance: that is, training effects are demonstrated. This may well be the case, but, because a coach describes what was set as the training stimulus does not mean that athletes exactly experience it. Figure 3.4 illustrates a possible explanation as to why performance improvements occur in a typical heavy-training, weekend-off segment cycle.

The first two days of training expose the athlete to a training stimulus that is of sufficient intensity to cause considerable fatigue. After Tuesday, fatigue accrues because of insufficient opportunity to recover. On the third day (Wednesday), the athlete 'cheats' on the program, probably as a survival ploy, by not following the programmed training stimulus. This can be done by not performing with the prescribed intensity, taking more rests than usual, and/or altering the program in some way so that the overload

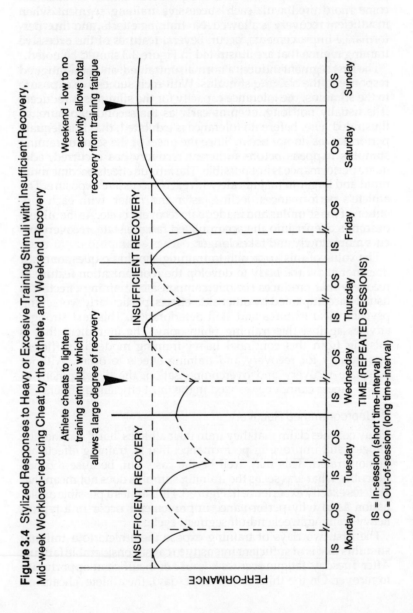

Figure 3.4 Stylized Responses to Heavy or Excesive Training Stimuli with Insufficient Recovery, Mid-week Workload-reducing Cheat by the Athlete, and Weekend Recovery

factor in the training stimulus is diminished. Coping behaviors of these types are frequent responses of serious athletes as they attempt to follow the wisdom of their own appraisals of their response to training rather than the excessive demands of a coach-determined program (Rushall and Roaf 1986). The reduction in the severity of the mid-week training stimulus allows the athlete to recover and, in some cases, even achieve a small training effect. On the Thursday and Friday of the illustration it can be seen that the two consecutive exposures of a heavy-training stimulus again produce accumulated fatigue. With no training on Saturday and Sunday, sufficient time is afforded the athlete to fully recover and incur a training effect for the whole week. Had the mid-week, athlete-determined reduction in stimulus intensity not occurred, then the level of fatigue that would have accumulated after Friday would have been excessive. It is possible that the two days off at the weekend may not have been sufficient for full recovery to occur if that had happened. Thus, the mid-week athlete-determined reduction in stimulus intensity 'saved' the outcome of the week's work.

Similar cases or variations of the features described in the above example explain why athletes exhibit training effects and performance improvements despite what coaches attempt to do to them with excessively hard training stimuli. It is contended that the more 'experienced' (wise) that an athlete becomes, the more subtle are the manipulations of the training stimuli which, in turn, avoid the state of excessive accumulation of fatigue.

☐ Training Stimuli Which Are Too Easy

Figure 3.5 illustrates the responses to training stimuli which are too easy. When no fatigue occurs the body does not have to recover and overcompensate. Consequently, there is no accumulation of training effects, only a minor amount of decay during the inactivity stage between exposures to the training stimulus. Thus, for each successive day, performance improves in the tolerance stage of the response, and then declines during the inactivity stage. Without sufficient stimulation, training effects do not occur.

☐ Training Stimuli Which Are Too Infrequent

Figure 3.5 also illustrates what happens when training stimuli are sufficient to cause a training effect, but the frequency of their occurrence is not sufficient to maintain the temporary training-effect state. Between exposures to the training stimulus, the effect decays back to the pre-exposure level and no performance change occurs.

Figure 3.5 Stylized Response Curves to Training Stimuli Which Are Too Easy or Too Infrequent

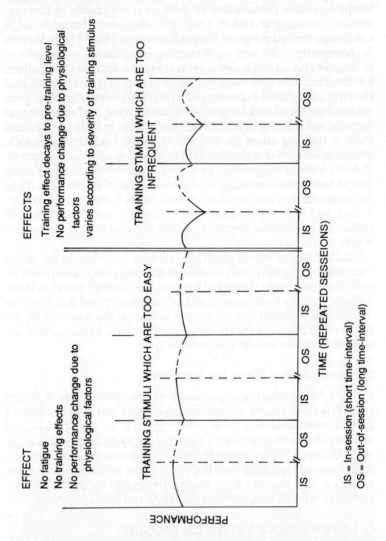

The last two features, highlighted above, indicate the need for the stimulus that accompanies a segment of training to be of sufficient overload (severity) to cause some fatigue to occur in the athlete. Repeated exposures to the same stimulus need to occur frequently enough to avoid having an athlete enter the decay stage of the response, while at the same time allowing sufficient time for recovery and overcompensation. Thus the timing of exposures to training stimuli and allowing sufficient opportunity to recover and overcompensate is one of the critical decisions that have to be made when developing and administering training programs. The alternation of training loads with recovery is commonly termed 'periodization'.

The programming of segment microcycles is predicated on there being definite objectives for training. A microcycle entailing a training stimulus should aim to produce some training effect in an athlete. The need for exposing the athlete to the stimulus should be balanced with the need for the athlete to recover. Since recovery occurs much more slowly than does the onset of fatigue, it is wise to conclude each microcycle with a phase of stimulus reduction, just in case adequate recovery has not occurred between each of the previous exposures. Figure 3.6 illustrates the segment microcycle model.

Figure 3.6 Basic Form of a Segment Microcycle

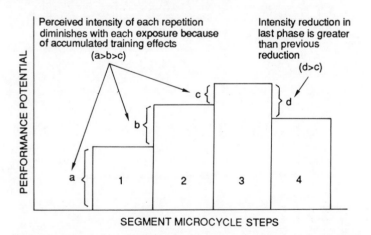

SEGMENT MICROCYCLE STEPS

Physical fitness is best developed through a step-like graduated program of segment microcycles rather than a linear form. Each step includes several exposures to a training stimulus followed by reduced exposure. The final reduction in stimulus intensity allows adaptation and recovery to occur. The feature that is important for coaches to understand in implementing this training model is that the recovery from a training stimulus is as important as the magnitude/type of the stimulus. In the past coaches predominantly focused on the work (training stimulus) to which an athlete should be exposed. Modern training approaches now require coaches to be as concerned with recovery as they are with workloads. It is not appropriate to expose an athlete to a training stimulus unless full recovery from the previous training stimulus has occurred.

The rest of this text will consider the use of forms of the microcycle, training stimuli, and training loads in formulating strategies for developing the physiological characteristics of athletes.

4
The Principle of Overload

This states that whenever an athlete is subjected to a training stimulus that causes fatigue (strain), the body will reorganize its capacities so that the next exposure to the same stimulus will produce less strain, given that sufficient recovery has occurred between exposures. Adaptation occurs through a gradual development of the capacities required to tolerate the stimulus (overcompensation or training effects). The level at which strain occurs is called the *threshold capacity*. Once that is exceeded, there is a certain amount of fatigue which temporarily reduces an athlete's capacity to perform. As a result of that physiological and neurological disruption, the body reacts to increase its stimulus-tolerance capacity. With repeated exposures to a stimulus, the cost of accommodating it will be reduced. For sports training, the implication of the overload principle is that with repeated exposures to successively more difficult, but similar, training stimuli, progressive improvements in performance will result. Performance improvement is higher the more frequently an athlete is exposed to a training stimulus, provided the frequency is not so great as to stop overcompensation (Bompa 1986).

The overload principle can be applied to both specific training stimuli and to the more general load of a training session.

Training Segment Overload

The training of a fitness component involves the repeated exposure to overload conditions followed by sufficient opportunity to recover to the point of producing a training effect. The level of overload which governs the usefulness of a training stimulus is inextricably yoked to the recovery requirement. Training benefits for athletes will occur only if both processes are allowed to occur in sequence.

The effects of the overload of a training stimulus in a segment microcycle diminish with each exposure to the segment. If there were too many repetitions of the same stimulus, the load intensity would diminish to the point where it did not exceed threshold capacity. From an athlete's viewpoint, at that stage the activity would be 'too easy'. Generally, the overload value of each successive segment microcycle needs to be progressively increased if further fitness improvements are desirable. However, there are limitations on the ultimate stimulus overload that can be presented to an athlete:

1. An athlete has a finite level of fitness that can be achieved. Once that is attained, further attempts to increase the fitness level yield little value and are potentially more harmful than beneficial.

2. The type of activity that is used to improve a fitness component affects the speed with which the component is increased. Simple activities which do not involve learning complicated skills produce changes quickly. For complex activities where intricate learning has to take place, physiological increases do not occur until neuromuscular reorganization has been achieved. In those activities, early gains in the fitness component stem from more efficient use of an existing capacity.

3. For each particular sport, there is a level of fitness that can be attained that can be fully used in the execution of its tasks. Above these levels, the extra capacity is not able to be used. For example, there are levels of strength and power that can be employed in swimming. However, it is possible to be very strong or powerful, but the activities of the sport are such that the extra capacity cannot be used. The consideration of this fact will be addressed in Section V, Methods and Effects of Training.

4. The programming of microcycles should be considered to be step-like. This differs from the common practice of gradually increasing the overload stimulus, usually with each training exposure. Each microcycle contains repetitions of the same stimulus, increases not occurring until the next one is introduced. In developing these stepped overloads, it must be realised that there is the possibility of accumulated fatigue effects, particularly those involving damage to the

body's structures. It is standard practice to provide an unloading microcycle that reduces the overload for the fitness component after a number of segment microcycles have been completed (Bompa 1986). Figure 4.1 illustrates this recommendation.

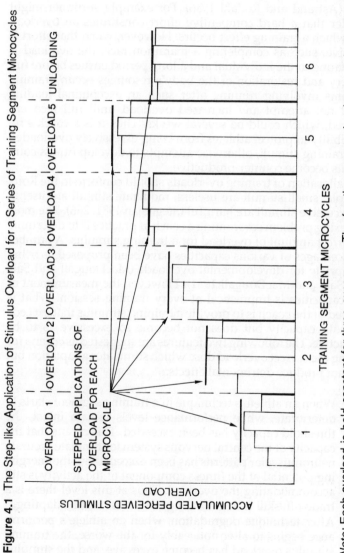

Figure 4.1 The Step-like Application of Stimulus Overload for a Series of Training Segment Microcycles

Note: Each overload is held constant for three exposures. The fourth exposure involves a reduction in the overload intensity. The sixth microcycle is the unloading one, where the degree of overload intensity is reduced relative to the preceding mircocycle overload intensity.

The amount of stimulus overload that can be beneficial to an individual athlete is limited. It is possible to exceed the adaptive capacity by setting stimuli that are excessive. Experiments have shown that training for an excessive duration in a segment does not contribute to any further increase in the development of a particular component of fitness. The initial loading produces the potential for training effects, while the excessive amounts are of no value (Astrand and Rodahl 1986). For example, a runner might consider that a hard competitive effort constitutes an overload from which a training effect occurs. However, when that effort is excessive, such as completing a marathon race, the overload is devastating to the individual and a long period ensues before full recovery and restoration of the body's resources occur. Training segments involving running after such an exceptional loading would not attempt any increased overload until full recovery occurred, which could be several weeks. Thus it is a coach's responsibility to protect athletes from being excessively overloaded with training stimuli, otherwise attempts to develop fitness components become counter-productive.

The allocation of training overloads should conform to the Roux Principle: small stimuli are useless, moderate stimuli are useful, and excessive stimuli are harmful (Stegeman 1981: 266). The most perplexing problem confronting a coach at practice is to determine the correct amount of overload for a training stimulus. A number of percentages of various capacities have been proposed as being appropriate for developmental overloads (MacDougall and Sale 1981, Sale and MacDougall 1981). However, the measurement of such capacities is impractical at every training session. What is required of the coach is to provide a training stimulus that exceeds threshold capacity but does not become so excessive as to be destructive. The following two features are suggested as criteria for judging the correct overload dose which stimulates adaptation but does not produce detrimental effects:

1. When an athlete's technique in a training segment starts to deteriorate, while performance levels remain intact, the threshold capacity has been exceeded. This means that the capacity of the central nervous system to stimulate accurate neuromuscular patterns has been exceeded but the energizing potential of the fitness component of the activity is still accommodating the overload. Thus at this level there is a trade-off: skill is deteriorating but fitness is still adapting.
2. After technique degradation, when an athlete's performance begins to alter noticeably for the worse, the training stimulus overload has become excessive, and the stimulus

should be stopped. At that stage neither skill nor fitness is adapting and any further training with that stimulus derives no benefit to the athlete.

Thus the guidelines for judging acceptable stimulus overloads encompass the monitoring of technique precision and performance levels. Diminished technique levels as a result of a training segment overload are often acceptable but disruptions of adequate performance levels are not. By maintaining training segment demands within these two bounds, it is believed that an adequate amount of overload will be produced to spur an optimum level of adaptation. These criteria are suggestions only and have not been verified in laboratory settings. Until better guidelines are produced, they remain these authors' best guess at a practical guideline for assessing the 'right amount' of physical work to produce the best training response. They should allow a coach to adhere to the Roux Principle.

When determining a training stimulus, the complexity of the activity needs to be considered. Generally, the more complex the training unit, the longer will be the time required for full physiological and neuromuscular adaptation. For example, one should expect that strength gains from doing arm curls (a relatively simple strength activity), would occur at a faster rate than would be achieved for doing a full clean-and-jerk (a complex strength activity). This has direct implications for planning training stimuli, microcycles, and progressions. It indicates that the greater the complexity of a training segment activity, the greater should be the number of repetitions within a microcycle. Complex activities require planning considerations that are different from simple activities (see Chapter 17).

The increase in performance potential that results from progressive overloads is gradual. The rate of the increase depends upon the way segment overloads are increased. There is a general principle that can be followed when planning segment microcycles. The amount that a segment load is increased is related to the length of time in the microcycle. Usually, the smaller the load increase, the shorter will be the time spent in a microcycle, while the greater the load, the longer will be the microcycle, provided the severity is not excessive. Figure 4.2 illustrates the reactions to two levels of segment overload. Some of the outcomes of each have been verified by research while others still remain hypothetical. The general features of a comparison of the two levels of overload:

1. When an easy training stimulus is experienced, the time spent in the tolerance stage is long, low levels of fatigue are incurred, the length of the recovery period is relatively

short, small training effects result, and training effects decay quickly.

2. When a heavy training stimulus is experienced, a short tolerance period is exhibited, high fatigue results, the recovery period is long, the size of the training effect is relatively large, and the training effect is more durable.

3. When overload stimuli are excessive, such as in the example of running a marathon or participating in 'hell weeks' in swimming, the effects on the athlete are destructive. It is possible to train too hard.

Figure 4.2 Comparative Effects of Hypothetical Easy and Heavy Training Stimuli

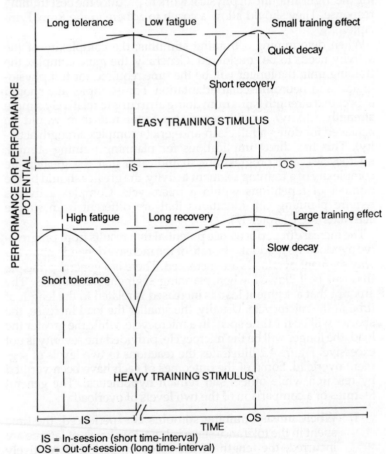

IS = In-session (short time-interval)
OS = Out-of-session (long time-interval)

One of the features of the art of coaching is to be able to estimate the correct amount of overload to develop an athlete at an optimum rate of progress. There is currently no exact answer to that problem. However, it can be assumed that the correct rate of overloading for an athlete will be peculiar to that individual. For one athlete it might be best to program many small load increases and microcycles, which would result in many small training effects. For another it might be more efficient to have an overall heavier training program which would cause fewer but larger training effects to occur. For others, a mix of heavy, moderate, and easy loads might be best. Unfortunately, there is no definitive principle that can be followed by coaches for developing athletes to their fullest potential in the most efficient manner. Coaches can only attempt to achieve the greatest level of efficiency through their knowledge of known principles of fitness training and the capacities of the individual (see Chapter 7 for a discussion on individuality).

Fitness components such as strength, power, and endurance respond to training loads at different rates. For example, the development of strength occurs at a faster rate than does endurance. This complicates the programming of training even further. If an athlete is to achieve peak levels of all necessary fitness components at the same time, then it will be necessary to adjust the segment overloads that develop each component, the length of time allocated to each segment microcycle, and even the time of commencing the component-development program. The challenge for the coach is to time the development of these capacities through appropriate training stimuli so that they 'peak' at the same time. This task is becoming more formidable and frequent as more sports involve multiple components and activities (e.g., decathlon, triathlon, medley events).

Following an overloaded session, the next overload should ideally occur during the overcompensatory phase of adaptation. Thus successive loadings in a segment microcycle should not occur until a training effect has been derived from the previous stimulus. Many common training practices violate this necessity. Coaches often feel that since training sessions have been scheduled for twice per day that training stimuli have to be presented on both occasions. Coaches must resist the temptation to program overloads according to the convenience of training schedules. They must be programmed instead according to sound principles of training. For many, altering the programming influence of schedules will be a difficult departure from usual practice. However, when that action is considered the folly of assigning overload experiences purely on the basis of, say, when pool times are scheduled, when facilities are made available, or when training can be programmed, will be realized.

There are two major variations of training stimuli which produce overload. They are segment volume (quantity) and segment intensity (quality).

Segment volume refers to the total quantity of work performed during the completion of a training segment. The purposes of assigning overloads through increases in volume are to increase the ability of the athlete to perform greater amounts of exercise of a particular intensity, and to increase recovery abilities between repeated exposures to the training stimulus. When a high number of repetitions of an exercise of moderate intensity is experienced, the training effect achieved is characterized more by maintenance of performance than by changes in performance amplitude. The determination of training volumes is modified by the specific requirements of each sport.

Segment intensity refers to the total amount of work performed per unit of time. The more work that is performed, the greater is the intensity of the training stimulus. The greater the intensity of a training stimulus, the greater is the muscular tension and nervous energy required. Overloads based on stimulus intensity tend to be more destructive of the athlete's systems than those effected by volume-oriented training. Consequently, when training is determined by intensity, longer recovery phases are usually required between each stage of the segment microcycle. The intensity of a training stimulus will affect the degree of fatigue that is developed, the size of the training effect that can be achieved, the time between sessions of repeated exposures to the training stimulus, and the capacity to engage in other training activities.

Successive segment microcycles can be constituted of variations of overload due to changes in both stimulus volume and intensity. The objectives of the segment activity will dictate when each factor is introduced and by how much it is emphasized.

There is a reciprocal relationship between segment volume and intensity. The harder the work, the less the volume, and vice versa. When the intensity of a training stimulus is excessive, the volume of work at that stimulus level should be reduced. On the other hand, high volumes of work require low levels of segment intensity. As a general rule, the following interpretations can be given to the two parameters of overload: intensity affects performance quality and magnitude, and volume affects performance stabilization and persistence. For improvements in fitness components other than forms of endurance, training overloads are better administered through changes in stimulus intensity, while endurance capacities are better facilitated through changes in stimulus volume.

The overload of a training stimulus is increased when the activity is first introduced. Novel activities not only require physiological work to be done, but there is also an added cost involved in learning and getting used to the new activity. Fatigue occurs more quickly when activities are new than when they are familiar. Thus the introduction of new training segments needs to consider the stress of adaptation to novelty as well as the stress of adaptation to the actual load of the segment.

When quick performance improvements are expected in an athlete by applying heavy to excessive training stimuli, the ultimate level of fitness that will be achieved is reduced when compared with other levels of loading. The reduction is caused by the athlete breaking down before full fitness potential is realized. As he or she becomes fitter, further improvements become harder to attain. Since the obvious results of training diminish, there is often a tendency for coaches to increase the level of overload to produce a 'more obvious' training effect. Such increases are counter-productive because they only hasten the onset of overtrained states or injuries.

The above considerations of overload are relevant to the institution of a training segment. Once a segment of a training session is completed, recovery starts to occur. If a segment is completed early in the session, recovery for that activity proceeds even though others are pursued. There is some possibility of a succeeding activity, which taxes a similar fitness component, retarding the recovery process. Thus the full recovery period includes time both in and between sessions. After a training session is completed, there is a general accumulated state of fatigue. The overall state affects the ability of an athlete to perform in subsequent training sessions, meaning that an athlete's response to a segment training load will be influenced by both the specific fatigue that resulted from the previous exposure as well as the state of general fatigue that exists. Generally, the greater the state of general fatigue, the worse will be the performance on specific segments of training. Consequently, coaches have to monitor both fatigue from specific training segments, and accumulated overall fatigue.

The above discussion has focused on the overloading of specific training segments. Segment microcycles employ the principle of overload to achieve certain training objectives. In some sports, training for different fitness components in one session can produce an added fatigue effect which must be considered when planning the magnitude of the session load. Therefore it is necessary for a coach to consider the general overload of a total training session if he or she is to prescribe a good program for developing sports fitness.

Training Session Overload

Each individual is endowed with a certain finite capacity to handle stress (Selye 1950). The stress-coping capacity is shared among all of life's stresses. The events of everyday living, such as fatigue from work, emotional involvement in interpersonal relationships, deprivation of rest, as well as the training stress of sports participation, all subtract from the finite ability of an individual to tolerate life's stresses. Thus the state of fatigue that results from session training stress and the demands of other life stresses all compete for finite resources in an attempt to produce recovery and adaptation. If total stresses exceed an individual's capacity to cope, then physical and behavior disruptions occur. Since the capacity to tolerate and adapt to stress is limited, the more stresses which occur outside sport, the less capacity there is for tolerating and adapting to the stress of physical activity. One's training capacity is reduced when the demands outside training are excessive.

A particular training program has its load modified by the strain that it causes in an individual. The product of the load–strain interaction is the training stress for that person. In order for an athlete to participate in the most beneficial training program, the training stress needs to be considered so that the overall stress-coping capacity is not exceeded. However, if the capacity is exceeded, temporary modification occurs. Adaptation results in much the same way as does the development of training effects. Thus the overall pattern of adaptation to training stresses needs to be considered.

The pattern of response to the accumulated effects of training fatigue is not new. Carlile (1955) proposed the adoption of Hans Selye's *General Adaptation Syndrome* — GAS (1950). Prokop (1963) also classified response 'cycles' to the stress of training. Selye's model is still popular and has endured the test of time.

Training loads have generalized non-specific effects superimposed upon the specific effects of training segments. Under the influence of loads, the body adapts itself by exhibiting a complex of symptoms. It has particular response patterns to each training stimulus, and a general pattern (GAS) to the combined effects of the training stimuli, that is, the training load. The GAS response can be differentiated into three stages: the alarm reaction stage, the stage of resistance, and the stage of exhaustion. Figure 4.3 illustrates the stages and shape of the GAS.

The *alarm reaction stage* is divided into two sub-stages, shock and counter-shock. Shock represents the athlete's initial response to a sudden exposure to unusual workloads. The most noticeable of these reactions occurs when an athlete starts to train after a lay-off.

In the first one to two weeks of training, work is difficult, fatiguing, inefficient, and low in total output. Performance potentials drop below those that were possible prior to the commencement of training. As in general shock, the body responds excessively and inefficiently to seemingly mild work demands. With consistent attendance at training sessions, these symptoms are gradually lost, as the body begins to adjust to the overall stress of exercise training. The initial adjustment is the counter-shock reaction. In counter-shock, the physiological changes of shock reverse and soon the adaptive mechanisms in the body proceed at a greater rate than the destructive processes. Performance potential begins to increase and returns to the pre-training level. Faulkner (1964) showed that when unfamiliar exercise stresses were encountered, the shock response of the individual was much greater than when the stress was familiar. For practical purposes, this means that untrained individuals exposed to moderate to high levels of exercise stress exhibit more of a shock reaction than do athletes who are untrained but have a history of training behind them. Training histories generally decrease the alarm reaction stage, resulting in quick specific adaptation. This phenomenon was evidenced by Prokop's adaptation syndrome for experienced athletes, in which a phase that resembled Selye's alarm reaction stage was omitted.

Figure 4.3 Stages of the General Adaptation Syndrome as a Response to Hard Training

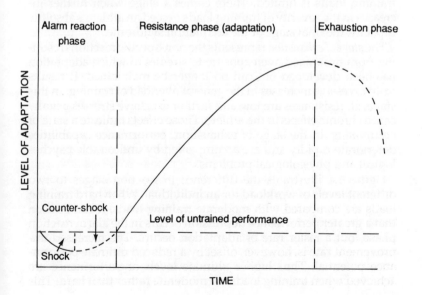

After the alarm reaction stage, a training athlete enters the *stage of resistance*. There is an increased resistance to exercise stress, and decreased resistance to all others. Performance potential increases during this stage. The duration of this second stage is dependent on training loads. Heavy to excessive training loads produce quick adaptation, but result in a diminished ultimate level. Moderate work loads do not produce as fast an adaptation rate but result in a higher ultimate level of performance. The individual variation that exists between athletes is great with regard to what training stresses can be absorbed.

While an athlete continues to resist the stress of training loads, vulnerability to other stresses is heightened. If the athlete's finite stress-coping capacity is exceeded through having other life-stresses increase, an alarm reaction may be superimposed physiologically on the resistance reactions. This phenomenon could be called 'phantom overtraining' because the symptoms are similar to those which occur in overtraining, but training is not the cause. Thus during a planned training program it is possible to have complete disruption of training adaptation due to other factors. In the training situation it becomes necessary to eliminate or minimize other stresses which could detract from the adaptation potential of the athlete, since every stress costs adaptation energy. The stage of resistance exhibits increased levels of performance while the demands of training remain within an athlete's stress-coping capacity. However, the ability of an individual to tolerate increased training loads is limited. There comes a stage when further increases in the severity of training loads exceed an athlete's absolute capacity, the final stage of the adaptation syndrome.

The *stage of exhaustion* represents the non-specific reactions resulting from prolonged overexposure to stresses to which adaptation has been developed but can no longer be maintained. It results from excessive increases in the general overload of training. In this stage, all resistances are low and further excessive stresses usually cause chronic effects in the athlete. Those effects indicate a state of *overtraining*. In the stage of exhaustion, performance capabilities deteriorate rapidly and are accompanied by undesirable psychological and physiological problems.

Figure 4.4 illustrates the difference in reaction stages to two different levels of workload for an individual. When hard training loads are compared with moderate training loads, it can be seen that a greater performance depression occurs in the alarm reaction phase, but a faster rate of adaptation occurs. The increased improvement rate is, however, offset by a reduced ultimate performance potential. Thus higher ultimate levels of performance are achieved when training loads are moderate rather than hard. This means that with regard to overloads, heavy ones may produce quick adaptation but the ultimate performance is lower. That phenomenon is in agreement with the overall implications of training, whether they be for specific training stimuli or for training loads. Moderate training demands followed by opportunities to recover produce the best training effects. Any attempts to accelerate the best programming of these factors reduce an athlete's ultimate performance potential.

Figure 4.4 Differential Reactions of the General Adaptation Syndrome to Two Levels of General Session Overload

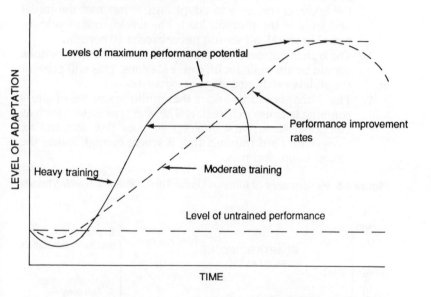

An implication of the general adaptation syndrome for training theory is illustrated in Figure 4.5. In training program A, the load is too light and the body has little reason to adapt. In training program B, the load is too heavy and the athlete reaches a stage of exhaustion where fatigue obscures any training effects. The result is one of failing adaptation, where many of the problems associated with overtraining are likely to be exhibited. In training program C, the load is ideal. Fatigue is minimized and the full benefits of training are demonstrated by improvements in performance.

There are several implications of the principle of overload as it applies to the general stress associated with repeated training sessions:

1. Training should commence slowly and progress gradually. An athlete would then be eased through the alarm reaction stage until some resistance and adaptation developed. On the other hand, if an athlete started from a low level of fitness, a high volume and intensity of training early in the program would cause fatigue and ultimate exhaustion. The overload principle would be better termed the 'principle of progressive overload', for that would better suit its implications for designing rational and sound training programs.

2. The training stress (volume/intensity) should be elevated gradually, in a step-like fashion, throughout the early stages of training. If it is kept constant, there will be no reason for the body to continue to adapt once it has met the initial demands of the training load. The weekly microcycle increase in workload should never exceed 10 percent.

3. The training stress should be cyclic in that harder sessions should be alternated with easier sessions. This will prevent the athlete reaching a stage of exhaustion.

4. The coach should be aware that multiple sources of stress combine to cause exhaustion. The effects of factors such as emotional stress, lack of sleep, or poor diet accumulate, along with hard training and, if severe enough, cause the athlete to break down.

Figure 4.5 Performance of Athletes Under Three Different Training Loads

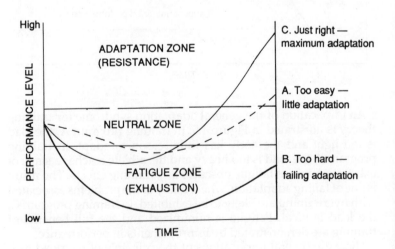

Selye's GAS offers the first hint that there might be some limits
to the ability of the body to adapt to training. There is a common
belief in Western sporting nations that if some training is good,
more training will be better. This probably stems from the 1930s
philosophy of training: 'miles make champions', and the more
recent emphasis on the quality of training efforts. In combination,
increases in both the volume and intensity of training can amount
to some extremely heavy training loads. It is not uncommon to see
modern swimmers training 10 to 12 times per week for a total of
more than 30 hours, during highly stressful episodes that are popularly known as 'hell weeks'. Elite distance runners usually cover
between 150 and 250 kilometers per week. Both these examples
usually result in athletes breaking down through overuse or over-
stress injuries. It is problematical whether such excessive exploit-
ation of the overload principle is needed for maximum adaptation.

Costill (1986) presented data on two marathon runners who
recommenced training after a six-month lay-off. Muscle biopsies
and treadmill VO_2 max tests were conducted as they gradually
increased their weekly distances. Figure 4.6 shows that there were
significant increases in VO_2 max when they increased their training
distance up to 40, and then to 80 kilometers per week. A subsequent
increase to 120 kilometers per week produced much smaller gains.

Figure 4.6 Changes in VO_2 max in Training of Distance Runners as a
Result of Increased Distance Overloads

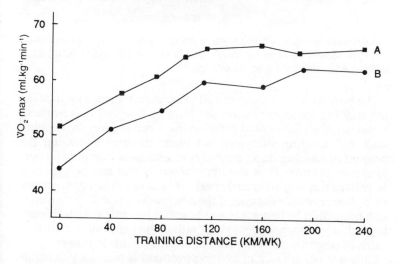

Further increases in training distance do not necessarily result in continued
improvement in aerobic power (after Costill 1986).

Running for distances beyond this, such as to 160 kilometers per week, resulted in greatly diminished returns. This led Costill to conclude that the running distance needed for maximum endurance training benefits was between 100 and 140 kilometers per week. That range of distances is less than the current popular practice of modern élite distance runners.

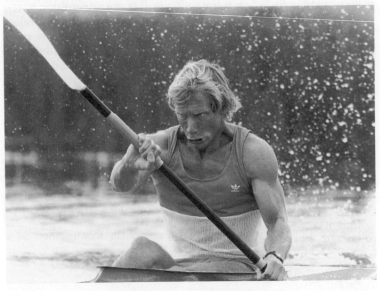

It is not necessarily true that if some training is good, more must be better. Athletes should become aware of their tolerance for coping with heavy training and adjust the load accordingly

The implications of the overload principle are correct for increasing training loads until a certain level of adaptation is reached. However, the relationship between the magnitude of the training load and sporting success is not linear. Despite increasing the amount of training done, there comes a stage of diminishing performance returns. Thus the improvements that can be expected from hard training in the early part of a season will be much greater than those towards the end of the season. As a season progresses, coaches would be better advised to spend more time on technical, tactical, and psychological skills rather than striving for further gains in performance as a result of improvements in fitness.

Only a small amount of training overload is necessary to maintain fitness once a high level has been attained. During the early part of 1965, the great Australian distance runner, Ron Clarke,

toured the world and produced a series of world record performances without involving himself in hard training. The competitive
efforts and a few training sessions between them were sufficient to
maintain the peak fitness he had attained prior to the tour. Another
example of the ability to maintain peak fitness over a lengthy
period without being involved in large amounts of hard training
was shown in the performances of the Russian national swimming
team in 1978. After performing creditably against the East German
team, the Russians travelled to the USA and two weeks later
recorded a number of Russian national records. These were
achieved without any demanding training between the two competitions. The same team then travelled to Canada and 10 days later
set 17 Russian records. These improvements in performances were
achieved without returning to sustained hard training. It seemed
that the stimulating effects of hard competitive efforts and reduced
interim training were sufficient to maintain previously attained
levels of fitness. After a high level of fitness has been developed,
the same amount of hard training is not necessary to maintain these
levels. A reduction in training frequency, but not intensity, to about
one-third is considered suitable for maintaining endurance capacity. It is suggested that even greater reductions could be tolerated
for strength and power activities. The relationship between Selye's
adaptation curve and the concept of fitness change and maintenance training is shown in Figure 4.7.

The stage of training A is the base level of adaptation and performance in an untrained state. B is the reduction in performance
capability that occurs in the alarm reaction stage in the early phase
of training. C is the performance change in the resistance phase of
the stress adaptation curve, that is, the stage where fitness is
changing ('change training'). Here the improvement in performance, within certain limits, seems to be directly related to the
magnitude of the training load. D indicates the phase of diminishing returns where further hard training does not result in commen-
surate gains in performance through fitness variables. E is the
plateau stage where fitness peaks: further hard training would not
result in greater fitness. This level of fitness is maintained by fewer
frequencies of hard training sessions ('maintenance training'). F
indicates the reduction in performance that would accompany
overtraining if maintenance training was not instituted. This
would have resulted if further elevations in the training load
occurred at stage D. The graph illustrates two important forms of
training. The first is 'change training', where the results of training
loads produce changed fitness levels. Since the amount of change
that can be achieved is limited, it serves no purpose to maintain the
frequency of loading that produced the change when no further

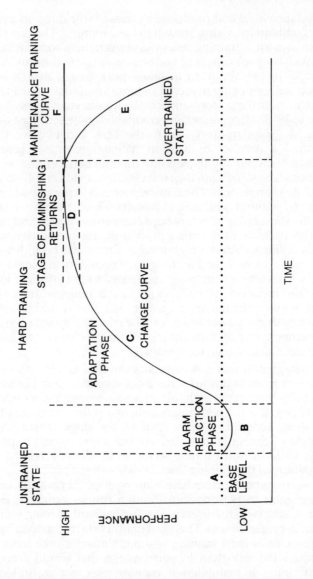

Figure 4.7 Training Progression Stages and Alternatives

Source: Rushall and Lavoie 1983

change is possible. Thus after as much change in fitness as possible has been achieved, the training emphasis is altered.

The aim of training should be to maintain the highest levels possible. Maintenance training requires different overloads from change training. The intensity of the workloads remain similar in both forms of training, but the frequency of training sessions devoted to maintenance fitness is reduced to about one-third of that required for change training.

The major decision that has to be made by a coach with regard to planning training overloads is whether to keep increasing the workload and run the risk of overtraining an athlete, or to reduce the workload and maintain the fitness states and benefits that have been attained. Symptoms of overtraining that will assist the coach to recognize when an athlete has been pushed into an undesirable state are discussed in Chapter 8.

5

The Principle of Recovery

An athlete's improvement is dependent upon the provision of adequate recovery so that training effects can be maximized. The Principle of Recovery implies that for maximum performance benefits and before a training stimulus is reintroduced, complete recovery from the previous stimulation must occur. To train without adequate recovery from previous fatiguing work does not produce any benefit to athletes, for they merely learn to cope with fatigue rather than improving in specific aspects of performance.

Recovery from three sources of fatigue is necessary: the fatigue of a specific training stimulus which is primarily physiological in nature; the general fatigue that results from the stress of a total training session and which is both physiological and psychological; and long-term fatigue that results from entering the stage of exhaustion in the overall stress adaptation syndrome. The latter form of fatigue is physiological, psychological, and biomechanical (the disruption of neuromuscular patterns) in nature. The importance of recovery and avoidance of extreme fatigue from each of these sources should be of central concern to coaches and athletes. The positive relationship between fatigue and recovery time is the underlying moderator of recovery planning. The greater the state of fatigue, the greater is the time that needs to be allocated to recovery. However, excessive recovery time could lead to the loss of temporary training effects. The timing of the regeneration/overcompensation reaction is critical for producing performance improvements.

The rate at which an athlete recovers from any source of fatigue determines the rate at which training can progress. Individual differences moderate recovery rates and so programming of training stimuli and sessions will depend upon each athlete's capacity. A failure to adapt training programs to each athlete's need for recovery represents poor coaching. Training programs need to be planned to accommodate the recovery requirements of each athlete.

If recovery between successive training stimuli and sessions is inadequate, fatigue will accumulate and adaptive training processes will not be evident. This results in delayed adaptation, performance decline, and an increase in the likelihood of injury and/or illness. The benefits of training and competitions are not achieved unless a coach emphasizes the recovery process with equal emphasis to that afforded overload. The most important factor that affects an athlete's health status is the alternation of overload stimuli with adequate recovery between each presentation.

Recovery from Training Stimuli Within a Training Session

After a training stimulus has exceeded an athlete's threshold capacity, the activity should cease. Recovery permits the re-establishment of all stressed systems to full functioning. Overcompensation involves the morphological reorganization of these functional systems to perform better during repeated exposures to the original stress. The functional systems are both physiological and psychological in nature. At one extreme, for pure physiological fatigue, the regeneration of physiological functions is emphasized. At the other extreme, in sports where psychological fatigue occurs, such as sailing, shooting, and archery, psychological capacities and their underlying physiological components are regenerated. Allowing the central nervous system to recover from stressful stimulation is often neglected in fitness-oriented coaching systems. Effective training allows time for both processes to occur (*Sports*, October 1986).

The adaptation to specific training stimuli is the result of the correct alternation between work/stimulation and regeneration/overcompensation. Regeneration is initially fast but then it slows. The absolute time for recovery depends upon the individual, the level of fatigue incurred, the energy systems involved, and a number of moderating factors. Some of those moderating factors are:

1.   Both fatigue and recovery will occur more quickly in simple than in complex activities, and performance will improve and reach its maximum level in a seemingly short period of time.

2.   Fatigue will take longer to occur if the technical proficiency of performance is high. This is because less energy per repetition of the exercise is used in more competent performers. Changes in technical efficiency partly explain why performances continue to improve after physiological capacities have reached their maximum adaptation level. Examples of this are clearly seen in running, swimming, and rowing. In activities where energy use is a primary factor, the efficiencies of techniques will be a major determinant of performance, and training emphases should accordingly reflect this. Training must be specific to produce the greatest rate of physiological and skill adaptation.

3.   The effects of specific volumes and intensities of training vary from increasing muscle strength and power to making both the central and peripheral adaptations that are important in endurance activities. The degree to which these effects occur depends upon the nature of the training stimulus. The particular mix of response components in the sport will dictate that different recovery times will be required for different activities and capacities.

4.   The nature of the work done affects recovery speeds. The time it takes to recover from exercise with a substantial component of eccentric work, such as running, is slower than that following the predominantly concentric work experienced in swimming or cycling (O'Reilly, Warhol, Fielding, Frontera, Meredith, and Evans 1987). Running places a higher degree of strain on the musculoskeletal system than do other activities. This explains why it is possible to complete twenty-two consecutive daily sprint and endurance stages of the Tour de France cycling event which would not be possible if running were the mode of exercise. Hence coaches of athletes who perform a lot of running need to be conservative when planning training, as opposed to what might be appropriate for cyclists, rowers, kayakers, and swimmers. Runners would need larger work/rest ratios than do those in other sports.

5.   Complex activities fatigue at slower rates than do simple activities. The complexity allows a family of neuromuscular coordinations to develop to achieve similar functional outcomes. It is not unusual for athletes to cycle through these alternative functional patterns while performing. Since each

pattern uses different muscle fibers, while one pattern is being used the fibers associated with another can recover. Minor alterations in techniques of sports which are cyclic in nature (e.g., swimming, running, rowing, cycling) occur as the activity progresses without any diminution in performance level. These technique alterations are also forced upon the athlete due to changes in terrain or activity demands. Thus fatigued sites incurred while running on a flat surface will partly recover on downhill or uphill sections. Although this phenomenon concerns muscle fibers, it also occurs on a much larger scale. For example, triathletes are able to shift the workload between different muscle groups according to the activity being performed. This alteration allows them to maintain high levels of work for very extended periods. The switch to 'fresh' muscles with each new activity rejuvenates their performance potential.

The one feature that delays recovery is the accumulation of lactic acid in muscles and the blood. Blood lactic acid levels can reach as high as 20 mmol.L^{-1}. The body can tolerate a certain level of acidity in the blood but, beyond that, unconsciousness results as a protective reaction to stop damage occurring. In certain sporting situations athletes occasionally incur unusually high levels of lactic acid in the blood and as a consequence they collapse during performance. This is a particular feature of weight-supported total body activities such as rowing. Training stimuli which produce high levels of acidosis may elevate resting oxygen consumption for several hours. When an athlete reaches maximum lactate tolerance at training, exhaustion occurs, and work must be terminated or at least sharply reduced. This suggests that only one exposure to a state of maximum lactic acidosis is appropriate for a training stimulus. Repeated exposures to maximum levels are not beneficial and detract from movement efficiency.

During a training stimulus, lactic acid concentrations in excess of 8 mmol.L^{-1} impair both training performance and the learning of new skills. Therefore in training for skilled (that is, most) sports, high levels of lactic acid should not occur.

Recovery procedures should be an integral part of a training session. Recovery can be facilitated by altering activities and scheduling them in particular sequences (see Chapter 18). It is not always necessary to wait for complete recovery before commencing a new training stimulus. By altering exercises and stimuli, substantial training demands can be made without compromising the recovery process for specific stimuli. Rest intervals cannot be considered 'true recovery periods' while parts of the body are still working.

Thus rest interval demands will govern the adequacy of recovery for specific exercises. Alternating activities does, however, allow some recovery to occur. The rate of recovery will depend on the degree to which the alternated activity generates lactic acid and the amount of use required of already fatigued muscle fibers.

Recovery from Training Sessions

Each training session has an accumulation of fatigue states and products that occur from the training stimuli experienced. Recovery after an exercise session primarily involves replenishing depleted energy stores, removing accumulated metabolites, and repairing damaged tissue. The stress of a training session is both psychological and physiological.

Serious and demanding training sessions cause a reduction in an athlete's ability to perform during and immediately after each training session. Thus the skilful manipulation of the training loads encountered during a session is usually one way of ensuring that excessive fatigue doesn't accumulate across sessions. Two ploys are used to guard against the accumulation of fatigue. The first involves a load reduction for each stimulus in the last step of a microcycle (see Figure 3.6). This will serve as a safeguard against overfatigue in each capacity and will reduce the accumulated stress of the sessions within the microcycle. The second strategy involves the consideration of the strain of each training session. The plan is that levels of strain occur, such as hard, medium, and light loads. Following a hard session with a light session at all times will allow recovery to take place, whereas one hard session followed by another may diminish the intended value of the second. Because of accumulated general fatigue from the two hard sessions it may even take longer to recover from two adjacent sessions than from each session conducted individually, interspersed with a light load session. The sequencing of different training session stresses will allow recovery to occur so that productive work can be conducted across the total microcycle.

It is possible to have training sessions that are too long and develop fatigue states which are more destructive than helpful, particularly in a neuromuscular sense. There comes a time when the accumulated fatigue within a training session is of sufficient potential harm for the session to be terminated. Coaches should avoid having athletes reach this critical state.

Recovery from fatigue induced by a training session can be accelerated by using recovery activities after training. The final activity of the training session (see Chapter 18) should serve to

disperse fluid and metabolites from the muscles and reduces residual soreness. A period of low intensity activity and muscle stretching exercises are ideal for this purpose. It is wise, from a
motivational point of view, as well as for physiological reasons, to
have athletes leave training or competitions in a partly recovered
state at least.

Recovery is more difficult if athletes train two or three times per
day. Light load or restoration sessions must be included to permit
recovery from the main specialized training session. It is important
to avoid closely-spaced sessions of intensive work of lengthy duration. Generally, the more training sessions conducted in a day, the
shorter the duration of each. Light-intensity sessions can be used
as strategy teaching sessions while the functional capacities of the
neuromuscular system are restored.

Diet is important in the recovery process. Protein, the important
nutrient in tissue building and repair, is required after prolonged
intensive efforts or in response to heavy strength training and
muscle-building programs. It is recommended that weight-lifters,
body-builders, and endurance athletes recovering from hard training or competitions, increase the amount of protein in their diet to
facilitate the requirements of tissue synthesis. This increase is
usually from the recommended daily intake of 1 g.kg^{-1} to between
1.5 and 2.0 g.kg^{-1} (see Chapter 9). This can be easily met from an
increased food intake and does not require the supplements (e.g.,
protein powders, pills) that are commonly used by strength athletes and body-builders.

The rate of muscle glycogen synthesis is increased by a diet rich
in complex carbohydrates. A study by Sherman (1987) showed that
an elevation from 50 to 70 percent carbohydrate in the diet during
successive days of hard training (16 km run at 80 percent $\dot{V}O_2$ max)
significantly improved muscle glycogen repletion rate. This strategy can normalize muscle glycogen within 24 hours, down from a
possible 36–48 hour time requirement (see Figure 5.1).

The time required for recovery of different physiological capacities varies a great deal as does the time for the replenishment of
biochemical substrates. Creatine-phosphate reserves are replaced
very rapidly. However, the replacement of glycogen stores and the
mending of damaged muscle elements take a markedly longer
time. Connective tissues (tendons and fascia) and supportive tissues (ligaments) take the longest time of all functions for recovery
primarily due to their decreased vascularization. The circulatory
system requires a moderate amount of time for recovery when
compared with other systems. Attempts to recover quickly must
be directed primarily at those systems which need more time to
recover. This requires a coach to modify the intensity and volume

of training by scheduling the occurrence of stimuli that are associated with different physical capacities at different times during training microcycles (see Chapter 18 and Figure 18.1).

Figure 5.1 Muscle Glycogen Depletion and Resynthesis during Successive Days of Hard Training under Two Different Carbohydrate Diets

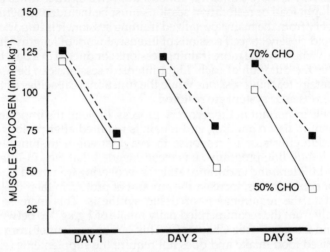

The 70 percent diet facilitated almost complete replenishment within 24 hours, whereas the 50 percent diet showed incomplete recovery producing a gradually worsening state.

Today's training loads are so demanding that 'natural' recovery alone can no longer provide adequate recovery. It is part of modern training lore that certain activities are needed to accelerate recovery, hence allowing a more frequent occurrence of training stimuli and stresses. An increase in volume of quality training has been effective in producing the elevated performance levels that are witnessed in modern sport. Methods for accelerating recovery are necessary to train today's athletes.

The recovery from training session stress is enhanced by active rest; sleep; alternation of working muscle groups in the training session; a positive psychological mental set during training and recovery; external stimulation such as massage and rub-downs; environmental stimulation from activities such as whirlpool baths and alternating hot and cold baths/showers; relaxation in flotation tanks and spa baths; and diet. Combinations of these activities accelerate recovery speeds even further. When active recovery (e.g., light runs, easy swims, a bout of surfing) is coupled with passive recovery (e.g., relaxation warm baths, massage) the speed of recovery is better than active recovery alone (*Sports*, February 1986).

Why recovery activities are helpful is not fully understood. When light exercise is performed in the recovery periods interspersed throughout a training session, the activity facilitates the use of lactic acid as fuel by the skeletal muscles, as well as rapid circulation to the heart muscle for the same purpose. Lactic acid removal is accelerated by active recovery (Belcastro and Bonen 1975). However, if the intensity of the effort in recovery is too high (> 60 percent $\dot{V}O_2$ max) it is likely that more lactic acid will be produced and recovery retarded. This process explains some of the effects of active recovery both within and between training sessions.

The alternation of active and passive recovery activities is not so well understood. The following hypothesis could explain this phenomenon. When activities unrelated to the training activity or stress are undertaken, the body mobilizes many resources in much the same manner as occurs in the alarm reaction phase of Selye's Stress Adaptation Syndrome (see previous chapter). This exaggerated response increases the body's functions and thus accelerates the recovery process. This means that recovery acceleration should be associated with non-specific activities that challenge the body's ability to cope with them. Alternations between various stimulus modalities increase alarm-reaction-type responses even further. For example, alternations of hot and cold baths/showers, passive/active exercise, rest/massage, upright/supine postural changes, jogging/swimming, have all been found to speed up the rate of recovery from fatigue.

There is no need to restrict recovery to only one form of activity. It would seem that a variety of recovery activities of a total-body nature are better than single isolated activities. It has been recommended that special recovery techniques should not be employed until 6–9 hours after either competitions or very intense training sessions (Talyshev 1977). However, more immediate recovery activities are popular in modern sports. Research needs to be conducted to discover the most desirable timing of these procedures.

The time that an athlete has available and the activities pursued outside the training environment should be monitored. If these activities are stressful they can impede the speed of recovery. Athletes have to be taught how to behave at such times so that there is no interference with regeneration and overcompensation. Time away from the sporting environment should be used to ensure physical and psychological regeneration before the next training session.

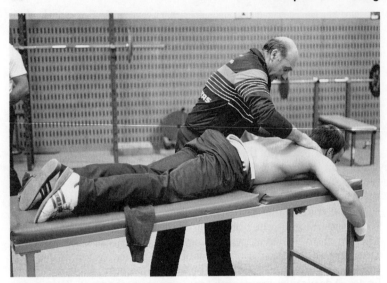

Massage is used as a means of hastening recovery from fatigue associated with hard training

The point behind recovery procedures between training sessions is that a greater number of intense sessions can be completed if recovery rates are accelerated. The means by which that acceleration is promoted vary greatly and depend on the preferences of athletes for each type of activity. Specific recovery work between training sessions is now an integral part of modern sports training.

Recovery from Long-term Exhaustion

The body can cope for only for a limited period with adapting to excessive levels of a specific stress. Performance improvements due to specific exercise adaptations occur and then reach a plateau. If the stress of training continues, performances deteriorate rapidly, as does the ability to cope with even light amounts of the specific exercise stress (see previous chapter referring to the 'stage of exhaustion'). The measurement of this state is discussed at much greater length in Chapter 8.

That fatigue accrues in the latter stages of exercise stress adaptation is demonstrated by the benefits derived from reduced workloads in the tapering process (the final step in peaking) in the competition phase of training. Both the volume and intensity of training stimuli are reduced prior to important competitions (see Chapter 19). Swimmers have produced 3 percent improvements in performance after a 14-day tapering period in which their total volume of training decreased from 7,500 to 3,500 yards (2,250 to 1,050 meters) per day and the volume of interval work decreased from 5,500 to 1,500 yards (1,650 to 450 meters) per day. These gains in performance were associated with a significant increase in power output measured on a Biokinetic swim bench and in a power swim test. This tapering procedure had no influence on the acid–base status of blood measured after a standard-paced 200-yard swim at 90 percent maximum speed (Costill, King, Thomas, and Hargreaves 1985). In tapering, the major targets for recovery are energy provision and the physiological state of the central nervous system.

Case studies of international track cyclists also showed that performance benefits can be achieved by tapering. Improvements in muscular power and mechanical and cardiovascular efficiency were measured in laboratory cycling tests throughout a 4–10-day tapering period. It was also noted that mood state variables tended to alter in concert with physiological variables. For example, the cyclists became less tense and depressed and reported feeling more vigorous as the taper period progressed (Pyke, Craig, and Norton 1988).

The mechanisms responsible for the benefits of tapering are not clearly understood but the consistent finding of improvements in muscular power suggests that neuromuscular events are involved. This supports the common observation that during periods of intensive endurance training, athletes experience a marked reduction in muscular strength and power which recovers with rest and detraining. Thus if athletes are to perform to their full potential, it is essential that the physical stress of training be reduced in the days leading up to a competition and be non-existent on the competition day. The challenge for the coach in programming such recovery is to avoid detraining, which could occur when too much rest is scheduled. The fear of this happening has even retarded the acceptance of tapering regimes in some sports.

Overtraining results from overlooking the work/recovery ratio. Its onset is accelerated by exposing an athlete to high-intensity stimuli when he or she is in a state of fatigue. The ability to tolerate exercise fatigue is governed by the accumulation of stresses from within and outside the sport setting. When outside stresses are increased, training loads must be reduced. Psychological demands and stresses can also hasten the onset of fatigue. Training loads must be moderated in the light of these extraneous effects.

When an athlete arrives at the stage of exhaustion (i.e., an overtrained state) a serious error has occurred in the planning of training. Unloading microcycles in the structure of macrocycles are supposed to be the insurance policy to avert long-term exhaustion. However, if overtraining does arise there are very few options for the athlete to follow in order to recover. If a stage of mild exhaustion has been reached, then extended periods of reduced volumes and intensities of training with increased amounts of rest may be sufficient to allow regeneration to occur. Having the athlete also engage in alternative activities that produce non-stressful physical demands and positive psychological states will also assist in recovery. Testing sessions and competitions should be avoided and psychological pressures reduced. With mild exhaustion it is possible that performances will recover after a relatively short time (perhaps one month, but this is dependent on the severity of fatigue).

When an athlete is thoroughly exhausted the prognosis is different. Then he or she is usually required to cease training. The period of recovery is quite lengthy even though other positive-experience activities are enacted. The major recovery procedure is rest and the avoidance of any intense specific activity. The time for such recovery to occur is individual and can often be as long as six months. Performance potential deteriorates dramatically during this recovery period because of marked detraining effects. The combination of physical fatigue and its negative psychological correlates could also thwart any complete recovery. There are many anecdotal cases of athletes being severely overtrained and never regaining previous levels of performance despite reduced workloads and seemingly more sane training programs after the occurrence. If one recalls one part of the Roux Principle, *excessive training loads are harmful*, then long-term exhaustion is to be avoided at all costs. The only options for recovery are, in order of preference, rest, irrelevant activity, and low-intensity and low-volume specific activity.

As a means of stress control, the proportion of training time devoted to recovery, the provision of unloading steps in microcycles, and unloading microcycles in macrocycles, are all critical. The stage of exhaustion should be avoided for it has no beneficial effects for an athlete.

Recovery and Reversibility

If recovery time is extended there is always the concern that detraining might occur. The rate at which it occurs is relevant for understanding the detrimental effects of enforced bed rest, limited movement as a result of injury, and detraining between competitive seasons.

Bed rest produces a marked deterioration in endurance performance with decreases in $\dot{V}O_2$ max of 6–7 percent occurring in one week and as much as 25 percent in three weeks. It then requires from four to six weeks of retraining to recover the 25 percent loss (Saltin, Blomquist, Mitchell, Johnson, Wildenthal, and Chapman 1968). A significant decrease in the endurance performance of runners has been noted after 15 days of detraining. This was particularly noticeable in the oxidative enzymes in muscle and was not recovered in the same period of retraining (Houston, Bentzen, and Larson 1979). Costill, Fink, Hargreaves, King, Thomas, and Fielding (1985) demonstrated significant reductions in the respiratory capacity of the shoulder muscles of swimmers and hence the amount of lactic acid produced in a standard speed swim, only one week after cessation of training. Brief lay-offs seemed to significantly reduce endurance performance and led to the conclusion that 5 months of endurance conditioning can be completely lost in 6–8 weeks of inactivity.

While muscular strength and power seem to be lost less rapidly than endurance, they are still only transient attributes (Berger 1962). The different time courses of the rate of deterioration of muscular power and endurance perhaps explain why the taper period for a sprinter is usually longer than that of a distance runner. However, with complete immobilisation in a supporting cast following bone fractures or joint reconstructions, the size and strength of the muscles can deteriorate very rapidly.

There are two implications of these findings. Athletes who are injured should be encouraged to maintain certain aspects of their fitness by using other limbs or modes of exercise. For example, footballers with ankle injuries may not be able to run but can cycle or swim to maintain their central aerobic fitness and some aspects of muscular fitness. During the break between seasons, athletes should remain active. This will allow them time to recover from the specific demands of the sport and to maintain fitness during the transition phase (see Chapter 19). They will then enter the basic preparatory phase for the next competitive season at a higher level of fitness and be in a better position to make annual improvements in performance. The possibility of detraining effects occurring during a season when physiological capacity demands are altered is discussed in Chapter 18.

Summary

Recovery is a critical factor in modern sports training. Coaches need to program recovery opportunities within training sessions (by planning the order, alternation, duration, and intensity of training stimuli); between sessions (by providing the opportunity to participate in active/passive recovery activities); and from over-training. If recovery within and between training sessions is adequate, then overtraining or 'burn-out' should be avoided. The Principle of Recovery should be considered to be of similar importance to the Principle of Overload.

⑥
The Principle of Specificity

The Principle of Specificity states that the maximum benefits of a training stimulus can only be obtained when it replicates the movements and energy systems involved in the activities of a sport. When a sport can be divided into particular components and tasks, the more they can be practiced, the better will be the performance. Research indicates that task repetitions should be as physiologically, biomechanically, and psychologically similar to the sport performance criteria as possible.

This principle may suggest that there is no better training than actually performing in the sport. However, it is not so simple in its implications. In intermittent sports such as tennis, volleyball, and netball, there may be only a few times during a game when the effort made by the player is of adequate intensity to generate a partial training stimulus. The few game repetitions may be sufficient to maintain the fitness component that is taxed, but they will not improve it. The coach needs to select specific samples of game-related activities for intensified attention in training. Training programs for these types of sports would, therefore, attempt to overload the fitness components that are required in a game by grouping repetitions of game-situation simulations. However, a similar approach does not work for other sports. If a runner or swimmer were to train merely by performing race efforts, the demand would constitute an extreme load that could not often be repeated in a training session. The training stimulus would then be applied too infrequently to produce any marked training effect. It would be better for a coach to select portions of the race distance and repeat these several times. The dissection of events into portions of distances (intervals) allows an athlete to be subjected to a higher quantity of high-quality work than is possible in continuous activity. The interruptions between the repetitions serve as rest periods and allow some recovery. Thus, with sufficient repetitions, an athlete is subjected to repeated exposures to stresses which approximate various stages of a continuous maximum race effort. This form of training allows an athlete to be appropriately loaded to improve on the specific energy and fitness demands of the sport.

The evidence in support of the principle of specificity is overwhelming. It relates to both the muscle groups being employed and the muscle fibers or energy system being used.

Muscle Group Specificity

It takes only a small change in the position of a movement to drastically alter the muscle groups involved in the action. For example, in a simple movement such as flexion at the elbow joint, the forearm could either be pronated or supinated. Electromyograph (EMG) studies have shown that when flexion is performed with the lower arm pronated, the smaller brachioradialis muscle is used to a greater extent than the larger biceps brachii. The situation is reversed when the forearm is supinated where the powerful biceps play the dominant role. This explains why more bar-chins can be completed with an underhand grip than can be done with an overhand grip on the bar.

The lesson behind this example is that the manner of the exercise determines the exercise training effect. The sport of rowing requires flexion at the elbow at the finish position of the rowing stroke. Since holding an oar or sculls requires the forearm to be pronated, it would be more beneficial to practice elbow flexion exercises (chins, curls, etc.) with the wrists in that position rather than with them supinated. Although flexion of the elbow is used to describe the exercise irrespective of the forearm position, however, that does not mean that the training effects derived from flexions with the wrist in either position are the same. It is crucial for efficient use of fitness training time that the muscle groups of an activity be trained in the same locus of movement and speed of contraction that will be used in the sport.

The postural position that is used in training also affects the type of training effect. Rasch and Morehouse (1957) reported that a training program that increased elbow flexor strength at the waist had no effect on the muscular action when the arm was overhead.

Another example of the specificity of the strength training response was shown in a study of leg-squat training. The muscles are used in different ways in squatting and pressing, so quite different responses exist for the two activities. A much greater improvement in leg-squat strength than isometric leg-press strength was obtained. The muscular strength adaptations gained through squatting only partially transfer to the action of isometric leg-pressing (Thorstensson and Karlson 1974).

Isometric knee-extension training at the knee-joint angles of 15 and 60 degrees also produced quite specific training effects (Lindh 1979). Training at the 15 degree joint angle produced a 32 percent increase in isometric strength measured at that angle. The improvement at the 60 degree angle was only 13 percent. On the other hand, training at a 60 degree joint angle produced a 30 percent increase and only a 10 percent increase at 15 degrees. A load is carried in a different manner by the muscles in the thigh when they function at different knee-joint angles. Hence, the training adaptations are specific to the degree of muscle involvement.

Another variable that affects the specificity of training is the type of equipment used. Pipes (1978) trained groups using the same movement pattern on Nautilus (isokinetic contractions) and Universal (isotonic contractions) weight machines. Strength increases of 25 percent on the training equipment were found to be only 10 percent increases if measured on the alternate equipment. Thus, even though the exercises were visually similar, the actions required by the two different forms of apparatus were more different than they were alike. Martindale, Robertson, Coutts, and McKenzie (1982) showed that training on rowing ergometers was very different, in terms of internal work, from performing in a real shell. There are a number of examples of would-be rowers who can achieve high power outputs on rowing ergometers but are less effective on the water. Thus ergometer performances are related only to a minor degree to actual rowing. The emphasis placed on rowing-ergometer training should be evaluated in light of this knowledge.

Most coaches claim to be aware of the principle of specificity yet violate it in training practices. For example, there is a widely held belief that training on one strength activity will transfer training effects to another even though the locus of movement and skill quality of the acts are dissimilar. Strength gained in resistance exercises supposedly can be re-educated into skill performance (for example, see Bompa 1986). Sale and MacDougall (1981) showed this assumption not to be supported by research.

It would appear that the many benefits of training fitness components reside in the neuromuscular patterning of activities, and this appears to be a critical feature when understanding the principle of specificity. Training activities should be analyzed to be qualitatively the same as those required for competition. Coaches are warned of the potential for supplementary training activities to produce competing and often dominant neuromuscular patterns which reduce or even hinder performance. Some originally highly-skilled, world-record-setting swimmers have slowed because they substituted resistance training movement patterns in their swimming routine, swimming with resistance-training patterns of movement which were less efficient than natural-stroking patterns. This has important implications for fitness training. There is the possibility that if supplementary training is sufficiently emphasized, artificial and inappropriate movement patterns will come to dominate the natural and efficient movement patterns of athletes, and supplant the natural desirable patterns; performance will then deteriorate. In effect, a swimmer could finish up swimming with pulley-obtained arm patterns as opposed to naturally correct swimming movements. Neuromuscular patterns for speed, strength, power, and balance are all dependent on the speed and pattern of movement of that activity. Costill, Sharp, and Troup (1980) concluded that swimming strength is best achieved by repeated maximum exercises that duplicate as closely as possible the skill of swimming. The most appropriate exercise that they suggested was a series of maximum sprint swims.

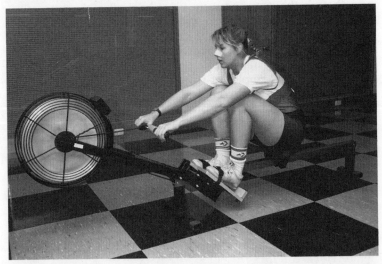

While athletes are encouraged to be specific in their training, care must be taken to avoid training on ergometers that do not exactly duplicate the movement patterns involved in the sport

The more the training and competition activities differ, the less valuable will be the training activities for affecting real performances. The gradient of transfer value loss of a training effect between two activities is particularly steep. For example, activities which look similar, but are performed at slightly different speeds, are most likely to be completely dissimilar in their training effects. This means that for every alteration of the speed of action — and the same applies to path of movement or apparatus used — there is a different neuromuscular pattern of movement developed. In essence, if the 'same' skill is practiced at 10 different speeds, an athlete will develop 10 different skills and training effects.

Several endurance training studies over a range of sports have found that non-specific training does not produce the same benefits as specific training. One of the first studies showed that on a running treadmill, rowers produced more lactic acid and performed worse than they did when rowing on a rowing ergometer (Brouha 1945). Another study of training specificity showed that kayak endurance performance was enhanced by kayak training but not by bicycle training. Evidence of improvements in mechanical efficiency, anaerobic threshold, and VO_2 max while kayaking showed that adaptations only occurred in the specific muscle groups employed in training (Pyke, Ridge and Roberts 1976). After a two-month period of swimming training, a group of swimmers significantly improved their training responses and performance times as well as their VO_2 max in tethered swimming. No improvements were observed in running VO_2 max. The specific adaptations of swimmers were also seen in the measurements taken on the former great Swedish swimmer, Gunnar Larson. During the two-year period leading up to his medal-winning performance at the Munich Olympic Games, physiological measures obtained in a swimming flume reflected his training status throughout this period, reflections not evident in treadmill assessments (Holmer 1974). Stamford, Cuddihee, Moffatt, and Rowland (1978) trained two groups, each on a different task of either hand-cranking or stepping. VO_2 max increased for each group in each activity but there was no transfer of training effects in either maximum or submaximum work. What these examples, and the literature in general indicate, is that training effects are task specific and appear to be based predominantly in the musculature.

A recent study showed that training energy systems on different apparatuses produced different training responses. Payne and Lemon (1982) conducted a metabolic comparison between tethered and simulated swimming ergometer exercise. For maximum exercise, some of the indicators (heart rate, ventilatory exchange, subjective assessments of similarity) were the same but the energy requirements were quite different. This suggested that simple measures may not be sensitive enough to discern more important energy requirement differences. Subjective assessments are influenced by many factors, including erroneous beliefs in the value of some forms of exercise. If these two forms of exercise are used as training activities for high-level swimmers, it must be asked, if both activities are so different, which of them is more valuable for training swimmers? The possibility that neither is valuable should also be considered.

In closely comparable activities, such as cycling and running, which predominantly use the muscles of the lower limbs, it has been found that cycling training produces gains in cycling performance that are not as readily noticeable while running (Pechar, McArdle, Katsch, Magel, and DeLuca 1974). Again, the load is carried differently by the muscles of the lower limb when running and cycling. Under most circumstances the gastrocnemius (calf) muscle is used to a greater extent than the quadriceps group in running than in cycling. The reverse is true for cycling. However, there are some examples of benefits transferring from one form of exercise to another. Hickson, Rosenkoetter, and Brown (1980) reported using heavy resistance training on the quadriceps, which along with gluteals are the prime-mover muscles of cycling. After 10 weeks, strength had increased by 38 percent. Time to exhaustion had improved by 47 percent on a bicycle test but by only one quarter as much on a treadmill running test. $\dot{V}O_2$ max improved only 4 percent. This suggests that strength training may increase endurance capacity even without an accompanying increase in $\dot{V}O_2$ max. This 'transfer' was qualified by indicating that the greater the concentration on the muscle group and action, the more likely this effect is to occur. One way of accounting for this phenomenon is that after strength training the same load is supported by fewer anaerobic muscle fibers because a person works at a lower percentage of maximum strength. Consequently, endurance is increased because it takes a longer time to exhaust all the strengthened fibers. Even though 'transfer' of training effects was evidenced, the amount was trivial and would have been achieved much faster and more efficiently by specific training.

Implications of Specificity for Coaching

There are several practical implications surrounding the principle of specificity for coaching. It is clear that the muscle groups involved in a sport should be those that are trained. While there may be some initial value in improving the size, strength, or endurance of muscles with non-specific training, ultimately the muscles must be engaged in the exact movements of the sport. Commercial resistance machines, in which movements such as the leg press and shoulder press are used to enhance the size and strength of certain muscle groups, have their greatest benefits for rehabilitation and body building. They have little specific value for sporting movements. Total-body free-weights, such as squats, cleans, and snatches, require balance and coordination. Other activities, such as medicine ball work and plyometric rebounding, also involve large groups of muscles in complicated actions. Integrated actions that are required by such activities may have greater value as a method of training for sport than do isolated simple exercises.

Particular care must be taken when using devices that attempt to duplicate the movement patterns of the sport. Interference with technique can occur when the movements are similar but not identical. For example, the Biokinetic swim bench uses isokinetic movements to overload the muscle groups throughout the range of movements involved in the swimming stroke. However, it does not allow *exact* duplication of the stroke. The pattern of movement in the water is different from that on the bench, and the contraction modes are dissimilar. These are two features which have been highlighted above as being critical for determining the value of training activities in terms of specificity. A coach needs to be very careful that a swimmer's technique is not disrupted by this type of training.

The use of some devices for training sports that require an ability to accelerate quickly, such as bowling a cricket ball or throwing a baseball, is even more questionable. Maintaining a constant speed throughout the movement is simply inappropriate for a sport that requires such rapid acceleration. A more useful method of specific resistance exercise for throwing activities would be obtained by using very light weights or medicine balls. However, even these activities need to be integrated carefully into a skill training program. As a ball is such a light weight, the need for speed and technique is more important than strength.

The early onset of fatigue in an endurance training session can produce movement patterns that are not specific. This is often seen in swimming, rowing, and kayaking. Exaggerated body movements requiring the recruitment of additional muscle groups are likely to interfere with the learning of skilled techniques. A coach should also ensure that the specific muscle fibers and energy systems required in a sport are used in training. Sprint and power athletes must engage the fast-twitch muscle fibers that are capable of quickly generating high tension. Low-power distance training will not involve the nervous and muscular systems responsible for generating speed and power. In fact, there is every possibility that excessive amounts of distance training will detrain adapted fast-twitch motor units that are responsible for exerting force and explosive power.

On the other hand, endurance athletes must concentrate on training activities that initially involve slow-twitch muscle fibers. The increasing involvement of the fast-twitch fibers, as an athlete tires towards the end of a training session, will assist to improve endurance potential even further. Hence the aerobic potential of both fiber types in the muscle will be improved by endurance training. Prolonged efforts that last longer than one hour will call on the provision of fat as the fuel for oxidation. Since marathon/triathlon athletes depend heavily on fat as an energy source, long-duration training will produce appropriate and specific training effects.

Coaches of high-energy team and individual sports need to develop elements of both speed and endurance in their athletes. Their training must include both aerobic and anaerobic work which involves both slow- and fast-twitch fibers. This can be done with a combination of distance training and specific high-intensity interval work containing the short work and recovery periods that are experienced in these sports. The most specific training is that of interval skill-drills, which place the skills of the sport within a high energy situation. Details of these drills are contained in Chapter 13, Endurance Training.

One of the most obvious signs of a lack of specificity in training is soreness experienced in muscles after unaccustomed exercise. For example, a regular jogger is likely to wake with sore buttocks the morning after playing a game of squash. The bending and reaching which is a large part of squash is not part of jogging. Even when the jogger is asked to do more sprint work, the recruitment of fast-twitch fibers, which is unusual, can produce tell-tale signs of a lack of specific training. Coaches should be aware of signs of soreness that result from competitive efforts. What signs do occur indicate that training has not been comprehensive enough to fully prepare athletes for all the activities required in competitions. There are four signs that also indicate non-specific or unrelated training. They are as follows:

1. muscular soreness in recovery
2. acute localized fatigue in the activity
3. a subjective appraisal by an athlete that the work being done is harder than usual
4. a quick occurrence of fatigue

Another alternative that must be considered as an index of non-specific training has to do with training effects and their enduring

status. For example, Carlile and Carlile (1961) reported that Australian swimmers trained with weight exercises prior to commencing hard swimming training in preparation for an Olympic Games.
During the swimming training, no weight training was performed.
After 10 weeks of swimming training that produced overtrained
states, thereby attesting to the intensity of the training load, it was
found that strength gains that had previously been achieved prior
to swimming had regressed back to untrained levels. If strength
gains had been valuable, then the intense swimming training
would have at least maintained some of that developed fitness
component. This suggests that the level of strength adaptation that
had occurred through resistance exercises was unrelated to the
sport of swimming. Another negative aspect of strength work in
swimming also occurs. The body density increases which alters
buoyancy resulting in increased resistance. This example raises an
intriguing question for coaches. Why train on activities which are
not required (stimulated) by the specific sporting activities themselves? There are some cases where non-specific activities can be
tolerated, for recovery, for diversity of training activities, and for
establishing a general activity potential in basic preparatory training. However, it would seem to be prudent to decrease the volume
and intensity of non-specific activities as the importance of specific
training increases. As training focuses more on specific developments, potentially unnecessary or damaging non-specific activities
need to be decreased. The only non-specific activities that should
be tolerated should be familiar, low-intensity activities, which
facilitate recovery. Thus, another index of specificity exists. When
training effects are incurred but are not maintained by the activity,
then these effects are generally not specific to the activity.

In light of what has been stated in the preceding paragraph, there
is one case where that index does not hold true. In some sport
competitions, important events occur but relatively infrequently.
The frequency is not sufficient to produce a training overload or
resultant training effect. For example, if one were to require flexibility on odd occasions, such as when a limb is forced into a
position that is not usually required in the sport, a lack of flexibility
would hinder performance or even result in injury. The same might
be true for high levels of strength. A basketball player may need a
high degree of specific strength when challenging for a ball possession or a position on the floor. If no strength training has been
done to increase the athlete's capacity in strength, then performance in those infrequent situations will be determined by strength
levels that are maintained by natural circumstances. However, if it
is decided that such situations are crucial, then training needs to be
undertaken to increase that infrequent need even if it does not

occur frequently in competitions or competition simulations. The fitness component needs to be developed and maintained at an artificially high level through training, until the odd occasion occurs when the capacity can be fully taxed. This requires a coaching decision to be made. How much training time should be devoted to training fitness components to unusual levels for general participation in the sport so that performance can be enhanced in rarely occurring circumstances?

Specific physical preparation should be guided by the characteristics of a sport. Specific training stimuli should lead to high levels of functional specialization which foster greater amounts of work in training and enhance recovery. Specific training stimuli should constitute the majority of activities in most training phases because they have training effects which are related to the frequency and intensity of their presentation. The challenge presented by the principle of specificity is to choose training stimuli which have the movement characteristics of the activities involved in a sport. This is very difficult to achieve since only minor alterations from an exact action change the characteristics of the systems that produce the altered action. Such changes are potentially harmful to a well-trained athlete.

Training increases the skill for an activity at a particular work intensity. Neuromuscular patterns are established which produce efficient use of existing resources. As well as a movement pattern, specific training has a specific action in relation to lactic acid production during heavy muscular work. The major physiological site of specific adaptations is in the muscles. Specificity applies between sports, between events within sports, between precise skills, rates of work, etc. What is trained is what is developed and if the activities of training do not replicate those of competitions, then the value of observed training effects will be decreased. Training effects can occur even though they will serve no purpose in a competitive effort.

The principle of specificity implies that specific training will only achieve desirable training effects that transfer directly to a competitive performance. Non-specific activities — and activities do not have to vary much to become non-specific — have the potential to interfere with good technique and the competent use of fitness components. Training activities which do not replicate the physiological and neuromuscular components of a sport have the potential to detract from performance through the phenomenon known as negative-transfer (Bompa 1986).

However, there are cases where non-specific activities do have value in training programs. Very non-specific activities may not load the muscle groups and fibers involved in the sport, and so in unloading the stress, may aid the recovery process and the ultimate training response. Non-specific activities could also serve as general conditioners in early phases of training and may serve to fill time between presentations of specific training stimuli. Unrelated activities might also provide variety in the sporting environment which could relieve boredom that would result from consistent overuse of the same specific activities.

In using non-specific activities, their volume and intensity should decrease as the period of major or important competitions approaches. The emphasis placed on them should never match that afforded specific training items.

Coaches need to decide the specific and non-specific activities of a sport. Non-specific or near-specific activities have a potential to be harmful. Unrelated activities can be used to assist in recovery and for program variation. The selection of specific training stimuli will determine the effectiveness of sport fitness programs. Only those activities which have direct positive transfer to competitions are those which should constitute the major portion of a training program.

7
The Principle of Individuality

The Principle of Individuality dictates that the decisions concerning the nature of training should be made with each individual athlete in mind (Rushall 1979a). A coach must always consider that each athlete should be treated independently (Bompa 1986: 17). Incorrect forms of training prescription result from all athletes in a team training with the same schedule and load. Attempts to copy the programs of champions, which is still a common practice among many coaches, will also result in incorrect loadings of the work of training for most individuals.

It does not take an astute coach long to realize that athletes within a team or squad are quite different. They have different performance and fitness attributes, life-styles and nutritional preferences, and they respond to the physical and social environments of training in their own unique ways. It is essential that training programs cater to these individual needs and preferences to optimize performance improvements. The factors which exist in the training process around which programs are designed are: the quality and abilities of the individual athlete, age, and the principles of training. This chapter discusses the major factors that need to be considered when individualizing training prescriptions.

Tolerance of Training Loads

The optimum training loads vary between athletes. Australian swimming coach Forbes Carlile often recounts the training performances of Shane Gould and Karen Moras, the best two distance swimmers in the world in the early 1970s. Shane Gould thrived on seemingly hard training, with her training performances being of quite a high level. On the other hand, Karen Moras exhibited training performances that were much slower than those of Shane. However, in competitions, the two recorded remarkably similar times. It was the training loads, as exhibited by training performances, which were different. It is conceivable that if either of the two athletes were made or encouraged to train closer to the other's performance level, her subsequent competitive performance would have suffered. Dr James Counsilman of Indiana University also described Mark Spitz as being a light trainer when compared with other swimmers in the same pool. His training load was less than that for other swimmers such as John Kinsella, although both were the best in the world at that time in freestyle swimming events. These are examples of different training loads being required for different athletes to produce the optimum training stress to record world-best performances.

There is no guarantee that an athlete who tolerates heavy training loads is going to be the best performer in competitions. They often set the 'training standards' imposed by the coach but are not capable of succeeding in contests against the peers whom they have beaten consistently in training. Their performances also suggest that fitness is not the only factor responsible for achieving sporting success. The tolerance of training loads also seems to be related to an athlete's history of involvement. It is simply not possible to withstand the rigors of a heavy training and competitive schedule if the foundation or basic training is weak and insubstantial. Gradual adaptation to training over a number of years provides an essential basis for absorbing later heavy loads. The coach must carefully monitor the capacity of the athlete to cope with the training load and adjust the training program when necessary. The signs, symptoms, and measurement of overtraining are discussed in some detail in the next chapter.

Responsiveness to Training

The capacity to respond to training is related to the initial level of fitness and the physiological characteristics of the individual. The potential for improvement is greatest when the initial level of fitness is lowest. This is clearly illustrated in the change-maintenance training graph (Figure 4.5). When an athlete is not fit, then performance improvements will be obvious and substantial with the onset of training. When an athlete is fit, performance improvements will be small and relatively infrequent. Once maximum fitness has been achieved, it requires much less training to maintain performance than to gain it in the first place. Thus the response of an athlete will vary depending upon the level of fitness and the training program content.

There are some athletes with higher sensitivities to the fitness component being trained. With regard to strength, this becomes very noticeable in males around the time of puberty when some have increased their secretion of testosterone while others have not. Early maturers develop muscle size and definition quickly and often dominate strength and power-oriented sports in a particular age-group. No matter how much weight training is completed, a late maturer has to await the arrival of puberty before significant gains are made. But even with the advent of puberty, individuals will differ in their response characteristics and performance levels resulting from programs. Some athletes just cannot become as strong as others.

A further strength training factor that produces individual responses is the proportion of fast-twitch muscle fibers in the muscles. Those athletes with a high proportion profit more from strength training than do endurance-oriented athletes (those with a high proportion of slow-twitch muscle fibers). This is because the high degree of tension created in the muscles during weight training exercises requires the fast-twitch fibers to become involved. After some time these fibers hypertrophy and, due to their abundance in the muscle, contribute significantly to increases in its size (Dons, Bollerup, Bonde-Peterson, and Hancke 1979).

Throughout this text, further features that cause differential responses to training between and within athletes will be discussed. A person of one age will respond differently from one of another age, such as in the example of strength training and the maturational factor of puberty. With regard to training loads, young athletes will break down and recover faster in training than they will when they become older, a feature discussed at greater length in Chapter 20. The practice of individualizing training programs requires consideration of the 'responsiveness to training' factors.

Figure 7.1 illustrates the training responses of five Canadian Olympic swimmers during the final stages of the 'hard' training phase prior to commencing a taper (peaking) period for the 1976 Canadian Olympic Team trials. Throughout the time of the observations, each athlete completed the same training segment on a number of occasions. What is depicted in the figure is the average time for each set expressed as a percentage of the time recorded in the subsequent competitive performance. The data can be interpreted as the percentage of effort when time is used as the basis of calculation. What is noticeable is the variation of performances within and between each individual.

Figure 7.1 Training performances of Five Canadian Olympic Swimmers for a Three-week Period prior to the 'Tapering' (Peaking) Phase of Training Leading to the Olympic Trials

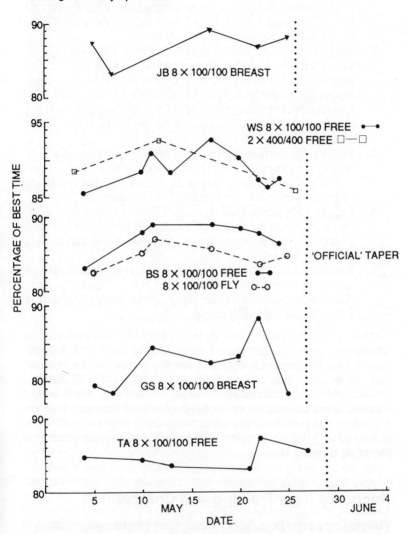

The repetition training segment is expressed as the number of repetitions by distance. The value following the slash character is the racing distance against which the intensity of the training efforts were determined. A data point constitutes the average percentage for the number of repetitions in the segment when compared with the subsequent competitive performance.

A summary of the data is as follows:

1. Subject JB completed four of five sets within an 86–89 percent intensity range. The remaining set was slightly over 83 percent. Except for the lone lower figure, the training responses were remarkably consistent.
2. Subject WS performed two events, one a 100 meter sprint, the other a more endurance-oriented 400 meter event. The intensities of training for both events fell within the same range, 86–93 percent. The commonality of the training intensities is surprising since sport science suggests that endurance event training should be performed at a lower intensity than sprints.
3. Subject BS performed two 100 meter sprint events. The freestyle performances were consistently three to four percent higher in intensity (range 87–89 percent) than were the butterfly performances (range 83–87 percent).
4. Subject GS's performances ranged 78–88 percent for the 100 meter breaststroke event. This included the lowest intensity of any training segment and widest individual variation of the five athletes.
5. Subject TA exhibited four consistent levels of performance with two subsequent performances being elevated prior to the commencement of the taper. Performances ranged in intensity from 83–87 percent.

What is evident from these data is that some athletes trained consistently while others varied considerably; most athletes produced little performance change over the period of observation; and the training intensities of two males (WS and GS) differed considerably. The individual variations in training responses of these athletes training in the same pool would warrant different programs and performance expectations. Such needs would not be met by having the athletes perform the same training program with the same training stimuli.

Recovery from Training and Competition

The recovery time from heavy training or intense competitions is longer in some athletes than in others. This is particularly the case with older athletes. Many players of contact team sports late in their careers find that they are only able to train lightly from one week to the next. Such light loads are required to facilitate recovery and negate the possibility of further overload training to produce altered fitness states. Coaches should recognize these differences either by reducing the training load or lengthening the recovery period in athletes who display the symptoms of chronic fatigue described in the next chapter.

Athletes with different physiological profiles also seem to require different tapering regimes. Strength-trained athletes show a level of maintenance of strength-related variables during periods of inactivity. Hence, reduced or tapered training loads can be extended without fear of deterioration in strength or explosive power performance. On the other hand, endurance qualities are lost quickly, and extended periods of reduced training in distance-

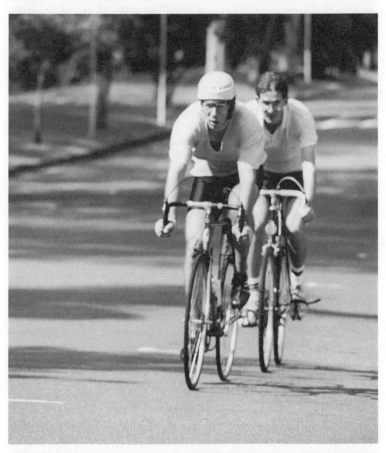

Within any sport there are wide individual differences between athletes, and the coach should be aware of this when prescribing training programs and competitive strategies that optimize their capacity to perform well under all conditions oriented athletes are not recommended. Thus an athlete's type of training will require different programming considerations with regard to what occurs in recovery periods. However, even within like sports, individuals will recover at varying rates.

Training Needs

The coach should aim to developed a balanced profile of attributes in each athlete that have been determined through objective measures. The individual case for fitness training must be weighed against the need for skill and mental training. More particularly, the prescription of fitness training should be based on known strengths and weaknesses in the physical profile of each athlete (see Chapter 12). For example, a pursuit cyclist with well-developed endurance capabilities but a weak sprint, would be best advised to spend training time on improving anaerobic power and capacity which would contribute to improved sprint performances. Another alternative for improving sprinting would be to develop a race strategy aimed at maintaining a fast pace throughout rather than relying on a sprint finish. Such an athlete would need to train with a program that was different from others with dissimilar needs.

Team game players should have individualized programs that not only round out their fitness profile but also allow them to meet the specific requirements of selected playing positions. For example, in soccer a set position player is more dependent on strength and speed than a mid-fielder who has a greater requirement for endurance. While modern team-game coaches increasingly encourage versatility in players they should still have, in the back of their minds, an ideal arrangement of personnel requiring specialized and individualized attention while training.

Training Preferences

In order to maximize the productivity of training, a coach should try to cater to each athlete's likes and dislikes. Some athletes thrive on the formal requirements of interval training accompanied by exact timing of distances and regular monitoring of heart rates. Others prefer a mix of continuous, over-distance, and Fartlek work. Although athletes should not be encouraged to work only on their strengths and ignore their weaknesses, it is important for them to develop and maintain a positive attitude and adhere strictly to a training schedule. Chapter 10 discusses the major factors that are associated with constructive programs and the atmosphere of training that encourage the best training responses. These factors require some understanding of athletes' training preferences.

Nutritional Preferences

The important role that nutrition plays in optimizing training was stressed in Chapter 5. While it is relatively easy to maintain a balanced diet in the Western world, it is important for coaches to understand that small deficiencies can become major obstacles to improvement in the hard-training athlete. For example, vegetarians need to take special care to ensure that they get enough minerals and vitamins in their diet. This can become a particular problem for the Vitamin B complex and iron and may require multi-vitamin and mineral supplementation. Coaches should be particularly aware of the potential for poor nutrition in young athletes who are living away from home for the first time. Some form of regular dietary counselling is advisable to keep track of and correct any dietary inadequacies. Poor dietary habits can cause differential energy responses and fluctuations in body composition. These variations will affect individual needs for training programs.

Environmental Tolerance

There are wide individual variations in response to physical features of the environment. Tolerance to heat and cold is partly related to body physique and composition. Body heat is more easily retained if there is an ample amount of insulative body fat, and the ratio between body surface area (for heat removal) and body mass (for heat production) is low. Hence, fatter individuals with heavier builds are more tolerant of cold than those with slighter builds. The reverse is true for hot conditions. Training responses and needs will vary depending on climatic fluctuations. A coach should be aware of these differences when exposing athletes to training in hostile and extreme climates.

It is also known that altitudinal and polluted environments affect some athletes to a greater extent than others. Symptoms of mountain sickness, such as headache and insomnia, can be debilitating for some individuals at quite moderate altitudes whereas others can tolerate more severe hypoxic stress without encountering problems. In a similar manner, some athletes experience respiratory distress in only mildly polluted air while others are unaffected. The negative psychological effects associated with the mere smell of ozone, one of the major constituents of pollution, and the irritation it causes the eyes, nose, and throat, can make training difficult for some. A coach must be able to adapt training loads according to the perceived tolerances of individuals for varying environmental conditions.

Physical Characteristics

Variations in body physique and composition can influence the capacity to withstand a training load. More heavily built athletes have a low tolerance for heat and are more prone to injuries in sports in which they have to fully support their own body weight. For winter sports, care should be taken during the late summer preparatory training phase to ensure that larger team-game players do not overheat. If distance running training is prescribed, heavy individuals are also at risk of incurring orthopedic injuries. Progressions in training intensity and duration should be gradual, and appropriate footwear should be worn to avoid injuries due to a sudden increase in one specific form/surface of training. There is less concern for heavy-bodied athletes when they engage in weight-supported sports such as swimming and rowing, since the environments of these sports usually facilitate the removal of heat.

Life-style Variations

Within a training squad there are often athletes from all walks of life. Some might be students, manual labourers, or office workers, while others may work different shifts. Since the demands of their working life often compete with those of their sport, the coach should be aware of such commitments when planning training loads. These commitments may change from time to time. Peak external stresses for a student may occur at the time of final examinations, for the office worker at the end of the financial year, and for a laborer at the deadline for a job completion. Life stresses are cumulative and so training loads should be adjusted to compensate for any variations in life-style that will affect the degree of stress imposed upon the serious athlete. Chapter 8 describes a measurement tool for assessing life variations and impacts.

Social Interactions Within the Group

Training squads usually contain an assortment of individuals with different interests, tastes, and personalities. Because of the stress of hard training and intense competitions, these differences can produce interpersonal frictions that have a negative effect on performance. It is the responsibility of a coach to monitor the development of such problems and to affect a program alteration that will alleviate their occurrence. Chapter 10 discusses some of the strategies for designing training situations that will prevent such problems.

This chapter has listed a number of factors that produce individual variations in training requirements. The individual needs of each athlete have to be met to maximize training responses. Each denial of an individual factor will lessen the training experience for the majority of athletes. Recognition and the accommodation of this principle will require radical departures from the common handling procedure of having all athletes in a squad follow the same program. It has been traditional to treat the training of all athletes as if they were clones. Such a singular approach to control is easy and the least time-consuming for a coach. However, because it is easy does not mean that it is the best approach; the deficiency was highlighted by Rushall (1975b). His advocacies are still largely unheeded but are reproduced below to illustrate what it might be possible to organize in order to satisfy the needs of individual athletes, and to produce an optimal training response (Rushall 1975b: 167–72).

... The thrust of this incontrovertible argument is that by using the same program for a group of swimmers the development of most of them is reduced.

The technological procedures exist for analyzing swimmers so that their suitability for particular swimming events can be determined. Once a swimmer's capacities and event suitabilities have been established appropriate training programs should be devised. This will require a complete reversal of orientation for developing swimmers, a change from general/group to specific/individual programs ...

[Figure 7.2] presents a flow diagram of the programming process for developing the specific/individual content. A computer is used to print each day's program of training for each individual. The coach monitors the swimmer's progress, adaptation, and behavioral reactions. The parameters for program content are altered at any time, but usually only when a change is required (taper, failing adaptation, etc.). The task of completing this information is not as great as one would think. It is assumed that in advocating this method, the common unproductive and inefficient time usage procedures of the normal coaching role do not exist.

The psychological features of this process are involved with the use of program boards. Rushall (1975a) described these as being motivational because of their direct effect on training work quantity and quality. The procedure of publicly registering a program unit completion generated social, performance information, material, and performance progress reinforcers. However, those boards were used for small groups. This can be improved upon by having separate programs for each swimmer, but still retaining the public recording procedure. This will provide individual training programs under motivated conditions. [Figure 7.3] illustrates such a board. The change that is required of coaches here is that they will have to be prepared to relegate the control of the training program to a psychological technology through indirect control rather than through direct personal control. The implementation of specific individual programs is designed towards optimizing the swimming development of all swimmers.

Figure 7.2 A Flow Diagram of the Steps for Producing Specific/Individual Training Programs by Using a Computer (Rushall 1975a: 171)

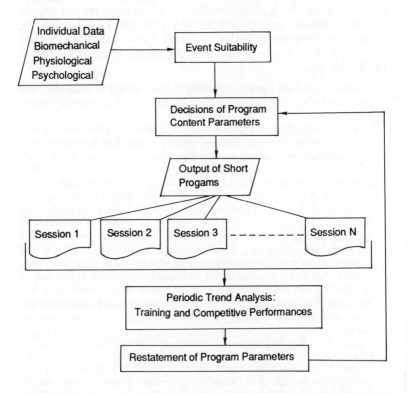

The critical feature is the number of decision parameters that need to be considered.

Figure 7.3 A Suggested Structure for Program Boards for Displaying and Using Individualized Computer-generated Training Programs

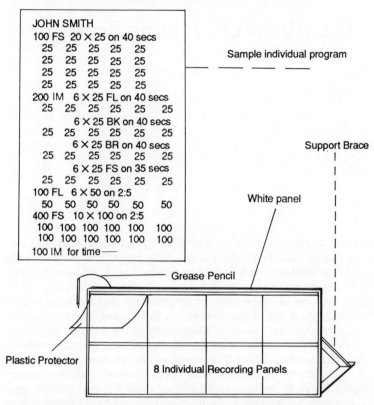

The computer generates an individual prescription for the training session. In this example, the output includes the event for which each training segment is targeted, the training segment, and each training unit for each segment (to be marked immediately after completion). The board itself contains panels for each athlete, is waterproofed with plastic protectors, and is constructed for easy access and use (Rushall 1975a: 172).

The individuality of training responses was demonstrated by Savage, Brown, Savage, and Bannister (1981) after they had assessed four physiological parameters over 75 days of intense training in a top collegiate swimming team. Group training produced different individual response profiles for ostensibly the same workout program. Different physiological and performance profiles also were evidenced during a peaking program. They concluded that to train an athlete appropriately, individualization in programming is essential.

8

The Abuse of Training Principles

Any failure to use sound training principles when coaching athletes can be construed as an abuse. This book is written with the hope that such occurrences will be minimized. At all times coaches should attempt to use established principles of training when designing and implementing programs. This chapter focuses more specifically on the abuse that stems from using training stimuli which produce accumulated fatigue and cause harm to athletes.

Training fatigue is caused by a number of components: performance depletion in the central nervous system which affects behavior, movement efficiency, and performance quality; energy depletion which reduces performance capacity; and morphological changes, such as tissue damage and altered blood states, which affect both behavior and performance. The nervous system is much more fragile than the body's physiology and so breaks down well before the physiological systems are taxed. *The state of the nervous system is what should determine training loads, not the state of the athlete's physiology* (Bompa 1986).

The onset of fatigue occurs in three general stages: psychological, performance, and physiological breakdown.

Fatigue Due to a Training Stimulus

Chapter 4 described the maximum level of fatigue that should be experienced when incurring a training stimulus. The 'training threshold' signals to the coach that the athlete is nearing the critical stage for beneficial effects from a training stimulus to occur. When the threshold is exceeded the stimulus should cease.

96

The first stage of training threshold attainment is reflected in an athlete's behaviors and mood. He or she can still perform at an adequate level, but symptoms of negativism, reduction in verbal behavior, mood changes from a smiling/happy countenance to one of serious concentration/concern, and acknowledgments of task difficulty all indicate that the threshold is being approached.

The second stage is that of performance breakdown. Skill deterioration occurs although performances, such as times swum and distances covered, are still maintained. This indicates that the neuromuscular patterns of movement are being disrupted by the level of fatigue that has developed during training. Extra psychological effort and the recruitment of more muscles might maintain the absolute level of performance although the efficiency of performance decreases.

The third stage indicates that the training threshold has been exceeded: that is, the training stimulus overload is excessive. Physiological indices of fatigue are obvious at this time. Incomplete or inadequate recovery between repetitions, performance deterioration despite honest attempts to increase efforts, increased ventilation suggesting lactic acid accumulation, and distressed behaviors are all physiological response signs which indicate that the cessation of training is warranted.

Most coaches are familiar with these symptoms and should be prepared to stop the activity once they appear and the functional benefits of training cease to be obvious. The common problem with this proposal is that many coaches believe that 'toughness' is taught by enduring excessive training overloads (sometimes called the 'hurt-pain-agony' syndrome). This is a belief that is not supported by scientific fact. Indeed, pain tolerance is developed by experiencing moderate but manageable levels of discomfort. Excessive pain often develops avoidance behaviors which actually sensitize the athlete and reduce pain tolerance. With regard to this proposal, part of the Roux Principle should once again be recalled: 'excessive training is dangerous'.

The coaching recommendation that is made here is that it is best to produce moderate amounts of fatigue, rather than excessive ones, in order to gain the maximum benefit from a training stimulus. Positive athlete behaviors and moods indicate that the beneficial level is being approached, and both skill and performance deterioration indicate that the level has been exceeded. Any further training efforts after these signs have been evidenced constitute an abuse of a sound training principle.

Fatigue Between Training Sessions

The severity of a training session stress governs the degree of the fatigue state. The more stressful a training session, the longer will be the period of between-sessions rest to ensure the occurrence of adequate recovery and training effects.

If inadequate recovery happens between training sessions, two kinds of effect can occur. First, sufficient time may allow recovery but is insufficient for training effects (overcompensation) to develop. In this case, the stress of training will be tolerated but no performance improvement will occur because no overcompensation has happened. Second, insufficient recovery means that an athlete will enter the next training session fatigued. This fatigue will inhibit the learning of skills, retard conceptual learning, and produce performance levels that satisfy neither athlete nor coach. Continual fatigued states and accompanying training dissatisfactions produce motivational problems and alter behaviors and attitudes.

Inadequate between-sessions recovery is evidenced by psychological, behavioral, and performance characteristics. Physiological symptoms also may accompany this undesirable state.

☐ Psychological and Behavioral Signals

When insufficient recovery has occurred, athletes display behaviors that suggest certain negative mood states. Their normal behaviors are altered. Usually, they are quieter, more hesitant to start warm-up activities, stay more in the background, rarely smile, and the quality of initial efforts is worse than normal. Generally a lowered willingness to train and altered attitudes are in evidence. If the coach looks closely, different modes of behavior will be perceived, although in large groups such close inspections are difficult.

☐ Performance Factors

Fatigued athletes do not exhibit quality work in warm-up activities. The techniques that are demonstrated during training stimuli might be reduced in amplitude, slowed in speed of execution, and/or performed with fewer trials than usual. Such performances could easily be interpreted as being caused by a 'lack of effort'. Once training stimuli are attempted, the period of tolerance of the training stimulus is either markedly reduced or non-existent. Athletes often start out with a worse-than-normal level of performance and deteriorate further. Techniques are also compromised in the early repetitions or stages. Actions are abbreviated or do not cover the normal full movement range. The onset of technique breakdowns occurs very early in the set of activity repetitions. If it is possible to measure the performance of an athlete during a training stimulus, fatigued athletes will decline in performance rapidly and attain lower standards. Such measures are an objective way of assessing whether adequate between-sessions recovery has occurred.

☐ Physiological Indices of Between-sessions Fatigue

Athlete complaints of stiffness, residual soreness from the previous session, elevated resting heart rates, sore throats, general discomfort or feeling of ill-being, and the need for more rest, are symptoms of inadequate recovery. The usual physiological measures that can be obtained in the laboratory are not sensitive enough to locate the physiological bases of residual fatigue. It is best for the coach to rely on psychological and performance indices to assess this state.

To require an athlete to train hard and perform to normal standards while in a state of incomplete between-sessions recovery constitutes a serious abuse. The merit of such an expectation cannot be justified on physiological, performance specificity, or psychological grounds. Any participation should proceed with a markedly reduced workload or with activities which are not affected by the fatigue. This may be difficult for some coaches to do because of the fear that it will display 'softness' or 'set a bad example for the other athletes'. That may or may not be true, but to demand extra training effort to offset the residual fatigue that exists in a particular athlete, is essentially unethical for it abuses his or her welfare.

Overtraining

The most troublesome aspect of coaching serious athletes is that of judging when, in the long run, they need an extended reduction in workload to recover the capacity required to adapt to the demands of training. Chapter 4 discussed the occurrence of the stage of exhaustion in the Stress Adaptation Syndrome. This occurs when an individual's capacity to adapt further to the psychological and physiological stresses of serious sports training fails and is accompanied by a noticeable performance regression.

From a coach's viewpoint, long-term fatigue is difficult to monitor because the subtle and minor changes that occur on a daily basis usually escape notice. A coach becomes accustomed to the small signs that indicate an athlete's deteriorating capacity to continue training in a relatively demanding fashion. It is not uncommon to see and hear of coaches attempting to push athletes through 'performance slumps' by rededicating their enthusiasm to even greater amounts of work. Reactions like this usually result in the modern phenomena of 'overuse injuries', 'staleness', 'burn-out', and/or 'stress injuries'. Chapter 5 discussed the options for recovering from this most undesirable state. It is definitely one that must be avoided when training athletes.

The onset of overtrained states is gradual and occurs in stages, the first level of degradation being psychological. The first characteristic that alters in young children due to excessive training demands is their emotional state. Tantrums, moods, and 'enthusiasm' are directly affected and usually noticed by coaches and parents, and should be taken as the initial sign that some opportunities to recovery and regenerate from the long-term stress of training should be provided. At least one unloading microcycle over about a week should be instituted for the athlete when this occurs.

☐ Psychological Factors

With high-level performers, psychological factors indicate the onset of overtrained states. Morgan (1980), Rushall (1975b 1981a), and McKenzie (personal communication)[1] have all indicated that psychological indices describe and measure the onset of overtrained states better than physiological indices. Rushall and Roaf (1986) showed that psychological self-report variables were sensitive to excessive overload changes in swimmers whereas physiological and performance variables were not. *As overtraining is incurred by athletes, psychological disturbances occur prior to the onset of the more serious and debilitating physiological breakdowns.* Stresses from outside the sport setting also contribute to failing adaptation. Thus, when considering long-term fatigue states, the accumulated stresses from all sources of an athlete's life must be considered.

For many years, individuals have attempted to measure the phenomenon of overtraining through physiological indices, which have largely been futile. Carlile (1981: 4), for instance, found:

> When testing overtraining no physiological indices have been consistently linked, and in most cases are normal, when performances are depressed . . . it appears that how the athlete feels may be the best guide for controlling overtraining and its consequent state of staleness . . . We may have to look to the 'head' rather than the body, and monitor such mood changes as tension, depression, anger, fatigue and confusion on the one hand, compared with vigor and a feeling of well-being on the other . . .

Since the only way of locating the early stages of overtraining is the assessment of psychological factors, the latter part of this chapter focuses on this. Indeed, for sports where there is no great physical demand, for example, shooting, baseball, sailing, and cricket, measurement of psychological variables is the only way of discovering when the psychological demands of a sport have become excessive. The point behind psychological measurement is that if the onset of overtrained states can be located before the more serious performance and physiological symptoms occur, an athlete's development will not be seriously hampered. Adequate rest and regeneration will usually suffice to produce recovery so that competion and training can once again be followed in a productive manner.

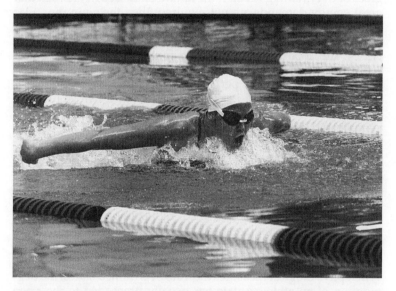

Studies of swimmers have shown that psychological indicators of over-training occur before the physiological symptoms of breakdown

☐ Performance Indicators

Psychological signs are the very earliest warning signals and indicate to a coach that more recovery is needed rather than continued hard work. Performances can still, however, continue at an acceptable level, even though psychological factors are deteriorating (Rushall and Roaf 1986). But adequate performance does not continue for long. The worsening psychological state of the athlete contributes to the onset of performance decline. Performance deterioration, then, usually follows quite closely from the onset of the psychological changes that mark failing adaptation.

Performance decline comes in two stages. The first is the advent of troublesome technique changes and errors. In sports where the nature of the performance is one of short and intense contractions and efforts, long-term fatigue tends to be peripheral, occurring in the muscle fibers and at the motor nerve end plate. With the extension of the duration of effort, as in endurance events, the causes of fatigue tend to become both central and peripheral. The physiology of the performance decrease will be determined by the nature of the activity. All sporting activities experience peripheral problems that affect technique refinements when moderate degrees of overtraining occur. If the nature of the activity is such that great energy demands are not required, then the neuromuscular disruptions remain the primary causes of performance degradation. In events where energy requirements and movement efficiency are important, some of the more obvious physiological functions are disrupted. It is proposed that even in these latter events, the first stage of performance deterioration is caused by deteriorating peripheral mechanisms and that if hard training is continued, and is a feature of the sport, the deterioration is further complicated by changes in central mechanisms that are usually related to cardio-respiratory functions.

When both psychological and performance factors change in an athlete after an extended period of time, the need for regeneration and recovery is greater than if only psychological factors have altered. Adequate recovery times usually take a number of weeks and should be coupled with marked reductions in workloads and the introduction of both rest and non-related activities.

□ Physiological Indicators

When physiological measures indicate overtrained states, the degradation of an athlete's state has usually proceeded to the stage where only extended rest and rehabilitation can return him or her to a healthy state. That form of recovery is accompanied by a marked detraining effect. Physiological problem indices can occur even in sports that do not have a highly demanding physiological component.

One of the first physiological signs of overtraining is a gradual increase in joint and muscle soreness as training progresses. This may become extreme after a particularly hard session or chronic if the overload is not lightened. Examples of overuse injuries include swimmer's shoulder, jumper's knee, and Achilles tendinitis in runners. The stress reaction can also decrease appetite and body weight. It is useful for the coach to have regular weigh-ins under standardized conditions as a means of determining if the athlete is overextended. Other medical symptoms associated with the lowered resistance that accompanies overtraining include head colds, allergic reactions, occasional nausea, headaches, constipation or diarrhea, and swelling of the lymph nodes in the neck, groin, and armpits. An elevated resting heart rate or blood pressure has also been used as an indication of overtraining. A useful guide to the level of adaptation of the athlete can be gained by taking resting heart rate at the same time of day (preferably before rising) and under the same conditions. When failing adaptation has occurred, the resting heart rate is elevated. The mechanism for causing that rise is probably due to the increased secretion of catecholamines as a response to the level of stress imposed. If the coach has access to more sophisticated testing and support services, it is possible to detect overtraining from changes in blood variables. These include lowered concentration of hemoglobin and hematocrit and an increased concentration of enzymes and myoglobin that have leaked out of the muscles as a result of damage to the membranes of the fibers.

When physiological indices substantiate that an overtrained state has been achieved, the level of overtraining has become excessive. This results in major disruptions to the annual plan, and even an athlete's career, in order to produce adequate recovery.

Prevention of Overtrained States

The principles of this text are designed to prevent the occurrence of overtraining. Some of the major guidelines for planning training so that this undesirable state is prevented are listed below.

1. Increase the training stimulus in graduated steps so that the athlete is prepared for each increment in workload. A sudden increase in the intensity, duration, or frequency of effort, particularly at the start of pre-season training or after an injury-enforced lay-off, is likely to induce an overtraining response.
2. Allow 24–48 hours of recovery time between hard training sessions. It is important to cycle heavy, moderate, and light workouts and give the athlete adequate opportunity to recover and adapt.
3. Eat a balanced diet containing all the basic nutrients, with particular emphasis on the carbohydrate component for endurance sports.
4. Ensure adequate rest and sleep between training sessions.
5. Individualize the intensity and volume of training being prescribed. This involves understanding the physiological

and psychological attributes and the state of fitness of each athlete in the training squad.

6. Be prepared to modify the training prescription to suit the environmental conditions. For example, on a hot day the effort required is much higher than normal, making it necessary to reduce the training load.

7. Be aware of any aspects of the life situation of the athlete that might impact on the ability to tolerate physical training. This includes any social, emotional, and work stresses that are likely to add to the stress of training. The coach must be aware of the life demands of each athlete in the squad.

8. Monitor the psychological, performance, and physiological responses of athletes during training and competition as a guide to their capacity to cope. If, for example, the heart rate does not return to its desired level in a consistent rapid fashion after a series of interval repetitions, the session might be ended or the intensity of training reduced.

9. Adjust training loads according to the implications of psychological and performance indices.

These preventive measures support the contention that there is a limit to the amount of training necessary to produce optimal adaptation. Skill and performance will continue to improve when the limit of physiological capacities has been reached. A high priority must be placed on rest and recovery to optimize the conditioning process. While it is obvious that too little training will not bring about the desired results, the negative effects of too much are often ignored. Coaches must try to find the middle road for each athlete and optimize training adaptation.

Measuring the Occurrence of Training Abuses

The first factors to be measured should be psychological, for they occur first in the breakdown of an athlete's capacity to adapt to stress. It has been shown that self-report measures of psychological reactions and changes are satisfactory for appropriate tools (Goodyear 1973). Two self-report measurement techniques have been widely reported as being useful for sporting environments. The *Profile of Mood States (POMS)* (McNair, Lorr, and Droppleman 1971) is popular. A number of scale scores are developed and increases in some of these are related to increased stresses and state changes in athletes. The major drawback with the POMS is that it is not sport-specific, although that does not appear to be a severe problem after athletes adapt to using it. For example, Pyke, Craig, and Norton (1988) found that POMS measures and physiological indices changed in concert during a tapering period with élite cyclists. However, the scale scores do not give specific information that can be verified by a coach's own observations of athlete behaviors and nor do they indicate the individual idiosyncrasies of athlete reactions. The generation of a number of scales that are not related to the phenomena of importance makes the device a little cumbersome. The POMS usually is not able to be directly interpreted by athletes themselves.

The *Daily Analyses of Life Demands for Athletes* (Rushall 1975a, 1979b, 1981a, 1981b) is a self-report sport-specific tool that has been used at events such as Olympic Games by several nations to refine the quality of coaching decisions about the stress reactions of individual athletes. It has the advantage of exactly describing the stress sources and characteristics of each person. Thus it allows the differentiation of the individuality of the stress responses as well as providing indices of what features are normal, worse than normal, and better than normal in an athlete's life and stress symptoms. This is reproduced in Appendix A, at the end of this book, and will be discussed at length below. It appears to be the most relevant and credible tool for use with athletes.

Dr Don McKenzie (personal communication), of Vancouver, Canada, researched topics associated with overtraining and attempted to locate those factors which best predict the emergence of overtraining symptoms. After exhaustive testing of blood, physiological, and psychological factors, the most significant indices that could be measured with predictive validity were psychological self-report measures. The measures contained in his final tool were quantified assessments of a number of items that yielded an overall score of stress severity. The higher the revealed score, the more stressed is the athlete. The scaled score loses information and individuality, the same drawbacks that are contained in the POMS. However, both tools are valid for predicting and measuring the stress of training.

The abuses of training principles cover a number of areas. They include exercising athletes who are in incomplete recovery, training when exhausted by jet-lag and travel fatigue (see Chapter 9), expecting high-level performances when a 'peaked' state has not been attained, and expecting normal hard-training responses in athletes who have their performance capacities reduced because of the accumulated effects of stressors which occur outside the sporting environment. The responses of athletes to these situations and the quantification of the severity of the stress is measured by the *Daily Analyses of Life Demands of Athletes*. Such measures can be the basis for making sound coaching decisions. The following in-depth discussion of the use of the tool is offered.

The response of an athlete to the matrix of life stresses depends upon the appraisal/coping capacity of the individual to each source of stress. The reactivity of an athlete to life stresses, including the activities associated with the sport, depends upon the number of stressors which exist at any particular time. If one accepts the assertion that one's tolerance for stress is finite (Selye 1950), then the accumulated stresses could exceed an athlete's capacity. It would be of advantage to both the coach and athlete to measure the sources of excessive stress which occur at any one particular time. Such knowledge would allow the training and handling of athletes to be appropriately modified.

Rushall (1975a, 1975b) published a *Stress Index* for swimmers. Consequent adaptation and use of that tool has verified its general utility for all athletes (Rushall 1981a). The inventory assesses whether an athlete is stressed and if so, what the factors are leading to the stressed condition. An athlete is required to consider a number of descriptions and determine whether his or her state is worse or better than normal. There are two parts to the inventory.

The validity of the *Daily Analyses of Life Demands for Athletes* (Rushall 1981a, 1987a) was established through content validity procedures after an item pool of 13 stressors and 44 symptoms was developed. The reliability of the tool was determined through test-retest procedures on 52 athletes repeated on 5 separate occasions, each at least 14 days apart. Items which were not reliable 80 percent of the time were deleted from the item pools. The validity and reliability screening procedure reduced the sources of stress to 9 areas and the symptoms of stress to 25 items. Thus a valid and reliable self-report inventory was established for use in sporting environments. Figure 8.1 illustrates the answer sheet for the tool.

The first part of the inventory (Part A) describes the general stress sources that occur in the everyday living of an athlete (diet, home life, school/work, friends, training, climate, sleep, recreation, and health). The individual is asked to indicate the pertinent sources which are stressful to him or her at the time of answering the test. The information that is generated indicates those areas of the athlete's normal daily activities which are perceived as being stressful.

The importance of this information is that it locates any general stressors which may be detracting from an athlete's exercise-stress adaptation potential. When extraneous stress sources are indicated, steps can be taken to alleviate them. Athletic performances can deteriorate when stressors other than exercise are incurred. Thus, this section of the inventory can be used to locate possible causes of poor performance. An athlete can also be stressed by a number of factors but still not have succumbed to them. A coach can take appropriate steps to reduce the possibility of failing adaptation by taking corrective steps to remove unnecessary sources of stress in an athlete's life.

Figure 8.1 A Sample Answer Sheet for the *Daily Analyses of Life Demands for Athletes* Booklet

---

ANSWER SHEET

Name: ....   Date: ....

RESPOND BY CIRCLING the appropriate response alongside each item.

     a = worse than normal   b = normal   c = better than normal

---

PART A				PART (right)			
1. a b c			Diet	8. a b c			Irritability
2. a b c			Home life	9. a b c			Weight
3. a b c			School/college/work	10. a b c			Throat
4. a b c			Friends	11. a b c			Internal
5. a b c			Sport training	12. a b c			Unexplained aches
6. a b c			Climate	13. a b c			Technique strength
7. a b c			Sleep	14. a b c			Enough sleep
8. a b c			Recreation	15. a b c			Between sessions recovery
9. a b c			Health	16. a b c			General weakness
				17. a b c			Interest

Total 'a' responses   ....

Total 'b' responses   ....

Total 'c' responses   ....

Record these values and the day's data
on the Data Log Part A

				18. a b c			Arguments
				19. a b c			Skin rashes
				20. a b c			Congestion
				21. a b c			Training effort
				22. a b c			Temper
				23. a b c			Swellings
				24. a b c			Likability

PART B

				25. a b c			Running nose
1. a b c			Muscle pains				
2. a b c			Techniques				
3. a b c			Tiredness	Total 'a' responses			
4. a b c			Need for a rest	Total 'b' responses			
5. a b c			Supplementary work	Total 'c' responses			
6. a b c			Boredom	Record these values and the day's data			
7. a b c			Recovery time	on the Data Log Part B			

Part A allows for recording self-perceptions of sources of stress in an athlete's life, while Part B lists possible symptoms of stress. The number of responses for each category is totalled on the answer sheet. These numbers are then transferred to a cumulative graph contained in the booklet.

The second part of the inventory (Part B) determines which symptoms of stress reaction exist in the athlete. Consequently, it can be used to conclude whether an athlete is or is not succumbing to the life stresses experienced. Questions concerning the symptoms of failing adaptation are evaluated as to whether they are worse than normal (negative), normal, or better than normal (positive). When the number of 'worse-than-normal' responses increases markedly, that is, the athlete reports an unusual number of negative stress symptoms, it usually indicates that he or she is unable to cope with the stress of life at that time. Coaches can then alter the training program and/or remove some sources of stress as indicated in Part A so that the athlete is given a reduced 'stress load' which should result in recovery.

The *Daily Analyses of Life Demands for Athletes* can be used periodically (possibly once every two or three days) throughout a period of training. It provides consistent, frequent evaluation of an athlete's stress reactions. Its use does not inconvenience the coach. It can be incorporated into a log book with a supply of answer sheets as was done with the Australian Olympic Swimming Team in 1980 (Rushall 1979b). The answer sheet requires the athlete to total all responses in each category for both test parts. The data are graphed. Thus, a marked increase in the total of either part for the 'worse-than-normal' category serves as a warning for coaches to take corrective action before more serious states are developed.

The administration, answering, and scoring of the inventory are all done by the athlete. He or she maintains the periodic progress charts. When changes in trends on the chart are evidenced the athlete then indicates to the coach that consultation is required. Alternatively, the coach can periodically scan the progress chart for trend changes. This process increases the coach's understanding of an athlete's specific reactions to a unique set of life stresses.

The inventory has a number of valuable benefits which warrant its adoption by coaches. It provides important information about an athlete's life that is not normally available under traditional coaching circumstances or recorded in other measurement tools. It locates both stress reactions and sources of stress. Apart from general use, it would also seem to have potential for beneficial use in the period before international competitions such as Olympic and Commonwealth Games and world championships. In that period, the levels of psychological and physiological stresses are increased for all sports while a peaked state is being developed. The complexity of that circumstance warrants special attention.

Uses of Self-report Stress Analyses

The relationship between psychological assessments and stressed states is the basis of the structure for the *Daily Analyses of Life Demands for Athletes* booklet. The following sections describe how to use the *Daily Analyses* booklet for monitoring features of athletes' personal states during training.

☐ The Training Response

Athletes in serious training usually attempt to attain a state of maximum adaptation to exercise stress. This is known as achieving the 'stage of resistance' (Selye 1950) where the majority of the body's resources are applied to coping with training loads. The cost of this specialized adaptation is that resistance to other stressors is lowered. Diminished capacities in other areas of living are often evident when an athlete trains intensely. This means that as he or she goes through cycles of fatigue and recovery, there are a number of 'symptoms' of the stress of adaptation that occur. The *Daily Analyses* booklet is a tool for measuring these.

The theoretical formulation for this assessment method is that during serious training there should be a number of symptoms that are reported by an individual that are 'worse' than if the individual were not training at all. When an athlete copes with the stress of training loads, and is adapting in a satisfactory manner, the symptoms of coping are relatively stable. If an athlete works too hard in a training session, consequently requiring a longer-than-normal recovery period, the number of symptoms that will be reported will be increased over what is normal. Thus changes in the number of self-reported symptoms of adaptation to training are the clues that indicate whether an athlete is training too hard (the number of negative symptoms increases) or training too easily (the number of negative symptoms decreases). The number of symptoms reported as being 'worse-than-normal', 'normal', or 'better-than-normal' indicates the training response of an athlete.

Monitoring Daily Training

When an athlete is able to cope with training loads that are not complicated by outside-of-the-sport stressors, the number of symptoms that are reported on a day-to-day basis are relatively consistent. This consistent response indicates specific adaptation to the stress of training. It will last for a period of time, that period being dependent upon the frequency of training sessions and intensity of training loads.

The demonstration of consistent self-assessments of training-stress symptoms over a period of at least two weeks is known as the training response 'window'. It is the baseline set of responses against which training assessments are compared. To establish the training response 'window', the following procedures are recommended:

1. Complete the *Daily Analyses of Life Demands for Athletes* assessment procedure on a daily basis for a period of 2–4 weeks. This period should start after the athlete has become used to training. It should not include the first 3 weeks of a training season.
2. Record the symptoms as required at the same time each day, preferably before an afternoon training session. This timing will give an index of the athlete's ability to recover from the previous training session.
3. Continue the assessments until the total number of 'worse-than-normal' symptoms that are reported are relatively stable. In the early assessments there may be some variability which results from 'getting used to' the measurement procedure. Stability occurs when the data points for the alternatives marked 'a' in Part B of the inventory appear to be of a restricted range. Figure 8.2 exhibits a set of stable data that varied for three assessments and then seemed to settle between a range of 3–5 symptoms. The 9 recordings in that range are then deemed to be the 'window' of the training response. It is suggested that 'windows' be considered after at least 10 data points have been collected. There could be considerable individual variability in the number of days it takes to establish a 'window', and the number of symptoms that exist in it. One should not be alarmed if the number of symptoms is high or low. It should be remembered that the data are self-reports and the criteria used by individuals for reporting states can vary greatly.
4. When athletes have entered training from an untrained state, or when they are young, it is possible for them to have several 'windows'. As they get stronger and their physical capacities change the symptoms of adequate training stress change in type and number. Thus, for a time after the commencement of training, a 'window' will be displayed. Then with a change in type of training to suit new capacities, a new 'window' will be likely to occur. With such athletes periodic tests should be made to see if they can tolerate different training loads and frequencies. Further, the stress of basic preparatory training will be different from that of

specific preparatory training: different 'windows' should be expected for each training phase. However, once athletes have entered maintenance training, 'windows' should be stable.

Figure 8.2 A Training-response 'Window' for 'a' ('worse-than-normal') Alternatives on Part B of *Daily Analyses of Life Demands for Athletes*

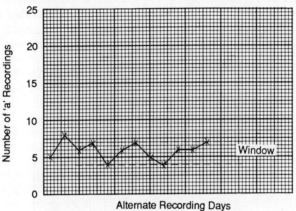

Alternate Recording Days

Data points were collected once every two days. When data points are obtained daily and training loads are carefully planned, the day-to-day variations in symptoms which are worse than normal usually will be less variable. This 'window' appears to contain two cycles of response, and the tool is sensitive to locating such cycles.

The frequency of recording in the booklet should be determined by the coach. If training loads are primarily of low intensity, then every second day should be satisfactory. If training loads are heavy, then daily analyses are recommended. The aim of coaching should be to provide training stresses which will result in athletes reporting symptoms which fall within the 'window'.

☐ Excessive Training Sessions

If a data point from a day's analysis is *higher* than the values included in the 'window', then it could be interpreted to mean that the previous session load was too hard. The extra symptoms that are reported mean a lack of adequate recovery. The subsequent training session should be of a lesser intensity to allow further recovery to take place. Increased training loads usually produce greater states of fatigue, require longer recovery periods, and cause an athlete to experience more training-stress symptoms that are worse than usual. Thus the monitoring of between-sessions recovery is possible with this measurement procedure. When symptoms are more numerous than those in the 'window', it can be concluded that previous training was too demanding and extra recovery is warranted. Figure 8.3 illustrates recordings that occur outside the 'window'.

Figure 8.3 A Training-response 'Window' for 'a' ('worse-than-normal') Alternatives on Part B of *Daily Analyses of Life Demands for Athletes*

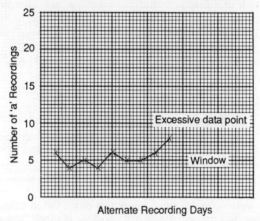

Alternate Recording Days

The last data point is outside the 'window', indicating that the next training session should be lighter than usual to allow the athlete to return to experiencing the number of symptoms associated with adaptation to exercise stress.

☐ Training Sessions Which Are Too Easy

When the number of symptoms that are recorded fall outside but *below* the 'window', then the athlete is not being stressed by training to the degree that produces optimum adaptation. The effects and fatigue resulting from training are not as much as could be tolerated. It could be interpreted to mean that too much recovery was being experienced and that the athlete was not undergoing an optimum level of specific training adaptation. The coaching response to an occurrence like this would be to increase the training load in the next training session.

The recording of symptoms yields an indication of how an athlete is reacting to the stress of training. Changes in the number of symptoms indicate changes in the training response. Subsequent training loads should be increased or decreased to return the number of reported symptoms back to the 'window' of training responses. Figure 8.1 indicates these features. There is considerable variability between athletes as to how much training can be tolerated and how susceptible they are to excessive training loads.

Monitoring Overtraining

After a period of time, athletes lose the capacity to adapt to training programs. Should this occur in athletes using the *Daily Analyses* booklet, it will be observed that the return to the 'window' does not occur as easily as when the athlete is adapting. When workloads are reduced on three successive occasions and there are no outstanding stresses occurring in other aspects of the athlete's life, but a reduction in 'worse-than-normal' symptoms does not occur, it can usually be determined that an overtrained state has been reached. At least one complete unloading training microcycle should be implemented immediately in this situation.

When athletes train consistently year-round, there comes a time when further performance improvement due to physiological adaptation is not possible. Increased workloads do not produce any further performance improvements. Athlete responses in the 'window' indicate adequate tolerance of training loads in a physiological sense. But the physiological capacities of an individual are limited in their potential for improvement. Thus 'windows' of stress symptom reports finally indicate the state of maximum physiological adaptation that is possible. Figure 8.4 illustrates recordings that indicate responses representing an overtrained state.

Monitoring Travel Disruptions

There are uses for this booklet other than the monitoring of training. A common one for serious athletes is the assessment of recovery from time-zone shifts ('jet-lag') and travel fatigue. The stresses that result from travel increase the number of 'worse-than-normal' symptoms reported. More symptoms occur but they are not necessarily those which are reported when training is excessive. This is because the stressors are different. A coach can monitor the type and number of symptoms that are reported as a consequence of travel. Light training sessions should only be considered until the number of negative symptoms returns to 'window' values. Heavy training sessions during this recovery and adaptation period would serve no good purpose. They would only delay the adaptive/recovery reactions of the athlete. Figure 8.5 exhibits the jet-lag responses of some Canadian Olympic ski-jumpers at the 1984 Olympic Games.

Figure 8.4 Sample 'a' ('worse-than-normal') Symptoms Associated with Adaptation to Exercise Stress

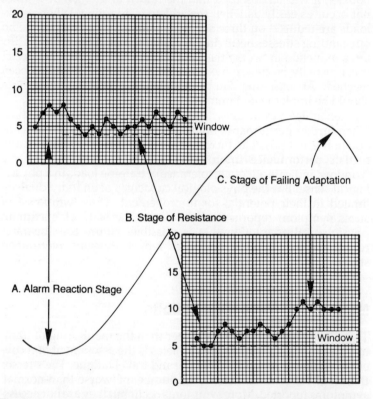

The first stage, with elevated symptom numbers, is related to the alarm reaction to the onset of training. The subsequent 'window' is associated with the stage of resistance (successful adaptation). Within these data plots, there were two occasions when heavier-than-normal training sessions caused responses to occur outside the 'window'. The separate graph depicts the transition from resistance ('window') to the stage of failing adaptation (overtraining). At that time, the data points remain outside the 'window' even though training loads are reduced. Undesirable responses usually decrease when recovering from overtrained states.

Figure 8.5 The 'a' ('Worse-than-normal') Symptom Daily Recordings for Three 1984 Olympic Athletes that Illustrate the Excessive Stresses Caused By Time-zone Shifts (Jet-lag) and Travel Fatigue

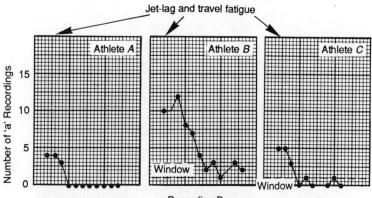

Note: For Athlete A the window is zero.

Monitoring Outside Stressors

The discussion above has generally assumed that exercise stress is the only factor that is excessive in an athlete's life. That rarely is the case. Since an individual has a finite capacity to handle life stresses, it is possible that symptoms associated with increased stress may be caused by the accumulated effects of training and other stressors. Thus it is essential that the possible incursion of other life stresses should be considered on a daily basis.

Before a decision is made about altering an athlete's training load because data have fallen outside the 'window', the number of life stresses that are reported as being 'worse-than-normal' should be considered. If they have increased, then it is possible that events other than training loads have caused them to be reported. If that is the case, then the athlete and coach together should attempt to reduce the outside stressors, for they detract from the exercise-tolerance capacity of the athlete. When outside-of-sport stressors are reduced, athletes can adequately handle heavy training loads, which in turn produce bigger training effects.

The above concerns are the reasons why Part A is included in the *Daily Analyses* procedure. The influence of outside-of-sport events on training responses is very marked and can now be measured. Coaching and training decisions should always consider such influences. Figure 8.6 illustrates changes in reporting symptoms of stress when the number of these stress sources increases.

Figure 8.6 The Relationship between Excessive Outside Stressors plus Exercise Stress and Self-reported Stress Symptoms for an Elite Age-group Swimmer

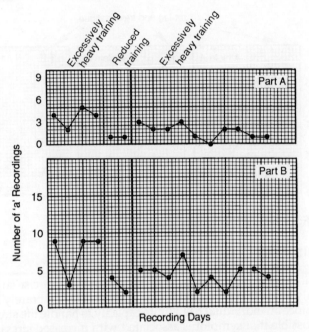

The 'worse-than-normal' recordings for both parts of the *Daily Analyses* booklet are represented (from Rushall and Roaf 1986). The lowest values were recorded when workloads were changed from excessively heavy to light.

Monitoring Peaking

One further valuable use of this measurement procedure is the monitoring of the peaking state. Athletes who record values in the 'window' are not capable of a maximum performance. A period of reduced training loads is necessary for peak performances to occur.

With this tool, peaked states are indicated when the number of 'better-than-normal' symptoms increases. This is why graphs of the three classes of response are maintained. Peaked states should prepare an athlete to feel as good as possible. Thus, an increase in the number of 'c' ('better-than-normal') symptom responses along with a reduction in the 'a' ('worse-than-normal') symptoms should be evidenced. Figure 8.7 illustrates recording changes that occur as the peaking state is developed.

Figure 8.7 The Relationship between Stress Symptoms Recorded as 'Worse-than-normal' and 'Better-than-normal' during Specific and Peak Training Phases for an Elite Sculler

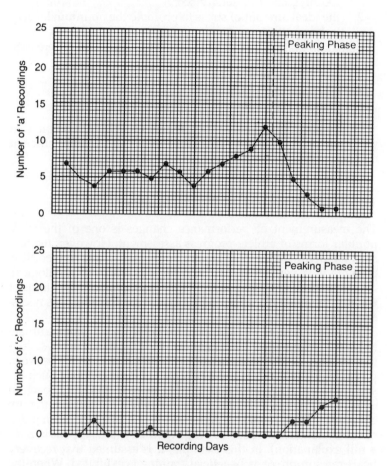

The increase in 'better' and decrease in 'worse' symptoms together indicate that a peaked-readiness state is being attained.

This analysis technique measures how athletes feel at any particular time. The appraisal of various symptoms of stress indicates responses to it: the greater the number of symptoms that appear to be worse than usual, the greater an athlete is stressed. It is on this basis that responses to training stress and life stresses in general are monitored.

It is now possible to measure the following features:

1. training responses which indicate that the athlete is either too stressed or understressed
2. the ideal amount of stress to promote the optimum level of training effort
3. the influence of outside-of-sport stressors that interfere with the training response
4. initial features of overtraining
5. reactions to travel fatigue and jet-lag
6. peaking responses

The use of this tool should promote better coaching decisions that will assist athletes to improve performances in a more efficient manner.

The Measurement of Performance

The measurement of performance changes is one of the more popular forms of athlete-progress assessment. However, the reasons for performance changes are not as easily determined. It is possible that performances could be affected by physiological, biomechanical, or psychological factors and even combinations of them. If there is a reason for performance change, then it is necessary to locate that reason.

The assessment of the relationships between physiological factors and performance is not new. The plotting of some physiological measure against performance indicates relationships between physiological efficiency and performance (Carlile 1964). Such assessments are still useful and provide information for a coach to determine training program content. Figure 8.8 illustrates the use of recovery heart rates and performance relationships as an index of the training response in rowing ergometry (see Appendix B for a full explanation). In this example, it is assumed that recovery heart rates improve as beneficial training is exhibited. When the recovery heart rates are plotted against low and high-effort performances, a baseline against which future comparisons are made is established. As training progresses, the general distribution of data points moves to the left on the graph. When no further progression to the left occurs, it is usually assumed that the ceiling physiological training effect has been reached. Of more importance is the migration of the points back to the right. This can be assumed to be a signal of overtraining because the cost of work for a particular level of performance is increasing whereas if beneficial adaptation were occurring it would continue to improve in efficiency. A decrease in the cost of exercise, even in the face of no change in physiological capacity, widens the comfort margin between cost and capacity and hence enhances performance. The size of the cost/capacity margin is a useful index of overtraining. The assumption behind such plotting procedures is that *changes only occur due to physiological functions*. There only needs to be a slight modification in technique which alters movement efficiency and, consequently, the cost of work, to make it impossible to tell if the performance changes are due to physiological and/or biomechanical events. This is a major concern for interpreting such phenomena. If field tests of this nature are coupled with laboratory tests, then the coach is better able to determine if any physiological changes have occurred.

Figure 8.8 A Training Effect Index, Recovery Heart Rate, and Performance in Rowing Ergometry

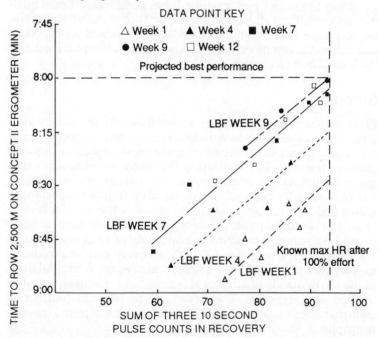

The frequent assessment of recovery heart rates and performances of various intensities allows a coach to assess whether the energy cost of a rowing performance is improving. If improvement, as evidenced by a shift to the left in data points, ceases to occur or reverses, then a ceiling-training effect, an overtrained state, and/or changes in technique efficiency have occurred. For greater details of explanation refer to Appendix B.

The above example used recovery heart rate (the total of 10-second counts taken immediately, 30 seconds, and 60 seconds after the performance) as the training effect measure. It is possible to plot other field test physiological measures, for example, lactic acid concentrations, single heart rate measures such as the number of beats between the 30- and 60-second time interval after performance cessation, and the number of breaths taken in 60 seconds. There are many variations on this form of field testing for adaptation states. They are best suited to cyclic activity sports, such as running, cycling, rowing, and swimming, where techniques become established and changes mainly come from fitness adaptation. However, it should be noted that when athletes undergo technique changes, the validity of these tests is markedly reduced. Their main use is with athletes who have established movement patterns.

It is not a great imposition for serious athletes to keep graphs of a training index and performance. It has good motivational qualities and sensitizes athletes to the importance of monitoring training responses and continually avoiding overtrained states. When this method is combined with psychological self-report methods, the benefit is even greater.

Summary

When sound training principles are not followed, the quality of an athlete's experience is downgraded. The accommodation of recovery requirements is perhaps the single most important need for effective training. The realization that early warning signs of a psychological nature are the first clear signals of excessive fatigue has only recently been validated. Altering training expectations within and between sessions to accommodate the need for further recovery is an appropriate coaching action. The avoidance of overtrained states is a paramount responsibility of an effective coach. The failure to provide for adequate recovery can be avoided if measurements of the athlete's stress reactions are made. Analysis of the life demands of athletes is necessary to effectively monitor their training responses. The correct interpretation of information from that assessment method will limit the abuse of sound training principles.

Note

1. Dr Don McKenzie of Vancouver, British Columbia, has recently completed a study on the measurement of overtraining in canoeists. Psychological self-reports are among the best indices for measuring overtraining and highly fatigued states.

Training Modifiers

⑨
Biophysical Factors Affecting Training

Heredity

Whether athletes are born or made has always been a controversial issue in sports. A number of research studies have determined the genetic contribution to performance primarily by comparing identical and fraternal twins. Because identical twins are composed of the same genetic material, any differences in performance can be attributed to the environment in which they are nurtured. On the other hand, variation in fraternal twins can be due to a combination of inherited and environmental factors. Despite differences in activity levels there is less variation in the physiological performance capabilities of individual identical twins than between fraternal twins (Klissouras 1971, Komi, Klissouras, and Karvinen 1973, Karlsson, Komi, and Viitasalo 1979). These studies have permitted estimates of the heritability of several physiological functions associated with oxygen transport, anaerobic power, and neuromuscular coordination to be made. The values proposed are maximum lactic acid concentration (81·4 percent), reaction time (85·7 percent), maximum aerobic power (93·4 percent), muscular power (97·8 percent), and muscle fiber type (99·5 percent).

There are many documented cases of the non-athletic offspring of former champions showing considerable physiological aptitude in laboratory and performance tests. While these observations underline the importance of the inherent physiological properties of the body, such a genetic advantage must be matched by intensive training before championship performances can be expected. Hence, both genetic and environmental influences are important in determining the ultimate level of performance attained. The trainability of an individual is also influenced by in-born characteristics. A person born with a muscle fiber composition suited to strength and power activities has more potential to profit from training those capacities than one blessed with endurance qualities. On the other hand, an individual with a high proportion of slow-twitch muscle fibers will have difficulty in being competitive in sprinting, jumping, and throwing events despite following an appropriate training program.

Age

The involvement of young children in hard training needs to be carefully evaluated. The period of mid-childhood (6–10 years) is a time of slow growth where there is a relatively constant ratio between height and lean body mass. This provides a stable environment in which to concentrate on skill development rather than fitness work. The potential for shaping the body is limited without the presence of sufficient quantities of androgens (testosterone) which act to hypertrophy skeletal and cardiac muscle and increase the oxygen-carrying capacity of the blood. While increases in strength and endurance can occur in response to training in children, these are not maximized until puberty is reached. The timing of an exercise program to coincide with peak height gain during puberty seems to offer some performance advantages.

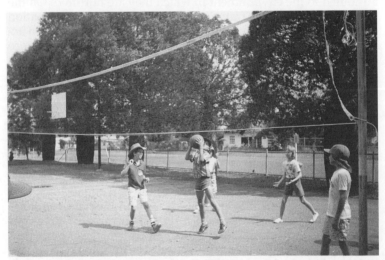

The period of mid-childhood is one of constant slow growth, which is ideal for the development of a wide variety of basic skills, rather than for concentrating on fitness work

The age of puberty varies greatly between individuals. In an early maturer the growth spurt is short and intense. The early gains that accrue in both size and strength initially offer physical advantages in many sports. However, coaches must be careful to attend to skill development or these children will be surpassed in performance by their late maturing peers. A late maturer experiences a growth spurt that is less intense but lasts longer than an early maturer. The ultimate result is a taller and potentially stronger individual. Coaches need to be patient and encouraging in order to optimize the development of a late maturer.

It should also be understood that the bones of young children are susceptible to injury associated with heavy training. In response to heavy repetitive loads bone-related problems such as stress fractures, epiphyseal plate fractures, and Osgood–Shlatter's disease frequently arise.

Peak function in most physiological attributes occurs between 25 and 30 years of age. After that the decline is at a rate of roughly 1 percent per year. While physical training may not prevent this decline in performance it does permit a higher level to be achieved at a particular age. The magnitude of improvement through training in veteran athletes is usually lower than that in younger individuals. Older male athletes have limitations similar to those of children in developing strength and endurance. A decrease in the secretion of testosterone with age restricts the potential for hypertrophy. Performance increases have therefore to rely more on neuromuscular improvements.

Anecdotal evidence suggests that older individuals take longer to recover from both injury and hard training than do younger athletes. This has obvious implications when prescribing training loads.

Sex

The successful emergence of hard-training women athletes in sport has provided convincing evidence that women can be trained as successfully as men. However, there are certain structural and functional differences between the sexes that deserve some comment.

Girls mature faster than boys. The hormonal changes of puberty affect the body composition of both sexes differently, boys showing a greater growth of lean tissue and girls a greater growth of fat. These changes have obvious implications for the training and performance of adolescent males and females. Young women find it increasingly difficult to perform in sprints and bounding events (e.g., gymnastics, running, and jumping). The extra body weight also increases the potential for injury. Higher levels of body fat in addition pose greater problems for removing heat from the body, which can be a limiting factor in prolonged training sessions. On the positive side, body fat improves buoyancy and insulation in water and can therefore improve biomechanics and thermoregulation in swimming.

As a result of increased secretion of the hormone testosterone, adolescent males become progressively better at activities that rely on muscular strength and power. Historically, females have been fearful of the masculinizing effect of muscle hypertrophy that might result from weight training. However, this concern has now largely subsided in the face of research studies showing that women who participate in resistance training increase significantly in strength without accompanying hypertrophy (Wilmore 1974).

The menstrual cycle of women can also be disrupted by hard physical training. Amenorrhea (absence of menstruation) is common in endurance athletes and gymnasts. This condition, which fortunately seems to be benign and is reversible, may be related to low levels of body fat, extreme weight loss, or an excessive training load. Women are also more prone to iron deficiency as a result of iron loss during menstruation. This can be corrected by increasing dietary iron intake and a sensible prescription of training loads.

There seems to be no harm to either mother or baby if a regular moderate exercise routine is maintained during pregnancy. In fact, this is regarded as a beneficial practice. However, it is not wise to engage in high-intensity, prolonged exercise, particularly during the final stages of pregnancy, since dehydration and high body temperatures should be avoided.

Otherwise, the responses of women to most forms of physical training are similar to those of men. However, it is fair to say that many research studies have been conducted on previously inactive women and less is known about the response of those involved in strenuous sports training. This a fertile area for future research.

The Physical Environment

The Olympic Games have drawn attention to a number of environmental influences on sports performance. During the time of the Summer Olympics it is usually hot and/or humid. On the other hand, the Winter Olympics invariably call for protection against the cold. The 1968 Mexico City Games, sited at 2,350 meters above sea-level, presented the situation of lowered barometric pressure and reduced air density. World records were set in the men's 100, 200, and 400 meter races and the long jump. Distance races were appreciably slower than in previous Games. In Los Angeles in 1984, concern was expressed for athletes possibly experiencing high levels of both heat and air pollution. While some athletes certainly suffered as a result of the climate, British middle-distance runner, Steve Ovett, and Swiss woman marathoner, Gabriela Anderson-Schiess, being the most obvious examples, the weather in Los Angeles during the Games was generally comfortable.

It is the purpose of this section to describe the physiological responses to a number of environmental conditions and to offer considerations that could be given during the performance of sporting activities.

□ Heat

During exercise a great deal of heat is produced by the body. In extreme circumstances this can elevate its core temperature from 37°C to beyond 40°C. When the surrounding air is cool heat can be lost from the body by the process of radiation (transfer of heat by electromagnetic waves), convection (by air movement), conduction (by contact), and evaporation (by sweating). As the surrounding temperature increases it becomes more and more difficult to lose heat by radiation, convection, and conduction. Hence, the predominant source of heat loss in warm to hot conditions is from the evaporation of sweat on the skin surface.

Sweat losses exceeding 6 liters have been recorded in marathon runners. These deficits constitute a body weight reduction of 8–10 percent and a body water loss of 13–14 percent (Costill 1979). Team-game players performing in warm to hot conditions can sweat at a rate of 2 liters per hour. During a game this can amount to a loss in body weight of 5 percent and a reduction in body water of more than 10 percent (Pyke and Hahn 1981). Losses in body weight of 2 percent have been shown to result in reductions in endurance performance as well as increase heart rate by 5 bpm.

The requirement for copious sweating places a heavy load on the circulation to provide blood flow to both the muscles to maintain work rate and to the skin for cooling. As the body progressively dehydrates the circulation is further compromised and heat storage exceeds heat removal. The resultant strain is indicated by increased heart rate, sweat rate, and core and skin temperatures. Collapse can occur if work is continued.

There are a number of factors which must be considered before individuals are exposed to work in hot conditions.

The Climate

Other than air temperature, both humidity and radiant heat should be assessed before athletes engage in hard training or competition in hot weather conditions. The most commonly used heat index in sport is the WBGT index which includes measurements of air temperature (dry bulb), humidity (wet bulb), and radiant temperature. These temperatures can be easily measured with a whirling hygrometer and a black bulb thermometer placed in a black sphere. The following calculations can be used to determine the WBGT index:

Outdoors
WBGT index (°C) =   0·7 × wet bulb temperature (°C)
                      + 0·2 × black bulb temperature (°C)
                      + 0·1 × dry bulb temperature (°C)

Indoors
WBGT=   0·7 × wet bulb temperature (°C)
                      + 0·3 × dry bulb temperature (°C)

When this climatic index exceeds 25 °C and the work rate is reasonably high, coaches should be aware of the potential negative effects on athletes. When it exceeds 28 °C the coach should abandon vigorous activities for poorly conditioned and unacclimatized individuals and be wary of signs of heat intolerance in others. In hotter months, training should be scheduled in the early morning or evening rather than at noon or mid-afternoon.

The impact that a hot, humid climate has on the physiological responses of a runner was well exemplified during performances in Darwin, Australia. Throughout a 30-minute run in cool conditions at a speed of 230 meters per minute, a man increased his rectal temperature from 37·7 to 39·3 °C and incurred a weight loss of 750 grams. This contrasted with an increase in rectal temperature from 37·2 to 40·6 °C, accompanied by a weight loss of 1,000 grams, when the run was repeated in the hot, humid conditions of Darwin. The skin temperature rose to nearly 38 °C in the heat whereas in the cool it fell to 31 °C. The reduced temperature gradient between the body core and skin experienced in the hot conditions meant that a large blood flow was required to transport heat from the core of the body to the periphery. This resulted in heart rates measured during the last 15 minutes of the run in the heat (190–200 bpm) being much higher than those measured in the cool (152–154 bpm). Hot, humid climates reduce endurance capacity in long-duration events.

Characteristics of the Individual

There are certain individuals who have a low tolerance to heat and need careful supervision by coaches. Those with heavier builds possess a lower ratio between skin surface area and body mass than those with more linear builds. This is a disadvantage for heat removal. High levels of body fat also encourage heat storage. Fat tissue has a lower specific heat than lean tissue and therefore, absorbs heat more readily. Individuals with a high level of endurance fitness tolerate hot conditions much better than those who are unfit. The average male has a higher level of endurance fitness than the average female and endurance fitness decreases substantially with age. This explains why males usually are more heat tolerant than females and younger adults more heat tolerant than older ones. However, when males and females and older and younger adults of equivalent levels of aerobic fitness are compared, these differences in heat tolerance disappear. One group that requires special attention in the heat is pre-pubertal children. They have poorly developed sweating mechanisms and overheat rapidly. Coaches should monitor them carefully for signs of heat intolerance during practice sessions. Risks should not be taken with them in hot, humid conditions.

Heat Acclimatization

It has been shown that physical training in cool conditions improves tolerance to hot conditions. However, full adaptation to heat can only be achieved by actually working in hot conditions. The adjustment is very rapid and is achievable in about 7 to 10 days if regular daily exercise for 90 minutes is undertaken. Heat acclimatization expands the blood volume which supports an increased capacity and precision of sweating. At a given relative workload a fit, acclimatized person commences sweating sooner, sweats more evenly over the skin surface and thereby loses less salt. An acclimatized person performs in a heat tolerance test with greater circulatory stability (lower heart rate) and lower core and skin temperatures than someone who is not acclimatized. However, the acclimatization process is retarded by dehydration. For optimal adaptation to occur, fluid balance should be maintained during the recovery periods between daily bouts of work in the heat.

It might also be noted that pre-pubertal children acclimatize more slowly than do adults. Elevations in the sweating response take longer in children despite their perceiving that they are adjusting. This makes it particularly hazardous to rely on the subjective response of children as to their reaction to hot conditions. Recovery breaks for cooling and fluid replacement should be regularly scheduled to counteract young athletes' inabilities to accurately discern fluid replacement needs.

The procedure of adding extra layers of clothing (tracksuit, windcheater, and head covering) while training during the winter months has been tested as a means of promoting heat acclimatization. Despite producing elevated thermoregulatory responses during each training session, the practice has been only partially successful in improving heat tolerance of well-conditioned team-game players (i.e., field hockey). If this procedure is used, particular care needs to be taken to ensure that players do not overheat during training, since heat will produce levels of fatigue that substantially erode the capacity to perform substantial volumes of skill trials (Dawson and Pyke 1988).

Clothing

During exercise in hot conditions, it is recommended that participants wear light-colored clothing made from open-weave natural fibers (e.g., cotton, wool). As much of the skin as possible should be exposed to the air to maximize the evaporation of sweat. Clothing made from synthetic fibers, such as nylon and polyesters, offers more resistance to heat removal and, in time, becomes uncomfortable.

Fluid Replacement

When fluid losses exceed 2 percent of body weight prior to exercising, a significant endurance performance deterioration occurs. It is wise to drink (hydrate) before exercising so that no dehydration occurs. However, during some high energy sporting contests, despite experiencing sweat losses of 4–6 kg, it is neither necessary nor advisable to attempt to entirely replace the amount of fluid lost. The body actually produces water during exercise. Most athletes only drink enough fluid to recover between 40 and 50 percent of the sweat lost. Partial fluid replacement has been shown to reduce the risk of overheating. During a series of 2-hour runs, marathoners who ingested 100mL of fluid every 5 minutes for the first 100 minutes maintained a lower rectal temperature than those who abstained. This occurred despite only absorbing 1,660 mL of fluid while losing 4,000 mL of sweat during the run (Costill, Kammer, and Fisher 1970). The sensation of thirst lags behind the state of negative water balance, and should not be used as the signal to drink. Drink breaks must be regularly scheduled and made compulsory during training and competitions.

Since the body loses more water than electrolytes during exercise, the body fluids become concentrated. Hence there is a greater need to replace water than electrolytes during periods of heavy sweating. The answers to questions concerning the frequency, quantity, and qualities of replacement fluids depend, to some extent, on the individual concerned, the intensity of effort, and the environmental conditions. The major concern is to replace water. Flavored drinks, commercial preparations, and other solutions are not necessarily the best forms of fluid replacement.

On hot days, fluid should be consumed before, during, and after training. This maintains the stability of circulation which is so important for endurance efforts. Water is the primary requirement and, in most circumstances, is the ideal replacement fluid. Fluids with high sugar and electrolyte concentrations empty slowly from the stomach for absorption into the blood via the small intestine. That slow emptying will actually delay the replacement of needed water. It is only when excessive sweat losses occur on successive days that small amounts of salt and sugar may be necessary in a replacement fluid. On cooler days, when fluid losses are less, a higher concentration of carbohydrate in the fluid assists in maintaining the blood glucose level. Whether the amount of carbohydrate ingested is large or small is not a critical factor in 'feeding' during events or training. It has been shown that more frequent feeds maintain more stable blood glucose levels. Therefore, if carbohydrate supplementation occurs during exercise, the frequency of feeding should be considered to be of the utmost importance.

In sports such as wrestling, body-building, weight-lifting, and rowing, where weight limits have to be achieved to perform in competition categories, the loss of weight at the right time is important. Such weight loss is best achieved through gradual dietary accomplishments. Attempts to 'crash diet' a short time before a contest can have debilitating effects on athletes by causing disruptions to internal well-being, feelings of distress, and reduced performance states through anti-carboloading. The even more harmful procedure of trying to lose 'water weight' through taking diuretics or dehydrating should also be avoided. The maximum safe value to lose, as has been pointed out above, is 2 percent of body weight. Values that exceed that will reduce the efficiency of the body's physiology, cause the circulatory system to work harder for a stated amount of work, and will reduce endurance performance. More often than not, unsound weight loss programs cause performances to decrease. Their value and benefit to the athlete should be seriously questioned.

The following are sensible fluid replacement guidelines for exercise:

1. The temperature of the fluid should be cool (8–10°C).
2. The fluid should be low in or lack sugar (carbohydrate) to enhance absorption of the water. The highest concentration of sugar should be 2·5 g per 100 mL of water.
3. During exercise, the volume taken should be no more than 0·5 liters per hour in doses of 100–200 mL every 15 minutes.
4. At least 0·5 liters of water should be consumed prior to exercise.

5. The loss of electrolytes in most activities is minimal in sweat and can be adequately replaced in the diet after exercise. The need for replacement during exercise is generally non-existent.
6. Keeping a record of body weight after waking in the morning is an easy method of monitoring hydration.
7. Forced regular fluid intakes are required. Do not rely on the feeling of thirst to determine when ingestion should occur.

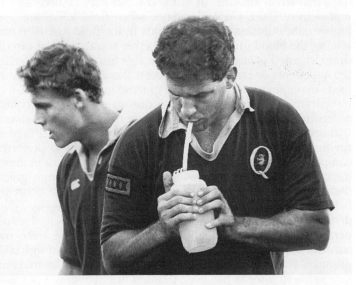

When the weather is warm, it is vital that athletes involved in prolonged and intensive training sessions replace some of the fluid lost in sweating and avoid the limitations imposed by dehydration

□ Cold

In cold climates the athlete continually tries to prevent heat loss and a fall in the core body temperature. A cooled state is referred to as 'hypothermia' or 'exposure'. In a fatigued person its symptoms are poor control of movement, disorientation, and poor judgment and reasoning. The two ways to cope with this problem are to produce more heat or reduce the amount being lost.

Increased Heat Production

Extra heat can be produced either by shivering or by exercising. Shivering raises the resting metabolism about fourfold but in the process interferes with the expression of skill. Nadel, Holmer,

Bergh, Astrand, and Stolzijk (1974) studied breaststroke swimming in water temperatures of 18, 26, and 33 °C and attributed the extra oxygen cost of performing in the cold water to the shivering response. Depending on the endurance fitness level of the individual, metabolism can be elevated twelve- or fifteenfold during intensive exercise. Fitness is necessary to maintain a high work rate and heat production during endurance sports. If a marathoner slows down towards the end of an event held on a cold day it is possible that heat loss will exceed heat production and that hyperthermic problems will arise. This is a particular threat in endurance winter sports (e.g., biathlon, cross-country skiing). Fatigue is the nemesis of the endurance athlete competing in cold conditions.

Decreased Heat Loss

There are several physical avenues for heat loss which must be considered if an athlete is to remain warm.

Radiation is the physical action whereby heat is radiated from the body to nearby cooler objects. This can be minimized by curling the body into a tuck and reducing the exposed surface area. Such a response is common when resting in cold conditions. Heat loss by radiation also can be reduced by limiting the blood flow through the skin. This is the first line of defence against cold and is managed by reflex constriction of the blood vessels supplying the skin. This mechanism is capable of improving the insulative capacity of the skin sixfold. Cooling the skin in this way reduces the temperature gradient between it and the environment and effectively reduces heat loss. However, this means of heat conservation results in the fingers and toes, with their large surface area to mass ratio, becoming particularly cold and losing their speed and dexterity. This is a problem in target and touch sports such as fishing, shooting, and golf. In extreme conditions, frostbite injuries can be sustained. Acclimatization to cold conditions promotes some improvements in local blood flow and enhances the capabilities of the extremities to perform with skill and precision.

The shutdown of blood flow to the skin of the head is much less than that in the hands and feet. If the head is exposed to the cold, substantial heat loss can occur. This has resulted in strong recommendations to wear headgear during sports played in the cold and to wear life jackets to prevent immersion of the head during aquatic rescues.

Another means of conserving heat by reducing radiation is to increase the insulative properties of the shell of the body by depositing fat under the skin. This has been observed in successful Channel swimmers (Pugh and Edholm 1955).

Thin pre-pubertal children with a high surface area:mass ratio are particularly susceptible to cooling while swimming in cold water. Central body temperatures below 35 °C have been commonly observed in children after swimming in 20 °C water temperatures (Keatinge and Sloan 1972). This is of some concern to swimming coaches who rely on the child's perception of cold to provide necessary protection. A lean and ambitious young athlete could easily become hypothermic while training enthusiastically in cool conditions (particularly when swimming) and should be watched carefully.

Convection occurs when heat is transferred from the body to free air. As cold air comes into contact with the body it is warmed, becomes less dense through expansion, and rises. The role of clothing is to trap warmed air close to the skin and develop a microclimate which is comfortable and heat retaining. Forced air convection occurs when the body is either fanned by or creates its own breeze in the process of movement. In external circumstances the 'wind chill factor' is such that a temperature of –1 °C in still air effectively becomes –18 °C if a 40 km.h^{-1} wind is blowing or if a skier or cyclist is moving at that speed. Windproof overgarments should be worn to avoid excessive heat loss in such conditions.

Conduction is the means by which heat is lost by direct contact with other surfaces that are cooler than the skin. Handling of ice axes, metal pitons, and ski poles with bare hands should be avoided since the temperature gradient between those pieces of equipment and the skin is usually very severe. Gloves and insulated boots are used to reduce the amount of conducted heat loss. The conductivity of water is 25 times greater than that of air. Much more heat is lost in water than in air at the same temperature. In one sense, the increased conductivity of water allows swimmers to perform greater volumes of work than runners since they are not inhibited by the build-up of heat.

Evaporation is the means by which heat is lost through sweating. Becoming inactive immediately after heavy sweating can invite rapid cooling and a dramatic fall in body temperature. This can occur on the bench after an intensive period of play in a team game or perhaps as a result of an enforced rest during an endurance event. It is important to have warm, dry clothing available to arrest the decrease in body temperature in such situations. The hiker or skier should try to avoid the situation arising where layers of clothing close to the skin become saturated with sweat. This destroys the insulatory value of the clothing and accelerates heat removal. Rain has the same effect. Clothing should be suited to the energy requirements of the sport, remembering that less insulation is needed as heat production increases. A doubling of the work rate from 3 to 6 Mets performed in 5 °C air temperatures requires only one-third of the original insulation (Burton and Edholm 1969). This is why it is appropriate to have layers of clothing in vigorous winter sports. The appropriate number of layers can be removed to maintain the proper level of heat loss while maintaining dry clothing. Clothing which permits insulation to be added or subtracted in accordance with the intensity of exercise is the most useful. Jackets that open down the front are more convenient than pullovers. Hoods that can be drawn back are ideal during intermittent activity. Drawstrings that allow clothes to be tightened or loosened at the collar, waist, and arm and leg cuffs conveniently vary the insulative value of garments.

It is important not to overprotect the hands and feet against the cold as the body will perceive itself to be very warm and not invoke the physiological temperature regulation processes which prevent a fall in core body temperature. It is better to insulate the trunk rather than the extremities. Three units for the torso, two units for the limbs, and one unit for the hands and feet has been recommended by Kaufman (1982) as the appropriate proportions of clothing distribution.

Should an athlete not follow these recommendations and develop hypothermia during a sporting contest it is critical to immediately start the rewarming process. After providing shelter, wet clothes should be removed and replaced with dry, warm ones. The individual should be warmed gradually under blankets or in a sleeping bag, administered warm, sugared drinks and kept awake until normal body temperature has been restored.

□ Altitude

As altitude increases, there is a decrease in barometric pressure which means that the air becomes less dense. Sprinters, jumpers, and throwers benefit from this phenomenon because they experience less resistance both for themselves and for their projectiles at moderate altitudes (1,500–3,000 meters). Their performances at altitude usually exceed those recorded at sea-level.

Lowered air pressure also results in lowered pressures exerted by respiratory gases, the gas of particular concern for sports performance being oxygen. As oxygen pressure in the air in the lungs is reduced, the pressure of oxygen in arterial blood is lessened, which reduces the oxygen carrying capacity of the blood (oxyhemoglobin saturation). Up to altitudes of 3,000 meters the flatter upper portion of the oxygen dissociation curve provides some, yet not complete, protection against individuals becoming hypoxic (starved of oxygen). Above 3,000 meters, substantial reductions in oxygen-carrying capacity occur. Human beings are equipped to compensate for reduced oxygen amounts relatively well up to certain altitudes. After these, performance capacities deteriorate rapidly. The lowest altitude that can be tolerated without adverse effects on performance is less than 1,200 meters. Performing at higher altitudes reduces the ability to produce sea-level-equivalent endurance performances. Altitude also prolongs the recovery from endurance activities.

Immediate Effects

For every 300 meters above 1,500 meters, maximum oxygen uptake is reduced further by 3–3¾ percent. Thus, at Mexico City, 10 percent reductions in endurance performances must be expected. Training intensities that can be performed at sea-level are reduced by 8 percent at 1,500 meters and 18 percent at 2,300 meters. The inability to maintain training intensities results in reductions in $\dot{V}O_2$ max and aerobic performance.

Apart from the pure physical alterations caused by altitude, there is also the added problem of mountain sickness. Its symptoms are headache, dizziness, nausea, insomnia, and loss of appetite. This illness seriously limits the capability and willingness of athletes to perform. Sudden introductions to sporting contests at significant altitudes and the onset of this reaction will severely hamper all types of performance.

Acclimatization

There are both immediate and long-term adaptation phases when adjusting to altitude. The early phase is completed within one to two weeks. The next phase is considerably longer, its duration varying markedly between individuals.

In order to offset the problems associated with performing at altitude, there are a number of adaptive changes which start to occur within 24 hours. The body responds to the initial increased demands for pulmonary ventilation by readjusting the acid–base balance of the body's fluids; increasing the red cell count and hemoglobin concentration; improving capillarization; and improving the concentration of myoglobin and oxidative enzymes in the muscles. As these adjustments occur, the initial changes in ventilation, heart rate, and cardiac output return to near-normal levels. Forced hydration prior to arriving at, and while acclimatizing to, altitude will partially offset the reduced blood plasma volume. That will reduce the initial detrimental effect of altitude on endurance performance.

These adaptive changes improve endurance performance capabilities at altitude but never allow them to reach what can be attained at sea-level. The time for full acclimatization to occur depends on the altitude and the individual. It would take two to three weeks at least to adjust to an altitude such as that of Mexico City or Bogota. Despite allowing for adjustment time, a 6–7 percent reduction in $\dot{V}O_2$ max below that obtained at sea-level can still be expected. Therefore, the adaptation only accommodates a 3–4 percent recovery when acclimatization is possible. At higher altitudes the adaptation time is longer. The capacity to improve performance at altitude is further increased when the psychological disturbances created by mountain sickness are also removed. Acclimatization affects both the performance and the health physiology of an athlete.

Altitude Training

A question that is often asked is whether endurance performance at sea-level is enhanced by altitude training. The reason for exploring this possibility is that the hypoxic stress of high altitude produces some physiological adjustments that are similar to those induced by physical training. While several studies have demonstrated that the sea-level performance of untrained subjects is improved after training at altitude, the same cannot be said for the well-trained athlete. The major problem with altitude training is that the intensity and volume of work must be lowered in order to cope with the environment. If a coach or athlete wishes to indulge in this form of training it is recommended that the selected altitude be a moderate one (1,800–2,000 meters) where the symptoms of mountain sickness are not as acute and the work rate can be maintained at a reasonable level. The reduced work volume and intensity that occurs at altitude may not be sufficiently offset by the gains in the oxygen-carrying capacity of the blood. Research some years ago suggested that these gains were beneficial but now that opinion is not strongly supported. Individual responses to altitude training and its timing before competition require further investigation.

However, there is an area in which training at altitude does contribute to enhanced performance. Karvonen, Peltola, and Saarela (1986) reported that speed production and explosive strength increased in élite sprinters when they trained above sea-level (1,850 meters) in the final period prior to competition. The improvements were more than achieved by a comparable control group which remained at sea-level. This suggests that altitude training may improve the performance of sprinters, and possibly strength event athletes, when it is performed as the pre-competition phase before serious competition. Such training should not be used to increase anaerobic capacities. More research needs to be done in this area, for it has promising possibilities.

A further suggestion, for which there is no scientific evidence, is to live at altitude but train at sea-level. With that regimen, the body will still be able to maintain training volumes and intensities, and also experience the overcompensatory aerobic adaptations of altitude. This situation would present the best characteristics of both sea-level training (big volumes and high intensities) and altitude living (exaggerated aerobic adaptations). In theory, under these conditions the level of endurance performance should increase.

There are a number of training principles that can be followed to allow altitude acclimatization to occur:

1. Build a high aerobic base ($\dot{V}O_2$ max) prior to going to altitude to allow a higher reserve and faster acclimatization.
2. To offset the debilitating effects of mountain sickness, ascend at a rate of 300 meters per day after 1,500 meters, consume large amounts of fluids to offset dehydration, carbohydrate load the diet, and use acetazolamide, if necessary, to alleviate the sickness.
3. Be prepared for colder temperatures by wearing layers of clothes that can accommodate greater temperature ranges than those which occur at sea-level.
4. Keep training intensities very low for several days, that is, until all symptoms of mountain sickness and environmental adaptation have disappeared.
5. Plan for increased lactic acid levels and recovery times in the training program.
6. When resting heart rates return to sea-level values, workloads appropriate for altitude training can be undertaken.
7. When prolonged exposure to altitude training is not possible, arrive one to two weeks prior to competing.

□ Pollution

Air pollution is the product of complex chemical reactions that occur in many different ways. The combustion of coal and fossil fuels in the large cities of Britain produces sulphur dioxide, which in combination with carbon monoxide, forms the main constituent of British smog. Los Angeles' smog is different. The city is the perfect location for the development of photochemical haze. The heavy traffic produces large amounts of nitrogen oxide which is converted by sunshine to form ozone. These smogs, along with carbon monoxide, produce problems for athletes performing in their presence.

Ozone

Low concentrations of ozone can affect breathing during exercise. Its presence is harmful in endurance sports. An ozone concentration of 0·20 parts per million, equivalent to a Stage 1 health advisory alert, affects endurance. In summer in Los Angeles, this condition occurs usually once every three days. A more serious concentration, 0·35 parts per million (Stage 2 health advisory alert), occurs on average once a week. It was fortunate that these levels were rarely experienced during the Los Angeles Olympic Games in 1984.

Athletes who already suffer from respiratory problems, such as asthma and bronchitis, are markedly affected by ozone. It has an irritating effect on the eyes, nose, and throat. There are also harmful psychological effects associated with the mere smell of ozone. An athlete's concentration and dedication to performing can be affected because of this. Sensitivity to ozone is an individual matter, some athletes being unaffected while others complain of throat irritation and suffer spasms of coughing.

Ozone has a direct effect upon an athlete's performance and willingness to perform. The awareness that it exists as a pollutant produces psychological disturbances (e.g., revulsion, objection) which further lowers physical capacities.

Carbon Monoxide

The other smog substance that affects athletic performance is carbon monoxide. By attaching firmly to blood hemoglobin, it reduces the capacity to carry oxygen, as much as 5 percent of available hemoglobin being removed in this manner. This can occur in smog-ridden cities and in smokers (cigarette smoking being the other major source of carbon monoxide). The detrimental effect can occur within two hours of being in a smoggy city, particularly in traffic, and will result in significant reductions in endurance performance. The presence of carbon monoxide can also produce a deterioration in visual acuity and mental functions. That reaction can result in judgmental errors which can be critical in certain sports. Carbon monoxide can also distress athletes by causing headaches, particularly in hot weather.

The combined effects of ozone and carbon monoxide pollution on exercising athletes in hot conditions can be devastating. The capacities to transport oxygen to the working muscles and to sustain efforts are reduced. The circulation contains less oxygen, and usually less fluid as a consequence of heavy sweating caused by the heat. This increases the dual responsibility of supplying blood to the muscles in order to keep moving and to the skin to sweat to keep cool. This double demand compromises the circulation and forces the athlete to reduce his or her work rate.

Athletes should not expose themselves to large doses of carbon monoxide in the three- to four-hour period prior to competition. They should avoid smoking, smoke-filled rooms, and areas with heavy traffic.

Acclimatization

There does not appear to be any functional adaptation to smog. While there is some evidence that the sensitivity to ozone diminishes with repeated exposures, this reaction is not true for all individuals. The major concerns are the irritations caused by exposure to smog. They may create psychological problems in athletes in the pre-competition period, particularly a worsened appraisal of readiness to perform. Prior to their events, the wisest strategy for athletes is to spend as little time as possible in areas where smog may exist. That was the usual procedure adopted to combat the potential Los Angeles smog at the 1984 Olympic Games.

Long-term Effects

Brief exposures to pollution are unlikely to have any long-term effects on athletes. However, the constituents of smog do have the potential to cause medical problems if they are inhaled on a regular basis. Ozone is a toxic substance which is known to damage cells. Medical authorities are concerned about the connection between the presence of air pollutants and respiratory ailments such as chronic bronchitis, emphysemia, and lung cancer.

□ Jet-lag, Travel Fatigue, and Life-style Shifts

Jet-lag is a problem commonly experienced by athletes who have to travel east or west across a number of time-zones to participate in competitions. The competitive edge can be lost even after crossing one or two time-zones and can be significantly affected if greater distances are covered. Jet-lag results from disruptions to the body's circadian rhythm, that of an internal clock that regulates the physiology, such as the secretion of hormones, heart rate, and body temperature and anticipates the activities over a 24-hour period. For example, a person regularly sleeps for a particular period at the same time each day. The body gets used to lowering its metabolism at that time for that duration. When individuals have a particularly regulated life-style, as is often the case with dedicated endurance athletes, cycles of activation, reduced activation, and deactivation become established. There are times when the body is predisposed to eat, sleep, and exercise, because of the pattern of life that an athlete has followed. Physical and mental performances are strongly related to the peaks and valleys of circadian rhythms.

The circadian rhythm is disrupted when time-zones are crossed so that preparedness to function in a particular manner is not in concert with the actual time of a new environment. This disruption is primarily an alteration in the sleep–wake cycle, but can be complicated by demands for energetic work. It affects the regulatory endocrine and nervous systems of the body, leading to headaches, gastro-intestinal upsets, and mental symptoms of fatigue.

If an athlete travels across as few as two or three time-zones, the internal clock will not be synchronized to the altered real time. It is most likely that an individual will be exercising when the body expects to sleep, or eating when the body feels it should be exercising. This disruption causes performance capacities to be reduced (LaDou 1979).

Fatigue is another effect of jet travel that can influence performance. The air in an aircraft is dry, somewhat oxygen deficient, and causes the onset of lassitude and dehydration. Reaction time, perception, mood, motivation, and thought processes can all be negatively affected by travel fatigue and/or jet-lag. Some athletes may also experience stiffness and constipation due to prolonged sitting. Sleep deprivation, prolonged periods of idleness, and restricted activity are travel stresses which add to the level of fatigue incurred.

Another feature of competing in distant places is the order with which activities are followed each day. Alterations in the normal sequencing of life-style events are known as life-style shift. If an athlete is used to training early in the morning and late at night, eating meals of various volumes in a set sequence, as well as only sleeping at night, then a reordering of those activities will be stressful. That reordering will also complicate the adaptation process. At major competitions, training is usually scheduled during the day, as opposed to training times in the morning and evening. Often an afternoon rest is scheduled when this has never been possible at 'home'. Big breakfasts are possible in village or hotel dining rooms as opposed to what is available in a busy home environment. Such disruptions to normal living habits and sequences will extend the time needed for full adaptation to occur in the new environment.

Life-style shifts are also complicated by the degree to which the culture at the competitive site differs from that which is normal for the athlete. Environmental signals that make an individual feel comfortable — for example, those which exist in a familiar home environment — often do not exist. Thus there is a need to adapt and learn the new customs, signs, and activities of a foreign situation. These added adaptive stresses further retard the adaptive responses of individuals. Adjustments to life-style shifts are facilitated by having life-style cues in synchrony with time-zone changes prior to leaving the normal environment.

The sum of the stresses caused by jet-lag, travel fatigue, and life-style shifts is called general travel stress.

There are great individual variations in response to the disruptions and problems associated with travel. For some, a two-hour time-shift can be drastic while in others it will not be noticed (Fleming, cited in Campbell 1979). The primary disruption to the athlete caused by travel is the reduction in the amount of rapid eye-movement (REM) sleep (Weitzman, Kripke, Goldmacher, McGregor, and Nogeire 1970). When a complete sleep phase (8-hour) shift is experienced, body temperature, alertness, concentration, and mental performance take about one week to adjust, although there is still great individual variation. Noradrenaline adapts relatively quickly from jet-lag and so endurance performances recover in a short period of time. However, adrenaline is slow to adapt, so there is a likely to be a longer period of adaptation required for athletes in sprint, power, and strength events (Akerstedt 1977).

There are a number of procedures for coaches and athletes to follow to reduce the impact of travel stress.

1. Establish the life-style routine activities at home prior to leaving. Rest, training, eating, and sleeping sequences should be followed in the order that they will occur at the distant site.

2. Create an artificial time change prior to leaving. Set all clocks and home activities to match those of the new environment. This will result in less shock and faster adaptation.

3. Attempt to arrive at night so that rest can occur within a relatively short time.

4. For professional teams that are constantly travelling across time-zones it may be best to disregard attempts at adaptation and live a demand life-style. Eating, sleeping, and playing are all done according to the athlete's feelings. There is no attempt to establish regularity.

Judging Adaptive Responses of Athletes

There are a number of cues that a coach can use to judge how well an athlete is adapting to the problems of travel. The amount of day sleep required by the athlete is the single best index (Goodyear 1973). While that amount remains unusually high, the coach can infer that the athlete is still adapting. It is not the total amount of sleep that is important but the amount of day sleep that is the index. Subjective measures of the need for rest is a good indicator of travel-stress effects. Alterations in an individual's attention span also indicate travel stress. A coach should look for reductions in the amount of enthusiasm when executing tasks to judge this factor. Cognitive errors, such as slips of the tongue, inattention to detail, organizational breakdowns, and errors, also indicate that adaptation is still occurring. A final symptom of the problem is reduced persistence in training. Athletes usually cannot perform the same number of quality repetitions of skills and tasks possible before travel. When the normal level of persistent performance is recovered, the travel stress has mostly been dissipated. The *Daily Analyses of Life Demands for Athletes*, the tool that measures stress adaptation in athletes (see Appendix A), is sensitive enough to measure the effects of general travel stress.

Overall Implications

There are six general implications from the research on jet-lag and travel fatigue:

1. It is more fruitful to consider the complete experience — travel, adaptation, training, and competing — as the stressor rather than competition or jet-lag alone.
2. The life-style cues, such as clocks, daylight, activities of people in the environment, and eating times, are very important for promoting adjustment. They should be controlled and provided as early as possible when arriving at the destination. This means that the new rhythm for all activities should be initiated immediately upon arrival.
3. Situational novelty increases adaptation requirements. If athletes can be educated as to what to expect at the new site and taught how to cope with unusual events, the impact of novelty will be reduced.
4. No quick adaptation process exists: one can only minimize it. It is necessary to consider the athlete with the worst adaptive ability when planning trips for groups of athletes. If this is not done some athletes will be expected to perform when they are not capable of a best application of effort, that is, when they are still adapting to the stress of travel.
5. If there is insufficient adaptation to remove travel stress, performance arousal, precision, and volume will be decreased.
6. The equation for determining how long to spend in a distant environment before competing has to consider circadian rhythm disruption, recovery from travel fatigue, and adap-

tation to novelty. Recommended are: 1 day for each hour or 1½ hours of time difference, depending upon the direction travelled; 3 days for travel that results in sleep disruption; and 2 days for environment adaptation added to the amount of time planned to accommodate the cost of travel.

General Guidelines

The following list is a compilation of activities that can be undertaken to reduce the impact of travel stress.

Prior to travel:

1. Attempt to adopt the times of the new area in the home environment so that adaptation to time will be achieved.
2. Attempt to adopt life-style activities in the home environment. At least train at the times that will occur in the new location.
3. Educate athletes about the customs, sites, and language of the new environment. This will reduce novelty and uncertainty about being able to cope with the new environment and will accelerate adaptation.
4. Alternate 2–3 days of fasting and eating prior to departure. This will sensitize the body to changes in time cues.
5. The meals for 2–3 days prior to travel should be very high in carbohydrates. This will assist better digestion and retention of fluids during travel.

East–west travel is the form of travel tolerated best because it is similar to the experience of going to bed late. The phases of the circadian rhythm are delayed in relation to the events of the new time-zone:

1. Plan to arrive in the evening so that the journey can be followed by prolonged rest.
2. Delay eating patterns until they are in concert with the times to be experienced in the time-zone.
3. Only sleep on the plane if travel is overnight.
4. The time for adjustment can be calculated by allowing one day for each 1½ hours of time change.

West–east travel is the form of travel hardest on athletes. The phases of the circadian rhythm are advanced in relation to the events of the new time-zone:

1. Allocate sufficient days for recovery as suggested above.
2. Choose a flight which will arrive before the usual bedtime in the new time-zone.

3. If a morning arrival is scheduled, sleep for an hour after arrival and then spend the rest of the day outdoors and in mild activities. Idleness should be avoided.

4. The time for adjustment can be calculated by allowing one day for each hour of time change.

Dehydration and travel stress may be minimized as follows:

1. Drink plenty of fluids (e.g., juices, mineral water, water, or clear carbonated drinks). Avoid caffeine-loaded colas, alcoholic beverages, and coffees, all of which have a dehydrating effect. Drink regularly and do not wait until feeling thirsty.

2. Eat foods which are high in fiber content. The amounts should be small to accommodate the reduction in energy demands caused by the inactivity of travel.

3. Fatty foods such as gravy, sauces, creams, fried items, and red meats should be avoided. The eating of fatty foods should also be avoided the day before travel.

4. During the journey, participate in planned bouts of activity. Frequent stretching, bouts of walking around the plane, and moving as much as possible will avoid or retard the onset of stiffness and leg-swelling.

5. Attempt to engage in light, pleasant activities during the flight. Avoid extended periods of doing nothing.

6. Adjust the light in the plane to match the light conditions of the time in the new time-zone. That cue will start the adjustment process prior to arrival.

At the destination:

1. Immediately investigate the location of important items such as the eating facilities, a pharmacy, exercise areas, amusements, and sites of essential services.

2. Avoid tap water. Drink only bottled beverages and water.

3. Eat fruits which can be peeled, and select pre-packaged foods.

4. Eat in reliable restaurants that provide high standards of sanitation. Avoid foods that are sold by street vendors.

5. Take pre-competition foods so that a normal pre-game regimen can be followed.

6. Participate in activities other than sporting activities. Prolonged periods of inactivity (too much resting, idleness) will promote listlessness and will retard adaptation.

7. Immediately adopt the times and life-styles expected in the new situation.

8. Eat high-protein meals for breakfast and lunch in order to stimulate adrenaline and activity during the day.
9. Eat high carbohydrate meals for supper. This will facilitate sleeping several hours after the meal.
10. Match sleep time immediately. Extra sleep the first night can assist in adaptation speed. A short nap during the day can help alleviate some of the travel fatigue, but should not be of such an extended nature that it interferes with night sleep.
11. If it can be accommodated, participate in a light aerobic workout as a means of removing the residual physical discomforts associated with the restricted positions endured during travel.

Nutrition

The history of sport is riddled with myths surrounding the nutritional beliefs and practices of well-known coaches and athletes. While research has not supported many ill-founded notions, there is continuing interest in food supplements and additives as possible providers of a critical performance edge. This section highlights some important considerations when prescribing a training diet and discusses the potential value of some selected ingredients.

□ The Balanced Diet

The overriding principle of nutrition is that the training diet should contain sufficient quantities of the essential nutrients contained in the major food groups to meet the demands caused by physical activity. These groups include cereals and grains, protein, diary foods, and fruits and vegetables. Dietary requirements will vary according to the age, sex, and body composition of the athlete as well as the type of training and the environmental conditions of participation.

The energy value of the ideal training diet should be geared towards maintaining an acceptable body weight and meeting energy requirements. As distinct from the typical Western diet which is high in fat, the diet of athletes should be high in complex carbohydrates (e.g., wholemeal bread, pasta, cereals, potatoes), low in fat, and with adequate amounts of protein and fiber. As a general rule, *carbohydrates should comprise at least 60 percent, protein 15 percent, and fat 20–25 percent of an athlete's diet.*

□ Carbohydrate

Endurance-trained athletes often suffer from chronic fatigue as a result of a combination of overtraining and poor nutrition. One of the reasons for this is associated with depletion of muscle glycogen which can occur when hard training is conducted on successive days. Low levels of muscle glycogen impair both sprinting speed and the ability to sustain an effort throughout a long contest. Severe glycogen depletion can be averted by interspersing easier training sessions between harder ones while elevating the amount of carbohydrate in the diet. Since lighter training sessions do not exhaust glycogen supplies, replenishment of stores can occur when they are alternated with heavy training sessions.

The diet should be high in complex carbohydrates rather than simple ones (e.g., sugar, honey, confectionery) because the former are absorbed and released slowly, providing a sustained high energy release. Since complex carbohydrates are high in minerals, vitamins, and fiber, and low in fat and cholesterol, they contribute to the requirements of a balanced diet.

The double value of a diet high in unrefined complex carbohydrates is that it will also be rich in fiber. This adds roughage or bulk to the diet without increasing caloric intake. Wholemeal cereals, pasta, brown rice, raw vegetables, and fresh fruit are foods high in fiber content. However, fiber can interfere with the absorption of certain minerals. Therefore athletes should pay particular attention to ensure that their diets contain adequate quantities of minerals, particularly iron and calcium.

It has been shown that muscle glycogen content can be doubled by increasing the consumption of carbohydrate in the diet. This offers a considerable advantage in endurance efforts lasting more than two hours. Dietary manipulations, known as carbohydrate loading, were the focus of several experiments conducted in Sweden during the 1960s. Bergstrom, Hermansen, Hultman, and Saltin (1967) showed that increases in muscle glycogen levels could be achieved if they were firstly depleted by severe exercise, then maintained at a low level by adhering to a protein/fat diet for three days, and then eating a carbohydrate-rich diet. However, this regime produced negative side-effects and discomforts associated with the high-protein/fat diet and has been replaced by one that involves the combination of a reduced training load (peaking) during the last week and a high carbohydrate diet (70–80 percent) during the three days prior to competition. This facilitates easier adherence to the program, is preferred by many athletes engaged in prolonged effort activities, and achieves the same 'loading' effect as the original research regimen.

It should be noted that significant quantities of water are stored in association with glycogen. This may induce a feeling of stiffness or heaviness in the muscles and could detract from sprinting and jumping performance. A substantial weight gain of from 1–1·5 kg could result from this effect.

With normal mixed diets (protein 15 percent, fat 30–35 percent, carbohydrate 50–55 percent) it usually takes up to 48 hours to fully restore muscle glycogen. This can be accelerated to 24 hours if the carbohydrate content of the diet is elevated to 70 percent at the expense of fat. As an example, the following series of meals will provide a total of about 20,000 kJ (5,000 kcal, containing 70 percent carbohydrate) per day and should support the energy metabolism of an athlete involved in a high-energy sport.

Breakfast:	4 cups of Corn Flakes
	4 cups of milk
	2 cups of orange juice
	4 slices of whole-wheat bread or muffins
	4 teaspoons of preserves or honey
	2 large bananas
Lunch:	8 slices of whole-wheat bread
	6 oz. (170 g) of sliced lean meat
	4 oz. (113 g) of low-fat cheese
	2 muesli bars
	2 cups of apple juice
Dinner:	3 cups of spaghetti cooked with lean meat
	or low-fat cheese
	2 bread rolls
	2 tablespoons of margarine
	2 cups of green beans
	2 large apples
	2 large oranges
	4 pieces of cake

It is recommended that two days before a competition day, training loads should be light and deliberate attempts should be made to add more complex carbohydrates and simple sugars to the diet. This should continue through breakfast and lunch on the day of the contest. However, it is unwise to eat sugar-based foods an hour before activity. The sugars increase the secretion of the hormone insulin which, with the onset of exercise, causes a rapid fall in blood glucose. Sensations of light-headedness and weakness usually occur early in the contest.

□ Fat

Fat can be stored in large quantities in the body. There are health risks associated with excess body and blood fat levels. Unhealthy levels of fat (obesity) detract from sporting performance potential. Fat intake can be reduced by trimming fat from meat, reducing cooking fat, using low-fat dairy products, and avoiding foods high in fat content. An absence of fat is particularly important in pre-contest meals where rapid digestion is required. Fat slows the absorption of nutrients which is counterproductive to adequate pre-competition preparations.

☐ Protein

Protein is an essential ingredient in the training diet. Its principal use is for repairing and building tissue. Animal sources of protein that are low in fat include lean red meats, fish, chicken (without skin), and low-fat dairy products. Important vegetarian sources of protein are cereals, legumes, leafy vegetables, and rice. The recommended daily requirement for protein is 1 gram per kilogram of body weight. In athletes involved in body development and repair, or in growing children or adolescents, the level is usually elevated to $1.5–2.0$ g.kg^{-1}. The increased amount is usually well within that contained in normal Western diets. Expensive protein supplements are not required by athletes, even though they may be engaged in heavy body-building and strengthening activities, or recovering from prolonged strenuous exercise.

☐ Vitamins

The most controversial area of sports nutrition concerns vitamin and mineral supplementation. In general, an athlete on a well-balanced diet requires no additional vitamins or minerals. However, there are individuals who can suffer deficiencies, including those on diets of take-away foods, restricted vegetarian diets, diets high in refined carbohydrates, high alcohol intakes, and diets which include drugs such as laxatives and diuretics. Rather than relying on vitamin supplements, athletes should try to improve their diets through better understanding of the nutritional value of the foods they eat.

There are two major classes of vitamins: those which dissolve in fat (A, D, E, K) and those which dissolve in water (B complex and C). These vitamins are essential for energy production, tissue repair, and mineral metabolism. They are important for sports performance. For example, Vitamin A (growth), Vitamin B (metabolism of carbohydrates, fats, and proteins), Vitamin C (tissue regeneration, iron absorption), Vitamin D (bone mineralization), Vitamin E (red blood cell production), and Vitamin K (blood-clotting) all have functional implications for the hard-training athlete.

While vitamin supplements will not correct a poorly balanced diet, some of the newer multi-vitamin preparations do ensure that the recommended daily intake of each is met. Their ingestion is a useful safeguard against possible vitamin deficiencies. However, there is some danger of overdosing, particularly in terms of fat-soluble vitamins which can be stored in the liver and fat tissue. Water soluble vitamins are more rapidly released via the excretory system and if taken in excess, are less likely to have toxic effects.

There is no convincing evidence that vitamin supplements are necessary for athletes who consume a high energy athlete's diet that contains mainly natural and unprocessed foods.

□ Minerals

Iron deficiency is a particular problem that can be caused by hard training and a poor diet. An iron deficiency in training athletes is called sports anemia. Iron is important for the synthesis of hemoglobin which is the principal means of oxygen carriage in the blood. It is a critical ingredient in the diet of an athlete involved in endurance-based sports. Hard training promotes a high degree of iron loss either through sweating or in the mechanical destruction of red blood cells. Female athletes have another significant source of iron loss, the bleeding phase of the menstrual cycle. Iron deficiency is usually associated with a general feeling of sluggishness, fatigue, and loss of appetite. The state of iron deficiency is best judged by the level of ferritin in the blood. The more commonly used hemoglobin levels do not always give an accurate indication of iron status. It is important that the sporting diet is sufficiently rich in both iron and the vitamins responsible for iron absorption and synthesis, to meet any deficiency that might occur. Sports anemia can be prevented by eating the following foods at least three times weekly:

> Lean red meat (an abundant source of readily absorbed
>   hem-iron which is found in liver, kidney, and heart)
> Green leafy vegetables (spinach, lettuce)
> Beans, peas, dried fruit
> Wheat grain

The vegetable form of iron (non-hem-iron), while still important, is not as easily absorbed as meat-obtained iron. Since high-fiber cereals may interfere with iron absorption it is beneficial to eat iron-rich foods at lunch and dinner rather than at breakfast.

Iron supplementation via tablets may be necessary. This should be done under medical supervision as excessive iron use may become toxic. It is wise to take a multi-vitamin, multi-mineral supplement to ensure that the full benefit of the extra iron is not being lost by poor absorption or synthesis. Iron from plant foods is better absorbed if it is consumed with foods rich in Vitamin C, such as citrus fruits. Temporary reductions in the intensity and quantity of training also assist in the recovery from sports anemia.

Calcium is a mineral involved in bone formation and maintenance. It is contained in large amounts in dairy products. Many young athletes involved in sports such as distance running and gymnastics, where leanness is encouraged, can over-restrict their diet and calcium intake, resulting in serious reductions in bone mass. A particular example of this is seen in the increasing incidence of stress fractures in the bones of young female gymnasts, dancers, and distance runners. When hard training is coupled with a low caloric intake and body fat, and inhibition of menstrual bleeding, there is the distinct possibility that bone weaknesses may start to appear.

☐ Alcohol

Unfortunately, alcohol is closely associated with sport and athletes should understand its effects. It is a central nervous system depressant and interferes with reaction time, coordination, and judgment. Even in small doses, it has a negative influence on skill performance. Alcohol is also a diuretic and causes dehydration which can lower endurance performance. Alcohol is highly caloric and, if imbibed excessively, can produce body weight problems and vitamin deficiency (Vitamin B_3). A hard-drinking athlete is rarely a hard-training athlete. Such excesses, in the long term, can also cause damage to the liver and other organs. Ingesting alcoholic beverages has no value for sporting performance.

☐ Pre-competition meals

From a dietary viewpoint, little can be done immediately prior to an event to enhance performance. Any nutritional benefits should have been obtained from the previous day's food intake. Therefore, the pre-event dietary strategy should aim at minimizing any harmful effects of improper habits such as low fluid intake, excessive eating, and inappropriate timing of meals. Two to three hours before the contest it is desirable to consume a high carbohydrate, low-fat meal accompanied by abundant fluid. A breakfast-type meal with bread and cereals, low-fat milk, toppings, and fruit juice is ideal. A light lunch of fish and lean meats, salads, and fluids is also suitable. The traditional steak meal is inappropriate as it is high in fat content and is digested slowly. It has the potential to disrupt performance.

As mentioned previously, foods or drinks high in simple sugars should not be taken immediately before a contest for they will induce a hypoglycemic response when exercise commences. However, during a prolonged effort of over two hours, the ingestion of sugars is useful for assisting the liver to maintain the blood glucose levels.

It is important for the athlete to be familiar with the foods included in the pre-event meal. Sudden dietary changes are often quite unsettling. In this respect, commercial liquid meals, such as Sustagen and Sportsuite, are useful low-fat, easily digestible alternatives that have become popular with athletes in recent years.

□ The Coach's Role

The coach has an important role in the nutrition education of athletes. This involves understanding the physiological demands of the sport and its appropriate food requirements. A sound knowledge of basic nutrition should be taught, particularly in relation to feeding before, during, and after competition. It is essential that athletes know the foods that are likely to have a negative effect on performance, and are aware of the consequences of not following sound nutritional practices. An informed approach to nutritional habits offers the athlete a considerable advantage when preparing for high-performance sport.

Several obvious principles emerge regarding the nutrition of athletes.

1. Replenish muscle glycogen stores between training sessions with a high complex carbohydrate diet.
2. Replenish muscle enzyme systems with a well-balanced diet adequate in mineral and vitamin content.
3. Limit fat intake — avoid fatty meat and fast-fried foods.
4. Eat adequate amounts of fiber — vegetables, fruits, cereals, and grains.
5. Eat adequate amounts of protein — lean meat, fish, eggs, low-fat milk.
6. Limit simple sugar and salt intake.
7. Ensure adequate fluid replacement with non-alcoholic beverages.

10
Social and Psychological Factors Affecting Training

The discussion of social and psychological factors and their effects on performance could be very lengthy. This chapter focuses on factors, behaviors, and situations which affect the training responses of athletes. It avoids excursions into theories and descriptions of postulated items that cannot be subjected to verification. The purpose of the chapter is to highlight actions and situations that can be altered to produce better training responses in athletes.

Features Which Affect Training Effort and Efficiency

☐ Positive Atmosphere

Taylor (1979) showed that the quality and efficiency of physiological responses are altered according to the psychological states of individuals. He compared the effects of potentially rewarding (positive) and potentially punishing (aversive) situations on subjects performing an extremely demanding physical training test. It was found that under positive expectations, maximum muscle power and the duration of sustained effort were increased. This contrasted with the characteristics of aversively influenced performances where psychological stress-type cardiovascular responses (e.g., tachycardia and hypertension in excess of changes in cardiac output) and associated deteriorations in awareness and alertness were observed. Thus, when a person performs physically under 'aversive' (negative) conditions, physiological capacities are used less efficiently and some performance characteristics also deteriorate. The effects of negative control situations on behavioral characteristics have been extensively documented (e.g., Rushall and Siedentop 1972, Skinner 1968). The effects of the psychological atmosphere on performance have a number of implications for structuring the training environment.

An athlete can worry about the adequacy of his or her ability to perform; can wish that a training item did not have to be completed; can train so that he or she will not feel guilty about missing a training item or session; and can train to avoid letting teammates down; these are all examples of aversive or negative orientations to training stimuli. Training response quality is reduced in such situations. If training consists of responses which are inferior because of a negative mental state then its benefits will be reduced. Thus an athlete's mental approach to training is an important determinant of the quality of training.

Coaches need to construct tasks and training stimuli in such a way that their completion is achieved in a positive environment. Athletes need to interpret the segments of training as positive experiences. Rushall (1987) reported features of training that champion athletes described as being desirable (positive experiences). It is recommended that coaches structure training sessions so the following features occur:

1. Let the athletes know the training program well in advance of the session.
2. Keep the athletes busy all the time.
3. Allow athletes to establish challenges for themselves at each training session.
4. Include variety in the overall training program.
5. Stress skill improvement, rather than error detection.
6 Provide opportunities to test for improvement and progress.
7. Program opportunities to improve in all aspects of the sport, not just a particular specialty.

Each training session should be interpreted as an opportunity to achieve positive outcomes. These should be under the control of the athlete so that responsibility can be assumed for their occurrence. For example, if athletes were taught how to reinforce their own behaviors, rather than waiting for coach appraisal, the frequency and relevance of positive outcomes would increase. The use of peers as performance evaluators has been shown to improve discipline-training characteristics, such as completing assignments, adhering to timed intervals, and attending to task features, to a much greater extent than that which could be achieved by coaches performing the same role (McKenzie and Rushall 1980). When athletes are given responsibility for evaluating the quantity and quality of responses, they train better (McKenzie and Rushall 1974). A training emphasis on doing things well, rather than concentrating on what is being done badly, produces quality and quantity increases in performance. Training should be constructed to provide rewards from a variety of sources including the athlete him- or herself, peers, and the coach. The number and sources of positive experiences associated with training need to be increased to a much greater extent than those which usually exist. The number of positive experiences affects the positive outlook of the individual. The amount of positive thinking that occurs in training will directly affect the forms and efficiency of use of an athlete's physiological capacities. Conversely, the amount of negative thought that occurs at training will be related to the diminution of training response quality and quantity.

☐ Achievement

When athletes achieve or are successful in training activities they are motivated to improve the quantity and usually the quality of their performances. Traditionally, training achievements have been restricted to performance features. Improvements are rewarded when a training segment is performed better. However, the total atmosphere of the training situation must be considered, rather than focusing on that one aspect of performance quality. There are other features of training that should be recognized when they are done well:

1. *Effort level.* Sustaining effort levels and applications should be rewarded even though performance quality improvements are not exhibited. Sustained increases in work levels indicate elevated levels of effort (e.g., sustaining a series of repeat sprints of a certain standard, or gradually wearing an opponent down through 'determination').
2. *Work volume.* The amount of work completed in a session or unit of time should be rewarded (e.g., the number of consecutive training sessions attended, the tonnage of weights lifted, total miles run, the number of baskets successfully made).
3. *Skill level.* As an athlete increases his or her proficiency in set skills and also increases the number of proficient skills, reinforcing events should be provided for these achievements. Most athletes are very interested in the skill-technique standards of their performance, so it would be advisable for coaches to emphasize this feature as the primary focus of training.

This point is worth stressing. Some impressive studies have shown that the majority of athletes, and in particular élite athletes, apply themselves fully at training: that is, athletes consider their levels of training effort to be satisfactory. This contrasts with the most common emphasis of coaches, who urge athletes to try harder and explain performance problems in terms of failures to 'try hard', 'provide sufficient effort', etc. Thus there is a common conflict exhibited in most sport situations, athletes being satisfied with their effort levels while coaches are dissatisfied with them. The conflict is further heightened when athletes, and in particular élite athletes, most frequently want to receive feedback for skill or technique features of their performances. This feature is rarely exhibited as a primary coaching emphasis, the exceptions usually being in aesthetic sports. The proposal made here is that skill factors be emphasized at training, while effort levels should also be stressed but not to the same degree.

4. *Task execution.* There are many behaviors that athletes have to perform to be able to train and compete. These supportive behaviors should be reinforced (e.g., attending regularly, punctual arrival, caring for self and equipment, participation in club projects, helping younger athletes, assisting the coach and officials, etc.).

5. *Athlete interaction.* One of the primary reinforcing events that sports activities offer athletes is that the situation becomes their social environment. When this feature is emphasized and good social behaviors are rewarded, the environment increases in its motivational potential. If athletes are taught how to interact positively, are given the opportunity to organize social activities, and are counselled to solve personal problems within the sport environment, then the socially rewarding characteristics of the sport will be increased.

These factors will expand the sources and frequency of rewards and achievements that occur in the training environment: the more rewards, the more attractive. Less able athletes will be given an opportunity to achieve in the sport in factors that are not performance related. Expansion of achievement possibilities produces a number of desirable outcomes. Participation in the sport is lengthened, friends stay longer in the sport, participation is more consistent, and is motivated by multiple factors rather than a single performance emphasis.

The implication for coaches is clear. Allow athletes to achieve in all things associated with successful functioning in the training environment. Do not restrict achievements to pure performance factors.

□ Advancement

Advancement refers to the elevation of status in the various activities associated with a sport over a long period of time. This is not to be confused with achievement which is usually associated with the attainment of short-term or immediate goals.

The central feature indicating advancement is the definition of some ultimate achievement or status — accomplishments such as winning a world championship, being selected for an Olympic team, becoming a club or team captain, or playing a full year as a starter. For most élite athletes there is a clearly established set of performance accomplishments which constitute ultimate goals. These are almost invariably set by the athlete and are very difficult to alter, advancement referring to an athlete's gradual development toward these remote long-term goals. Periodic knowledge of progress indicates that continued participation will be accompanied by performance improvement in both training and competition. Testing sessions should be included in program development so that they can be used to indicate advancement in the physiological components of a sport.

The general concept behind advancement is frequent indications of progress towards higher levels of achievement in any of the diverse activities of a sport. For want of a better description, advancement is recognized when intermediate goals are attained. Thus, for long-term motivation, the succession of accomplishments would be as follows:

1. A number of achievements are recognized which eventually lead to an intermediate goal.
2. Intermediate goals are periodically achieved which indicate that an ultimate goal is still a possibility for attainment.
3. The ultimate goal is achieved.

What is experienced when advancement occurs lasts for long periods of participation, and so is a necessary ingredient for long-term motivation. Periodic testing of fitness component improvements works as a motivator.

The feature that must be considered with regard to sports fitness is that one can advance in physical measurements up to the point where growth and/or developmental capacities reach their limits. From that stage on advancement cannot occur. The task is then to use fitness maintenance, usually as indicated by component testing, as the basis for further performance improvements. Technical, tactical, and psychological skills should be built on a consistently established energy base. These skills can also be measured periodically as indications of the attainment of short-term and long-term goals.

☐ Training Activities

The physical tasks to be completed in training must have a number of features in them to make them add to the motivation to participate: they must be challenging. The following features contribute:

1. A goal should be established for each training segment. If the goal is set by the athlete it will be even more meaningful and effective.

2. Some method of evaluation should be made available to assess the adequacy of performances in training segments.

3. Tasks must be credible. There should be some obvious purpose and relevance behind each item. The principle of specificity is most appropriate for determining the nature of the tasks. The coach should be able to justify the value of the task in relation to the athlete's goals.

4. The major outcomes of all training segments should be positive.

5. Training tasks should be varied to produce novelty effects and avoid boredom. This means that coaches have to devise sets of different activities, each producing the same training stimulus. For example, bounding 4 sets of 8 double-leg jumps over a distance of 18 meters, 2 sets of 12 jumps over 25 meters, and 4 sets of 6 double-leg jumps to and from a 60 centimeter box are examples of plyometric training which could be used to develop muscular power in the legs. An athlete could experience these activities in the same microcycle on the assumption that each activity stimulates an equivalent overload factor in the same physiological capacity. As was mentioned in Chapter 3, determining equivalent activities is not an easy task and may well be a challenging area of research for sport scientists. The point behind constructing such sets is that an athlete can experience various training tasks, which will contribute to motivation, while the body is subjected to the same training stimulus.

6. Training segments should be constructed in tolerable amounts. The interaction of quality and quantity expectations will lead to an athlete's determination of self-efficacy

for performing a task. When this is negative, reduced performance levels occur.

Training tasks also need to be acceptable to an athlete. Athletes have to want to do the task, accept its need, and include some intrinsic assessment of its value. If athletes are made to perform training segments against their wishes, the quality of work that results will be inferior, and the experience will reduce the positive characteristics of the environment.

The way training segments are presented to athletes also affects the physiological efficiency of a response. In a study of the physiological factors that are associated with subjective feelings of fatigue, Michael and Horvath (1965) found that work tolerance decreases were associated with increased physiological costs. Thus, when training segment interest wanes, poor psychological states such as uncertainty, anxiety, and/or depression occur, all features which reduce effort tolerance. Consequently, less work will be done and the value of that work will be decreased because of the inefficiency of the response mechanisms. Rejeski and Ribisl (1980) presented two running tasks to athletes. After a 20-minute performance on a treadmill under standardized conditions, physiological measures were taken. The same task was later repeated but with the subjects believing it had to be performed for 30 minutes. The difference between the tasks was therefore one of accommodating different durations. In the longer run the subjects were stopped at the 20 minute mark, the same as in the shorter task. It was found that some of the important physiological measures were lower in the perceived longer task even though both tasks were the same. This suggests that athletes have a tendency to consider the tasks that are required of them, and then allocate their resources over their duration. This phenomenon is one of the reasons why athletes should be made aware of the total activities of a training session before it commences. If they are not aware of what is required, then all responses will be less than optimum, for some measure of capacity will always be held in reserve to accommodate unexpectedly demanding tasks. It also means that when a program is given to athletes, no further activities should be added, no matter what the reason. This is particularly important and is contrary to the frequent coaching practice of punishing athletes by requiring them to do extra work at the end of a session. Such a practice makes no physiological or psychological sense.

□ Self-improvement

The most powerful source of motivation for the participation of athletes in a sport is self-improvement (Rushall 1987b, Wankel and

Kreisel 1982). This factor embraces the topics of internal control and internal motivation. The effect that athletes have on their own training responses has only recently been recognized.

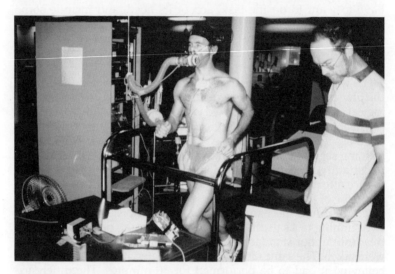

During an experiment in running on a treadmill it has been shown that athletes allocate their energy resources according to their knowledge of the duration of the task, which is why they should be made aware of all the activities of a training session before it starts

The main feature is that athletes have to perceive themselves as being in control of the majority of situations in their training experience. This is characteristic of élite athletes (Chalip 1980, Rushall 1987b), is associated with higher levels of motivation and consistent goal achievement, and is a major feature which yields sporting experience satisfaction (Andrisani and Nestel 1976). Self-controlled individuals handle stress better and solve problems more effectively than those controlled or directed by others. Authoritarian and coach-dominated environments generally do not produce the best responses in athletes. The development of self-control in a sporting environment requires coaches to gradually remove themselves from being the directors of athlete behavior. Athletes should change from coach-dependent individuals at the beginner stage, to self-dependent individuals when they perform at high levels.

The production of self-controlled athletes who monitor their own functioning and improvements will require some drastic alterations in traditional coaching models. It means that athletes will have to be coached to the eventual point where a coach is no longer the controlling agent or even the most significant individual in the athlete's sporting life. The decision-making processes surrounding training content, behavior control, and goal-setting, gradually have to be transferred to athletes through a series of appropriate teaching and developmental experiences.

Athletes need to be taught how to evaluate and reinforce their own behaviors in training. There are three major teaching tasks that befall a coach if this capacity is to be developed in athletes:

1. *Teach how to set standards.* The content of the education about a sport that is provided by a coach will determine how well this is done. Once self-standards are set for a training segment, they should not be altered. Self-reinforcement should only occur when the standards are equalled or surpassed.

2. *Teach the athlete self-reinforcement.* Athletes need to be taught what to say to themselves by developing a rich vocabulary of positive responses and emotional reactions. Most individuals are reticent to use a large variety of words that convey a positive meaning. The word 'good' was used more frequently than any other word in one subject (Rushall and Smith 1979). Thus synonyms such as 'fantastic', 'terrific', 'great', 'marvellous', 'grand', 'super', and many others should be developed in an athlete's vocabulary to expand the content of reactions. The verbal content of self-reactions should be varied in order to maintain impact.

3. *The coach should model the behavior.* The coach's verbal and emotional responses to training efforts should mirror what is expected of athletes in their own reactions. Positive evaluations should occur very frequently. This will require much behavior change in many coaches for it has been shown that, in general, coaches are more negative than positive in their reactions to athlete behaviors (Rushall 1981c), and the variety of positive responses that are offered is particularly limited (Rushall and Smith 1979).

Methods that promote self-assessment have to be devised for introduction into the training environment. Self-evaluation and recording of performance adequacy (Rushall 1975a), public posting of performance achievements (McKenzie and Rushall 1980), and methods of self-evaluating progress are important. Perceptions of improvement in training motivate further increases in competencies (Rushall 1987b). By having athletes always assessing their own participation efforts in training, reinforcement will always be available. The consequential increase in reinforcer frequency will add to the motivational qualities of the training experience.

☐ Social Situation

The social situation of training can directly influence the quality of participation. Cooperative associations, as opposed to having fellow athletes compete against each other, are preferred by champion athletes (Rushall 1987b). The development of strong friends is a desirable feature as are constructive and positive athlete interactions when working on training segments. It has been shown that social reasons are strong motivators for sports participation (McPherson, Marteniuk, Tihanyi, and Clark 1977, Reitter 1982, Rushall and Fry 1980, Rushall and Garvie 1977). A strong social activity program associated with sport training will add to the attractiveness of participation. This factor pervades all levels of sport and not just lower levels as is commonly thought.

Coach–athlete Relationship

This will directly affect the type of participation that athletes follow in a sport. The way the coach–athlete relationship should develop has already been discussed, but there are a number of areas within the relationship that, if not administered properly, will cause athletes to develop negative approaches to a sport:

1.   *Rules and procedures.* The conduct expectations of the training situation need to be clearly stated. This is best done in writing since word-of-mouth education often results in vague or ambiguous understandings of what is required for adequate and acceptable behavior. Rules need to be concise. If they are too long, they are too confusing for full comprehension to occur. What is expected of athletes should be made available to all of them. If rules are written as a contract or booklet, there is no excuse for an athlete pleading ignorance of their existence or a coach not applying them consistently. Athletes should be made aware of behavior expectations before they come into effect. This means that coaches do not make up new rules in response to isolated instances. The role expectations for athletes and coaches should be agreed upon by the athletes, coaches, and officials of an organization. Once rules and procedures are implemented they should be applied consistently. These features require the administration of training to be done under clearly defined expectations. This will reduce uncertainty and apprehension, two factors which reduce the work capacity of athletes.

2. *Coach supervision.* The manner in which athletes are supervised by a coach can be a cause of athlete problems. The coach should be fair, treating each athlete according to the same rules. Athletes should be treated equally at training. Favoritism towards particular athletes should not be evident. The coach should be credible: that is, reasons should be given for all directives. When determining and presenting the content of training sessions, a coach should be objective, not favoring beliefs but basing decisions on established facts.

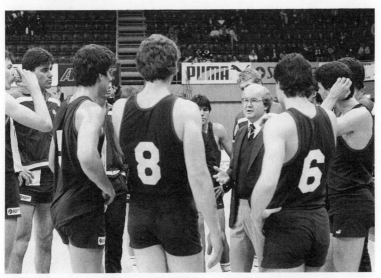

When dealing with players, the coach should ensure that all are treated equally at training, and communication should always be a two-way process

3. *Athlete's relationship with the coach.* The association should be viewed as having two-way communications. Athletes should have some input into the decisions that concern their participation in the sport. The amount of input should increase as the athlete develops. The interactions that occur should be fair, that is, the coach should observe some wisdom in the athlete. The association should be positive. Positive leaders are attractive to those being led. Negative leaders reduce the likelihood of interactions with a resulting reduction in productivity. Criticisms or admonishments should be administered privately.

These features should produce a relationship that develops the following responses in athletes:

1. They freely ask questions about the sport.
2. Coaches are trusted with regard to the validity of information offered about all aspects of the sport.
3. Coaching instructions are followed with enthusiasm.
4. When asked to try new things, athletes apply themselves fully.
5. Athletes will let the coach know when they disagree with any decision or directive.

The characteristics and behaviors which have been described above indicate an athlete–coach relationship that should exist with senior and/or experienced athletes. This means that coaches should gradually evolve a relationship that becomes a mutual association rather than one individual dominating another. Dictatorial coach models do not allow athletes to develop to their fullest potential because the associated suppressive atmosphere does not allow investigative, innovative, or exploratory behaviors. Consequently, athletes only develop in the manner that is dictated. They are not encouraged to use individual talents that are outside the scope of the coach's vision and understanding.

What has been described is a relationship that is different from the majority of the athlete–coach relationships which exist in sports. The time has come for change to take place. If sporting situations include the features that have been described, then the quality and quantity of training responses that will be exhibited by athletes will be improved.

Life Demands

In Chapter 4, The Principle of Overload, a brief discussion was given about the influence of events outside sport on training participation. It indicated that the more stressful an athlete's life outside sport, the less will be his or her capacity for adapting to sports training. Thus the quality of training responses and the level of adaptation potential is directly related to events in an athlete's everyday life. The life-demands that can be measured reliably to indicate possible problem sites, and the substance of the questions that are used to provoke responses in athletes, are indicated below.

1. *Diet.* Is the athlete eating regularly, in adequate amounts, missing meals, and/or liking meals?
2. *Home life.* Have there been any arguments with parents, brothers or sisters? Is the athlete being asked to do too much

around the house? How is the athlete's relationship with his or her spouse? Have there been any unusual happenings at home concerning family?

3. *School/college/work.* After considering the amount of work that is done in the appropriate environment, is the athlete required to do more or less in his or her own time? How are grades and evaluations? What are interactions like with administrators, teachers, or bosses?

4. *Friends.* Has the athlete lost or gained any friends? Have there been any arguments or problems? Are they complimenting the athlete more or less? Is he or she spending more or less time with them?

5. *Training and exercise.* This item is included so that it can be evaluated in the context of the athlete's life as a whole. How much and often is the athlete training? Are the levels of effort that are required easy or hard? Is there adequate recovery opportunity between efforts?

6. *Climate.* Is it too hot, cold, wet, or dry?

7. *Sleep.* Is the athlete getting enough sleep? Too much sleep? Can the athlete sleep when he or she wants to?

8. *Recreation.* This is in reference to activities that are done outside the sport. Are these activities taking up too much time? Do the demands of recreational activities compete with the efforts required to train for the sport?

9. *Health.* Does the athlete have any infections, health problems, or injuries?

The self-reporting of these factors is directly related to the quantity and quality of training. Rushall and Roaf (1986) found that when training loads were excessively heavy, factors outside training were also perceived as being worse. When training loads were reduced for a short period, it was found that athletes' perceptions of the stressfulness of outside factors were also reduced. This suggests that excessive training loads and their undesirable outcomes influence athletes' functioning in other features of living.

The training response is directly affected by social and psychological factors. The finite capacity of an athlete for tolerating all of life's stresses is the central concept for understanding training responses. If factors within or outside training become stressful, that is, are negative or too burdensome, then training responses will deteriorate. Some forms of deterioration are subtle. For example, an aversively controlled athlete will perform but the efficiency of the physiology that supports the performance will be reduced. When factors outside the sport are stressful, their effects will 'migrate' into the sporting environment and reduce the overall capacity of the athlete to train. When outside factors are also negative, they can be transferred into the sporting situation, reducing both the quality and quantity of the training response. The psychological and social situations of an individual's life will affect training capabilities. When the social and psychological atmosphere of training is positive, the fitness response components that are stimulated will be best, and an athlete's capacities will be appropriately stressed to produce an optimum training response.

IV
Analysis of Training Requirements

11
Analyzing Physiological
Requirements of Different Sports

The first step in planning a training strategy is to describe the physiological requirements of a particular sport. It is the purpose of this chapter to outline the means by which this can be done. Examples from different sports are given. However, it is not feasible to deal with the physiology of each sport in detail. There are four general approaches to discovering the physiological needs of sports.

Measuring Performance Responses

Assessments of the physiological responses to continuous sports, such as running, cycling, rowing, and swimming are relatively common. The development of a number of different ergometers, which closely simulate activities, has provided the capability to estimate these responses in some sports. Evaluations of oxygen uptake, heart rate, blood lactic acid concentrations, and muscle glycogen utilization, during actual and simulated efforts, have produced close estimates of the total energy expenditure of these types of performances. However, it is much more difficult to obtain similar information on high energy team and individual sports which involve intermittent efforts. In these situations, with the aid of video recorders, it has been necessary to undertake time–motion analyses in an attempt to estimate the duration and intensity of exercise. Researchers have measured certain indices of work effort, such as the total distance covered and the time spent in various levels of exercise intensity (e.g., walking, jogging, and sprinting). These estimations have provided coaches with some concept of the energy demands of particular games. For example, Mayhew and Wenger (1985) estimated that the average duration of a sprint in soccer was 4·4 seconds and the sprint/recovery ratio was 1 : 7. Other data obtained from time-motion analyses of soccer were summarized by Colquhoun and Chad (1986) and are presented in Table 11.1. Ekblom (1986), in his review of the physiology of soccer, showed that midfielders covered more ground in a game (10·2 to 11·1 km) than either half-backs (9·1 to 9·6 km) or forwards (9·8 to 10·6 km). These data all provide useful guides as to the demands of the game and therefore, the type of training that should be employed by a soccer coach. Time–motion analyses, particularly where meaningful categories of analysis are measured, yield indications of the proportions of activity classifications that can be used for planning training strategies. They are appropriate for many intermittent team sports. Comparisons between player positions also yield valuable information.

Table 11.1 Distances Covered and Intensity of Effort Maintained in Soccer Matches

Reference Source	Walk	Jog	Run Cruise	Run Stride	Sprint	Total (Km)
Brooke and Knowles (1974)	35·2%	54·0%			10·7%	4,833
Reilly and Thomas (1976)	36·8%	24·8%	20·5%		11·2%	8,680
Saltin (1973)	27·0%				24·0%	12,000
Whitehead (1975)	67·7%			17·3%	15·0%	11,692
Withers *et al.* (1982)	31·4%	47·1%			18·8%	11,527

Physiological responses to continuous efforts have been assessed frequently. It is now well known that a sustained sprint, such as a 1 km cycling time-trial, heavily involves the glycolytic-energy pathways and produces high levels of blood lactate (15–19 mmol.L^{-1}). The long-distance efforts, lasting 2 to 3 hours, are almost alactic (blood lactate levels of 2 to 4 mmol.L^{-1}) but severely glycogen-depleting. Hence, training programs for these two activities should differ markedly.

The direct measurement of the physiological responses to intermittent exercise presents some difficulties. It is seldom acceptable to weight players with cumbersome monitoring equipment while they perform. Energy expenditure during a game has mainly been estimated from heart rates monitored by telemetry which is one of the least disruptive measurement techniques. In this method, a small transmitter is attached to the player and an ECG signal is relayed to a transmitter placed off the field of play. In a running sport, the heart rate measured during the contest is then referred to an oxygen-uptake/heart-rate graph which has previously been established for the player during a series of treadmill runs at different speeds (see Figure 11.1). However, even with these measures there are problems. It is likely that the heart rate in the contest will be considerably higher than that obtained in the laboratory. Consequently, the energy expenditure (oxygen uptake) of a game will be overestimated. This discrepancy could be due to many factors: for example, a hotter environment or a greater level of excitement experienced during the game will elevate heart rate. Also, the stop–start nature of the activity does not closely resemble a continuous treadmill run that is used to generate the equivalent estimates of work.

The overestimation of oxygen uptake from heart rates measured during a 20-minute weight-training circuit has been evaluated. The hemodynamic response to weight-training circuit activities elevates heart rate to above 70 percent of maximum and yet oxygen uptake remained below 40 percent of maximum (Hempel and Wells 1985). Thus the use of estimates of exercise energy costs should proceed with caution.

Figure 11.1 Estimating the Energy Cost of Playing Soccer from the Heart Rate/Oxygen Consumption Relationship on a Treadmill Task

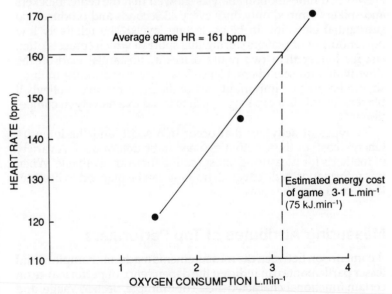

During breaks in play it has been possible to take blood and muscle samples which have indicated the degree of involvement

of certain energy systems. Cochrane and Pyke (1976) monitored blood lactate responses of a midfield player and a defender during an international soccer match and training session. The data in Table 11.2 show that training emphasized lactacid energy development that did not seem to be important in the match. However, the involvement of this energy system in soccer is likely to depend on the style of play employed by the team and the type of game in which it is involved. This study illustrates the feasibility of obtaining useful information during the non-activity portions of games.

Table 11.2 Blood Lactate Responses of Two Soccer Players at Training and in an International Match

Situation	Defender	Midfielder
Game	1·65 mmol.L^{-1}	2·20 mmol.L^{-1}
Training	9·90 mmol.L^{-1}	8·80 mmol.L^{-1}

Conlee, McGown, Fisher, Dalsky, and Robinson (1982) reported interesting findings about the muscle glycogen depletion patterns of volleyball players. Surprisingly for an activity regarded as intermittent and explosive, the depletion of glycogen from the slow-twitch fibers was greater than that from the fast-twitch fibers. However, a time–motion analysis showed that the center blockers and spikers jumped only once every 43 seconds and produced no substantial elevation in blood lactate levels. The relatively low power output of players during this sport in which contests often last for longer than two hours places a substantial load on the slow-twitch muscle fibers. Hence low-power endurance training should become an important part of the preparation of volleyball players for this is a capacity which is taxed extensively in competitions.

The types of activities that occur in a sport, and the intensity (energy cost) of those activities, need to be determined. A variety of methods for measuring or estimating them are available. When this information is discovered, training can be planned to best suit the demands of the sport.

Measuring Attributes of Top Performers

A comparison between the measurements made on champions and lesser participants can indicate the dependence of performance on certain functional characteristics. For example, Secher, Vaage, and Jackson (1982) compared the $\dot{V}O_2$ max of a winning crew at the 1971 European Rowing Championships (6·1 L.min^{-1}) with that of the sixth place crew (5·7 L.min^{-1}) and twelfth place crew (5·1 L.min^{-1}) in the same event. These data strongly suggest that aerobic power is important in a competitive rowing performance lasting about six minutes, that is, the better the aerobic power, the better the oarsman.

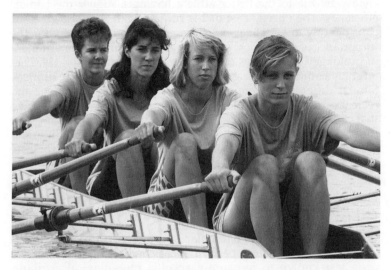

There is a high relationship between maximal oxygen uptake and rowing performance that has been established from comparisons of international rowers

Comparisons of scores made on sprint and endurance tests by the top performers in a variety of sports can also indicate the relative importance of these factors. Data presented on the maximal oxygen uptake of national and international caliber athletes in different sports in different countries show quite clearly the increasing dependence on this attribute as the duration and intensity of the competitive effort increases. For example, male middle-distance and distance runners usually have values (70–80 mL.kg^{-1}.min^{-1}) that exceed players in high energy intermittent sports (e.g., soccer, ice-hockey, squash — 55–65 mL.kg^{-1}.min^{-1}) who in turn exceed players in more skill-oriented sports (e.g, volleyball, golf, baseball — 45–55 mL.kg^{-1}.min^{-1}). Values for females are in the same direction but between 5 and 10 mL.kg^{-1}.min^{-1} below those for males engaged in each category of sport.

It has been observed that some outstanding long-distance runners do not necessarily have an exceptionally high maximum oxygen uptake. Other factors, such as the ability to run economically at high speeds without producing significant amounts of lactic acid (that is, they have a high anaerobic threshold) have been shown to be equally, if not more, important. Costill and Winrow (1970) provided evidence that supported this contention. Two ultra-marathoners had similar values for their $\dot{V}O_2$ max but one runner always finished ahead of the other. The performance difference was due to the better athlete having a higher mechanical efficiency. The energy cost of his running gait was shown to be considerably lower at several submaximum running speeds. The importance of mechanical efficiency as a performance determinant in prolonged efforts was also shown by Fox and Costill (1972) in an analysis of outstanding marathon and middle-distance runners. Similar differences were also found between élite, trained, and recreation swimmers (Holmer 1972). The measurement differences that are found between top and lesser performers indicate two things: first, the features which need to be stressed in training, and second, the qualities which are required by individuals if they are to be successful.

Determining Relationships Between Physiological Attributes and Performance

Important factors in a particular sporting performance can be identified by correlating performance scores with those obtained on a test known to measure a specific physiological attribute. Studies of kayakers and rowers have been conducted using specifically designed ergometers. In a study of 25 kayakers, tested on both a kayak ergometer and a treadmill, it was possible to account for 42 percent of 1,000 meter kayaking performance on the basis of $\dot{V}O_2$ max measured on the kayak ergometer. $\dot{V}O_2$ max and anaerobic threshold accounted for 57 percent of 10,000 meter kayaking performance. However, the non-specific treadmill test performance bore no relationship to flat-water kayaking performance (Pickard and Pyke 1981). The relationship obtained between $\dot{V}O_2$ max and work done on a sweep-oar rowing ergometer in a group of national level oarsmen, suggested that $\dot{V}O_2$ max accounted for about 40 percent of performance in a 6-minute rowing test (Pyke, Minikin, Woodman, Roberts, and Wright 1979). These studies provide some indication of the attributes necessary for success in these particular sports because they were measured using devices that were closely related to actual performance.

However, the consideration of ergometry as being the best sports test should be tempered with caution. There are many different types of ergometer, several very different ones being available for one sport. For example, a variety of machines have been developed for rowing. A study of rowers using a sweep-oar pull machine was referenced above as yielding impressive results. Martindale (1982) compared instantaneous segmental and total-body energy patterns of rowing in a racing shell versus a stationary and a wheeled Gjessing rowing ergometer. They concluded that the stationary ergometer was less similar to rowing in a boat than was an ergometer mounted on wheels. Since the ergometer itself was a direct center-pull machine, it required arm movements that were not like any done in a racing shell or scull. Also, the requirements for balance and timing that exist in rowing were not required for the ergometer tests. The correlations were not as high as those reported by Pyke (1979). These discrepencies highlight a requirement of tests for determining physiological attributes: that tests must be valid. They must replicate the sporting action, should 'feel' like it, from the athlete's viewpoint, and must have convincing established levels of empirical validity. There are good and bad tests currently being used with athletes. Practitioners are advised to be cautious when consenting to be tested or when using test results as a guide to performance improvement.

Measuring Effects of Improvements in Attributes on Sports Performance

The best evidence available to confirm the physiological requirements of different sports is obtained from experiments. By carefully controlling all the extraneous variables the effect on performance of an improved physiological status variable can be measured. For example, a group of swimmers undertook a 4-week isokinetic strength training program that simulated swimming and produced a 19 percent increase in watts generated in the arm pull on a swim bench (Sharp, Troup, and Costill 1982). This translated into a 4 percent improvement in sprint swimming performance. Similar experiments, indicating the performance benefits that can be obtained from improvements in variables such as strength, endurance, and flexibility, serve to underline the important physiological requirements of the sport. Experimental techniques require considerable sophistication. Often there is a tendency to attribute 'effects' to one factor when they could be caused by one or more others. Qualified sport scientists are perhaps the best individuals to accept the responsibility of conducting experiments in applied sport settings.

Summary

The physiological requirements of an actual competitive performance need to be determined. Four strategies for discovering the physiological features of a sport have been suggested. Measuring performance responses is perhaps the preferred option but is difficult to achieve because of the interference caused when taking measurements within the competitive environment. Indirect methods exist as viable options to direct measurements. Measuring the attributes of top performers suggests the most important qualities for successful performance. When these attributes are shown to decline in their values with a decline in performer standing, strong inferences about the association of the attribute and performance can be drawn. The measurement of characteristics on tests, simulators, and other machines or devices is a promising avenue for discovery. However, the measurement devices must be carefully evaluated according to strict criteria before their implications are embraced by athletes and coaches. Finally, experimental verification of the effects of changes in attributes on performance offers the most conclusive information. However, experimentation is difficult due to the number of factors that must be controlled in the competitive sporting environment. Many sports still exist for which there has not been a clear definition of what attributes need to be trained. The discovery of these factors is germane to the development of a sound training program.

12

Measuring Physiological Attributes
of Athletes

After determining the physiological requirements of a particular sport, the next step is to evaluate the physiological attributes of individual athletes. This will enable the coach to identify the extent to which each athlete is equipped to meet the demands of the sport. An individualized fitness program can then be prescribed.

An assessment of physical fitness can be obtained from laboratory tests that use quite sophisticated equipment, and from simpler tests that can be conducted in field situations. It is important for the coach to understand the potential benefits of a testing program and the criteria that should be applied when selecting suitable tests. The value of a testing program is governed by the quality of the results that it yields.

Reasons for Testing

☐ To Identify Weaknesses

Testing can be used to establish an individual's strengths and weaknesses. For example, a football player may score badly on a 35-meter sprint and a vertical jump. Since these tests assess explosive power, an important capacity for football, his training program should then be aimed at improving this feature. Another player may display a deficiency in endurance in both the 15-minute run and an interval-sprint test. The weaknesses exposed by those two tests could be rectified with a combination of continuous and intermittent training. The results from tests which assess the physiological capacities of a sport can be used to plan important aspects of a fitness program.

☐ To Monitor Progress

The effectiveness of a prescribed training program could be evaluated by repeating a series of appropriate tests at regular intervals. The results of evaluative testing on a cyclist are shown in Figure 12.1. Weaknesses in leg strength and explosive power were remedied with specific strengthening exercises and high-power bicycle training. The second test revealed a significant shift of the physiological performance profile to the right in the areas that originally had been 'below average'. The value of testing is greatest when it is repeated and used to monitor training progress. Essentially, it can be used to objectively verify the effects of training.

Figure 12.1 The Physiological Performance Profile of a Cyclist

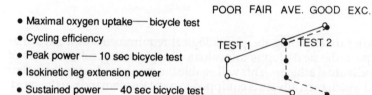

Several tests remained relatively constant while others changed in the direction of the objectives of training.

It is common practice to subject athletes to a 'one-shot' testing experience. Singular observations provide very little benefit for either the athlete or coach since they yield only status scores which have limited interpretive value.

☐ To Provide Incentives

The incentive for an athlete to improve on a particular component of fitness is often provided by a test score and the knowledge that the test will be repeated at a later date. The opportunity for members of a training squad to periodically compare their performances on objective and relevant tests is a motivational tool that can be used by a coach to encourage athletes to strive for improvements. When tests which are relevant to training are used, there is an increased incentive to participate in training.

☐ To Predict Performance Potential

The prediction of sports performance on the basis of fitness test results has not been very successful in a range of sports. This is hardly surprising in view of the many other factors, such as skill, tactics, and psychological preparation, that play an important role in performance. Even though there is a popular surge to establish talent-identification programs for young athletes, it seems particularly hazardous to predict adult performance potential based on the physiology of children measured before their growth has finished. There are wide variations in the maturation rates of young athletes. The consistent successes of late-maturing athletes in many sports is of sufficient occurrence to suggest that the prediction of performance potential is likely to be wrong when rates and patterns of growth are not known. Prediction of potential is the least useful reason for testing.

Criteria for Test Selection

☐ Relevance

In order to accurately measure physiological states, it is important that athletes respond to fitness tests in a positive manner. The recognition of the relevance of a particular test to the sport in question is critical. Tests should be selected in accordance with the known energy requirements of the sport. For example, a pursuit cyclist exerts a maximum effort for about 5 minutes in a 4,000 meters race. Maximum explosive and sustained power, using both aerobic and anaerobic energy pathways, are involved in such a performance and therefore should be part of a testing program. On the other hand, a field-hockey player requires both speed and endurance in efforts that are both continuous and intermittent in nature. Hence, a short sprint (20 to 40 meters), a series of interval sprints (6 to 10 repeats of 20 to 40 meters), and a longer run (5 to 15 minutes duration), all provide useful guides to field-hockey fitness, for they assess factors which are relevant to the sport. A basketball, rugby, or Australian Rules player may have energy requirements similar to that of a field-hockey player, but vertical jumping is an extra important factor. Consequently test batteries may have similar components between sports, but the components of a particular testing program must be relevant to as many of the fitness features of the sport as possible.

☐ Specificity

Fitness tests should assess the performance capabilities of both the muscle groups and the muscle-fiber types involved in a sport. For example, distance runs and treadmill tests should be used for measuring endurance in running-oriented sports. Bicycle, kayak, swimming, and rowing ergometers should be used for assessing physiological performance variables in the specific sports for which they were designed. Scores on non-specific cardio-vascular fitness tests (e.g, the Astrand bicycle test for swimmers), have little value for assessing the effectiveness of a training program aimed at improving the endurance of specific muscle groups used in a particular sport. Similarly, strength testing should not only relate to the specific muscle groups involved in the activity, but also to the patterns and speeds of movement involved. Tests need to be specifically adapted to replicate the movement patterns and intensities of sports. The usefulness of a physiological test is directly related to the degree to which the movements in the test replicate the activities of the sport.

□ Quality Control

The coach and athlete should be aware that test results are affected greatly by the conditions under which they were obtained. Repeated testings should employ the same conditions and procedures on each testing occasion. A tester should allow the time of day, warm-up, order of tests, recovery between tests, and the environmental conditions (heat, humidity, and air movement) to be consistent. Testing should be preceded by a set regime of fluid and food intake. The adequacy of rest and the absence of injury and illness needs to be controlled on each testing occasion. If factors such as these are not controlled, then changes in fitness test scores may be caused by one or more of them. Test score changes may have nothing to do with the prescribed training program. Not only does the test conductor have to structure similar and consistent testing conditions, but it is also the responsibility of athletes to present themselves for fitness testing so that they will be capable of giving a performance that reflects their peak physiological status at that point.

Before electing to participate in a testing program, the adequacy of testing control needs to be established. In Canada, the variations in testing procedures within and between laboratories, that is, the lack of quality control, was of sufficient concern for strict testing protocols (MacDougall, Wenger, and Green 1982) and certification of high-performance-athlete testing centres to be established.

□ Validity

An acceptable fitness test should be valid. It should measure what it claims to measure. The degree of validity of a test can be gauged from a close inspection of its content, from its relationship with another accepted test of the particular fitness component, or from its relationship with actual sport performances. For example, if a test is to measure aerobic power, it should be of sufficient duration to maximally involve that energy system. A test lasting longer than five minutes places sufficient emphasis on the aerobic energy pathways for it to be called an aerobic fitness test. However, performance in a test lasting only 60 seconds, or even as much as 2 minutes, relies heavily on the provision of anaerobic energy sources. It would lack sufficient content validity to be called a test of aerobic power because of the degree to which other energy systems are employed. The high correlation ($r = 0.94$) between performances on 5- and 15-minute runs in national-level field-hockey players substantiates the shorter run being a valid and acceptable measure of aerobic running fitness for these players (Aggis 1985).

□ Reliability

In order for a test to be valid it has to be reliable. A reliable test is one which yields similar results on two separate occasions. Test reliability is dependent on a number of factors remaining constant within both the subject and the testing situation. Reliability is closely associated with quality control and is enhanced if tests are administered under standardized conditions by trained and competent testers. The use of stopwatches and skinfold calipers appear to be simple processes but they are only perfected after considerable training and experience. Most laboratory tests have standardized instructions and procedures established for them which were part of the scientific development process. These steps need to be followed to produce results which truly indicate the status of an athlete on a test. It should be possible for a coach or athlete to obtain copies of the standardized procedures for the conduct of tests. With that knowledge, an individual can make his or her own judgments about test reliability.

□ Interpretable Procedures and Results

A test should be described fully to the athlete before it is conducted. The level of participatory effort will be enhanced if the athlete understands the reason for the test, its relevance to performance, and the physical commitment that is required. Test results should be communicated to the athlete in a meaningful way. This is part of the educational value and intent of a good testing program. Test results should also be supplied as soon as possible after testing has been completed. The greater the period of delay between testing and test feedback, the less valuable are the results, and the less relevant they become to both athletes and coaches.

Field and Laboratory Fitness Tests

The purpose of this section is to describe, and briefly comment upon, the tests that are in regular use in sport fitness programs. Tests that coaches can conduct in the field situation are emphasized. Some mention is made of laboratory-based testing. Fuller descriptions of each field test, and the standards against which athletes should be gauged, should be sought from experts in controlled athlete-testing centres.

☐ Aerobic Energy Tests

The maximal oxygen uptake of an athlete is best measured in the laboratory using rather expensive respiratory gas analysis equipment and ergometers specifically designed for the individual's sport. The absolute uptake value, expressed in liters per minute, is the preferred limit of measurement in the case of sports such as rowing, cycling, and kayaking where body weight is supported. In sports where athletes have to support their own weight, the value should be expressed relative to body weight ($ml.kg^{-1}.min^{-1}$).

Estimates of VO_2 max can be made by measuring the heart rate response to submaximum work loads on a bicycle ergometer. Two of the most common tests are the Astrand and the physical work capacity at 170 heart rate (PW_{170}) test. Two problems with these tests are the sensitivity of the heart rate to internal and external influences, and the difficulty in determining each individual's maximum. Heart rate recovery tests, such as the Harvard Step Test, also suffer from similar limitations. The applicability of these cycling and bench-stepping tests to sports that involve other movement patterns is questionable, because of a lack of relevance, specificity, and validity.

In a field situation where running constitutes a major portion of the sport activity, VO_2 max can be estimated from either the distance covered in 15 minutes or the time taken to run 1·6 kilometers. How that is done is illustrated below.

To estimate from a 15-minute run:

$$VO_2 \text{ max} = 33.3 + (\frac{\text{distance covered}}{15} - 133) \times 0.172$$

For example, if a soccer player runs 3,800 meters in 15 minutes, the estimated VO_2 max can be calculated as follows:

$$VO_2 \text{ max} = 33.3 + (\frac{3800}{15} - 133) \times 0.172$$
$$= 33.3 + 20.6$$
$$= 53.9 \text{ mL.kg}^{-1}.\text{min}^{-1}$$

To estimate from a 1·6 kilometer run:

$\dot{V}O_2$ max $= 133\cdot61 - (13\cdot89 \times$ time for run)

For example, if a distance runner covers 1·6 kilometers in 5 minutes and 6 seconds, the estimated $\dot{V}O_2$ max can be calculated as follows:

$$\begin{aligned}
\dot{V}O_2 \text{ max} &= 133\cdot61 - (13\cdot89 \times 5\cdot1) \\
&= 133\cdot61 - 70\cdot84 \\
&= 62\cdot8 \text{ mL.kg}^{-1}.\text{min}^{-1}
\end{aligned}$$

While these tests have problems associated with the variability of outdoor weather and track conditions, they are highly relevant to sports with a large component of running. The simplest procedure is measuring the time taken for a given distance (e.g., the 1·6 kilometre run). However, as performance time decreases with training, an athlete will involve an increasing energy contribution from anaerobic sources. Thus, in highly-trained states, the short-distance test may not accurately reflect the power of the aerobic system. The distance covered in a set time, such as 5, 12, or 15 minutes is usually preferred because the influence of anaerobic resources remains relatively minor no matter what the state of training.

Movement efficiency and the anaerobic threshold are most accurately measured in the laboratory using facilities for monitoring respiratory gas exchange and assaying blood lactic acid concentration. The laboratory environment limits the exercise mode to ergometers that attempt to duplicate the movements involved in different sports. Field estimates of cardiovascular efficiency and anaerobic threshold have been greatly facilitated by the manufacture of portable devices for monitoring heart rate (Sport Tester) and measuring blood lactate in micro-samples taken throughout a contest. Examples of data obtained in this way are presented in Figures 12.2 and 12.3.

Laboratory data obtained on the average oxygen cost of running various speeds have made it possible to estimate performance in prolonged running efforts. For example, if the fastest time for running 15 kilometers on a level course is 65 minutes : 33 seconds (4:37 per kilometer), reference to Table 12.1 shows that this speed requires an average oxygen cost of 46·0 mL/kg/min. An athlete with that performance level should be capable of running a marathon in 3:15. This involves running at 74 percent of $\dot{V}O_2$ max for the distance. An élite marathoner (best time 2:12) may have a $\dot{V}O_2$ max of 80 mL/kg/min and be capable of running at a speed of 3:15 per kilometer, which is equivalent to 68·0 mL/kg/min and represents 85 percent of $\dot{V}O_2$ max. Such estimates are useful for establishing target levels for training quality and performance goals. It should be possible to establish similar conversion tables for other sporting actions.

Figure 12.2 Typical Blood Lactate Responses in a Swimmer Before and After 10 Weeks of Endurance Training

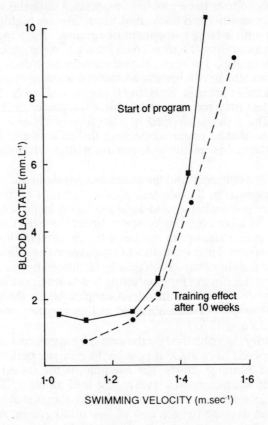

The shift to the right of the data points indicates a gain in aerobic power.

Figure 12.3 Typical Heart Rate Responses in a Swimmer Before and After 10 Weeks of Endurance Training

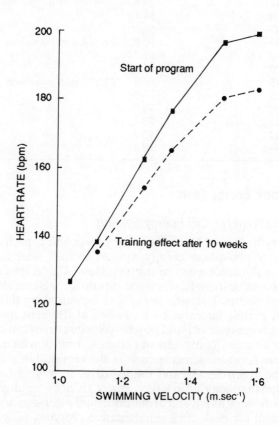

The lowering of the rate for a given velocity indicates a gain in aerobic power.

Table 12.1 Oxygen Cost of Running at Different Speeds

Kilometer Pace (min:sec)	Oxygen Cost $(mL.kg^{-1}.min^{-1})$	
6:00	34·5	
5:27	38·5	
5:00	42·2	
4:37	46·0	3 h : 15 min marathon
4:17	49·8	
4:00	54·1	
3:45	57·9	
3:39	60·0	2 h : 34 min marathon
3:32	61·7	
3:20	65·9	
3:15	68·0	2 h : 12 min marathon
3:09	70·3	
3:00	74·5	
2:51	78·7	
2:44	82·9	
2:36	88·3	

□ Anaerobic Energy Tests

The Alactacid (ATP–CP) Energy System

Laboratory tests used to measure the power and capacity of this high-energy phosphate energy system include various force-measuring dynamometers and ergometers. Cable tension tests measure *isometric strength*, where maximum force is exerted but no movement occurs. *Isokinetic strength* is measured by dynamometers that permit forces to be measured at different movement velocities. Force–velocity and power–velocity curves can be established for a variety of movement patterns, some of which attempt to simulate sport movements such as the arm pull in swimming (Biokinetic Swim Bench) and the leg drive in rowing (modified Cybex dynamometer). However, many devices employ simple movements, such as leg and arm flexion and extension and, while being useful for evaluating rehabilitative progress, offer little in terms of assessing the complex forces generated in specific sporting activities.

Two laboratory tests of alactic anaerobic power are the Margaria–Kalamen Stair Climb and the 10-second bicycle-ergometer sprint. The stair-climb test measures power from the product of the body weight of the person (force) and the speed of the climb (velocity). However, it is a mode of activity that is not commonly experienced in sport. It suffers through a lack of relevance, specificity, and validity. The bicycle test uses an air-braked ergometer and a calibrated work-monitor that provides an assessment of both the total work done and the peak power generated in a maximum 10-second leg-cranking effort. While there is a lack of specific applicability to arm and shoulder-oriented sports, the involvement of the major muscle groups of the thighs and buttocks in a simple movement pattern offers some useful information regarding the explosive qualities of those muscle groups. These tests would be useful for activities that emphasize upper-leg power (e.g, cycling, speed skating, jumping).

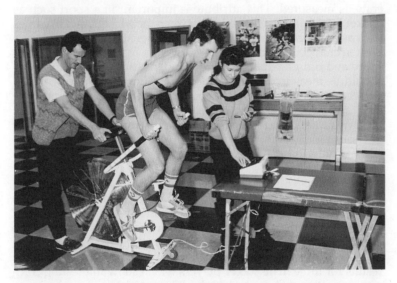

The front access, air-braked bicycle ergometer allows the subject to adopt an upright position and use the major muscle groups that extend the knee and hip joints. It has applicability to sports such as cycling, skiing, skating, jumping and sprinting

Field tests of this energy system offer a number of possibilities for the coach involved with running-oriented sports. The main criterion is that the sprint should take less than 10 seconds. Hence, a straight sprint over a distance of between 20 and 40 meters is appropriate. To substantiate this viewpoint, it is interesting to note that American football coaches have had an enduring interest in player performances in a 40-yard (36·6 meter) dash where a good time is considered to be less than 4·5 seconds.

Agility sprints, where the athlete has to accelerate, decelerate, and change direction, also provide important information about the explosive qualities of a games player. One of the tests used with cricket players in Australia is to run up and down the pitch three times, a total distance of just over 50 meters. This usually takes between 9 and 10 seconds. Something akin to this in baseball would be to run from first to third base. Similar agility tests have been devised in squash and tennis (Pyke, Elliott, and Pyke 1974). Agility tests should involve the movements of the sport in question.

A recent addition to the list of agility tests is the 5-0-5 Test (Draper and Lancaster 1985). This test is conducted over a 15-meter up-and-back course with the 5 meters before and after the turn being timed. Turning speed, as a product of the ability to accelerate and decelerate, is measured. This attribute is important in a sport such as cricket, which involves running between the wickets, and in games such as basketball, netball, and soccer, where the direction of play is often changed rapidly. Cricket studies have shown that turning-speed and running-speed are independent attributes and that both should be measured as a means of identifying the specific weaknesses of players in running between the wickets (Draper and Pyke 1988). It would seem that specific tests for other sports which involve rapid changes of direction and running could also be devised.

In many individual and team sports, not only is it important to sprint and change direction quickly, but this must be repeated several times. This makes it essential to have athletes use some form of interval-sprint test. For example, this can be done by having athletes perform eight maximum 35-meter sprints, one every 30 seconds. The average time for the first two trials is the speed score, and the total loss of speed over the next three pairs of trials constitutes the measure of speed loss. Table 12.2 lists the results for three male soccer players which show interesting comparisons. Player A ranked highest in speed but was shown to fatigue rapidly. On the other hand, Player B had a poor rating in terms of speed but did not fatigue appreciably. Of the three, Player C had perhaps the most suitable combination of speed and endurance for high-energy intermittent sports. He had good speed which could be sustained for a number of repeated efforts. The test could also be performed using a series of agility sprints rather than straight dashes.

Other tests of alactic anaerobic power that are in common use in sports fitness profiles include the vertical jump, the standing long jump, and distance throws. The selection of these tests should be based on their relevance to the particular sport in question.

Table 12.2 Performance Characteristics of National Level Soccer Players in the Interval Sprint Test (8 × 35 Meters Every 30 Seconds)

Player	Speed			Speed loss in seconds					
	Trials 1, 2	Rank	Trials 3, 4	5, 6	7, 8	Total	%	Rank
A	5·10	1/20	0·07	0·17	0·43	0·67	13·1	14/20
B	5·45	16/20	0·01	0·01	0·16	0·18	3·3	1/20
C	5·24	5/20	0·11	0·06	0·03	0·20	3·8	2/20

The Lactacid Energy System

There are a number of laboratory tests which can be used to assess the capacity of this energy system. Several tests involving maximum efforts for periods between 30 and 60 seconds are available. The Wingate Test is conducted for 30 seconds on a Monark bicycle ergometer. It provides an assessment of both peak-power output and power loss for each 5-second segment. Other tests use the Repco air-braked bicycle ergometer and last between 30 and 60 seconds. Again, both peak power and power loss are recorded (Telford, Minikin, Hooper, Hahn, and Tumilty 1987). One of the major drawbacks with these tests is that it is often difficult to encourage athletes to sustain peak power for such long periods.

It is possible to measure the capacity of the lactacid energy pathways by having athletes attempt a sustained sprint up a steep-grade treadmill (e.g., 15 km.h^{-1}, 15 percent grade). Determination of both blood lactate concentration upon completion of the task and during the recovery period after this test as well as the determination of oxygen debt can provide additional information.

In the field situation, activities in which a maximum effort is sustained for 30–60 seconds can be used to assess the endurance of local muscle groups. The number of sit-ups completed in 60 seconds or press-ups performed in 30 seconds are examples of such tests. However, since such tests require specific techniques, if the movement pattern is not carefully standardized, the test results become less reliable.

A 30-second running, cycling, or swimming sprint, and a 60-second rowing sprint are examples of tests that can be used to measure the capacity of the lactacid energy system. It is important to encourage athletes to sprint maximally for the full duration of the test. By taking sectional times, it is then possible to measure the magnitude of power loss that is occurring. The critical feature of these tests for yielding valid and accurate information is to motivate the athlete to perform maximally from the start of the test. If this is not done, inaccurate scores will result which will lead to incorrect coaching decisions.

☐ Flexibility

The degree of joint flexibility is most commonly measured with a protractor which assesses the range of movement possible when following standardized procedures. The sit-and-reach test of lower back and hamstring flexibility provides a reasonable assessment of general flexibility that is useful across a wide range of sports that require bending and reaching movements. The reliability of flexibility tests is increased if the muscles around the joints to be measured are thoroughly warmed up before the athlete is tested.

Table 12.3 illustrates two examples of test batteries that could be used to establish sports fitness test profiles.

Table 12.3 Examples of Sports Fitness Test Profile Regimens

Laboratory Testing
    Subject: Cyclist; 4,000 m pursuit; best time = 5 min; male
Day 1
    Physical characteristics: height, weight, body surface area, body fat
        (skinfold thickness at 8 sites)
    Mechanical efficiency: 10 min ride at 300 watts
        ($\dot{V}O_2$, HR, blood lactate)
    Aerobic power: 5 min ride to exhaustion
        ($\dot{V}O_2$ max, HR max, blood lactate max)
Day 2
    Alactic anaerobic power and capacity: 10 sec ride (peak power, total
        work done)
    Lactic anaerobic power and capacity: 40 sec ride (peak power, power
        loss, total work done)

Field Testing
    Subject: Field-hockey player, national class, female
Day 1
    Physical characteristics: height, weight, body fat
        (skinfold thickness at 7 sites)
    Running speed and agility: short sprint 35 m, 5-0-5 test
    Running speed and endurance: interval sprints 8 × 35 m every 30 sec
Day 2
    Flexibility: sit-and-reach test
    Aerobic power: 5 min run
    Muscular strength and endurance: 60 sec sit-ups

The batteries of tests for each sport will depend upon the requirements of the sport and testing capabilities. The selection of tests is an important decision. Given the criteria which have been explained in this chapter, a coach must decide which tests should and should not be used to provide information that can enhance coaching decisions by describing the physiological attributes of athletes.

Some standards for men and women for several of these tests are given in Appendix C, at the end of this book.

V
Methods and Effects of Training

13

Endurance Training

The objective of endurance training is to improve the ability to sustain a particular level of physical effort. The precise nature of a training program depends upon the duration and intensity of the activity. Brief thirty-second efforts, a prolonged one of more than three hours, and a game that lasts a number of hours but features intermittent periods of work and recovery, all have different demands for endurance. In all cases, both aerobic and anaerobic energy mechanisms are required, their importance being dependent upon the speed and duration of the activity. Most activities can benefit from both aerobic and anaerobic training, the coaching challenge being to train each in the appropriate proportion to produce the best energy capacities in athletes.

In sprint activities lasting from 10–60 seconds, the objective is to minimize speed loss. Sprinters aim to increase the rates of high-energy phosphate and glycolytic energy release by expending as much energy as possible in the shortest time in the most efficient manner. The predominant energy source for the actual activity is anaerobic, but an enhanced aerobic capacity is also important. The aerobic capacity increases the volume of training that can be done, it speeds recovery from anaerobically induced fatigue, and it delays the onset of general training fatigue. In longer duration activities (middle- and long-distance events) lasting from 2–10 minutes, there is a gradually increasing commitment to the use of the aerobic energy system during the activity. However, once again both energy systems are vitally involved in competitive performances and both must be considered when planning training programs.

Middle-distance athletes adapt muscles so that they are more resistant to lactic acid accumulations. More prolonged continuous efforts lasting between 30 minutes and 3 hours rely heavily on the athlete being able to work at the highest rate possible without accumulating lactic acid in the blood. This is not a simple task because when the task load is increased beyond that which can be supported by aerobic mechanisms, for example, when running uphill, into the wind, or on a soft surface, lactic acid is produced to meet the extra demands above that accommodated by aerobic capacities. In these prolonged activities, the ability to store glycogen in muscles also becomes a limiting factor for sustaining effort levels. Long-distance runners must shift the lactate turnpoint to a higher speed, increase the capacity for fat oxidation so they can 'spare' carbohydrate stores during racing, maximize the ability to store liver and muscle glycogen before exercise, and increase the capacity to absorb carbohydrate during competition (Noakes 1986). Finally, the intermittent activity characteristic of most team and court games requires anaerobic energy for the high-power component and aerobic energy for its restoration during periods when activity demands are lowered during the contest. The finite level of muscle glycogen stores can also be important in intermittent activity contests that extend beyond one hour. The nature of the physiological attributes for activities of various durations and type are listed in Chapter 2, in Table 2.1.

There are two major energy systems for exercise, one functioning in the absence of oxygen, the other in its presence. The more usual description for endurance pertains to the aerobic (cardio-respiratory, cardio-vascular, oxidative) energy system which is dependent upon the supply of oxygen. Aerobic training involves functional changes in both the central circulation and in the peripheral musculature. The anaerobic energy system comprises two subsystems, both of which also need to be trained to endure, that is, to sustain their form of energy provision for as long as possible. The first subsystem is the alactacid (ATP–CP, high-energy phosphate) energy system. The ability to improve the endurance of this system is very restricted but effects can be achieved. The site of its adaptations is only in the musculature. The second subsystem is the lactacid (muscular endurance, glycolytic) energy system which uses stored glycogen in the absence of oxygen as the source of energy. The site of its adaptations is also in the musculature. Coaches must consider methods for changing the enduring qualities of the three energy systems if higher quantities of performance are to persist in competitions. This chapter looks at the general forms of presenting training stimuli that develop endurance in all three systems.

Effects of Endurance Training

The effects of endurance training can be seen both in the central circulation and in the muscles themselves. The specific site of any changes through training depends on the intensity of effort undertaken in its various forms.

□ Central Changes: The Oxygen Transport System

Aerobic endurance training improves the mechanical ability to move air in and out of the lungs, increases the blood flow through the lungs, and enhances the rate at which oxygen diffuses across the lung membrane into the blood. This allows an athlete to undertake increased training intensities without lowering the oxygen content of arterial blood. There are also changes in the nature of the blood. Both the total red blood cell count and blood plasma volume increase in roughly the same proportion. This results in no overall change in concentration of hemoglobin in the blood but provides a greater overall transporting capacity of oxygen to the peripheral musculo-skeletal system. There is also an increase in the capacity of the heart to pump blood which results primarily from a larger stroke volume rather than from an increased heart rate. The heart pumps more blood per beat in a trained state than it does in an untrained state. This increased cardiac output can be attributed to either enlarged ventricular cavities and/or an improved ability to empty blood from them. These changes in ventricular structure and function are responsible for the lower heart rate seen at rest and during submaximal exercise following a period of endurance training (see Figure 13.1). Maximum stroke volume is reached at an intensity of 40–50 percent $\dot{V}O_2$ max. The contractile force of the heart is stimulated maximally at about 75 percent $\dot{V}O_2$ max. Continuous exercise at that intensity provides the greatest number of contractions of the heart, resulting in the maximum stimulus for aerobic training (MacDougall and Sale 1981). For a few activities (e.g., running) those central changes can be transferred, but only in trivial amounts, to other activities. However, specific activity training still remains the most productive form of aerobic endurance training (Peterson, Holding, Morrow, and Wenger 1981). Associated training (also called multilateral or cross training) is not supported by scientific evidence as being a viable principle of training.

□ Peripheral Changes: Musculo-skeletal System

All forms of endurance training promote changes in the musculature. Several changes occur in muscle fibers which aid the extraction of increased amounts of oxygen from the blood and, in more intensive work, facilitate the production of anaerobic energy.

Aerobic changes include increases in: the density of capillaries; myoglobin for transporting oxygen from the cell membrane to the mitochondria; the oxidative enzymes in the mitochondria involved in carbohydrate and fat metabolism; mitochondrial number and size; and the size of muscle glycogen and fat stores. When an athlete trains in a predominantly aerobic fashion the enzymes for anaerobic energy production are reduced through lack of stimulation and the capacity for sustained sprinting deteriorates. The number or type of muscle fibers does not change, but the size of fast-twitch fibers is increased by intensive high-powered training stimuli. The peripheral adjustments that occur for oxygen extraction are very specific for the exercise. Mitochondrial adaptations occur only in trained muscles and only in the muscle fibers that are active during that exercise. The adaptations are specific and do not generalize. For example, training for running on the flat does little for hill running. Both forms of running need specific training for adequate training effects to occur (Noakes 1986). A great deal of the strength of the principle of specificity resides in the selective adaptation of the muscle functioning for particular actions. This suggests that enhancement of oxygen extraction in muscles can only be trained by using the form, speed, and intensity of the targeted competitive activity as a training stimulus.

Figure 13.1 The Gradual Decrease in Sub-maximum Work Heart Rate Resulting from a Four-month Period of Training

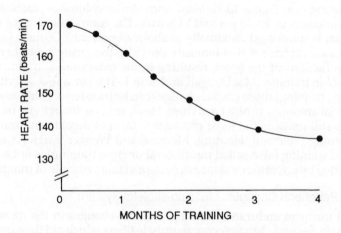

The latter stages indicate a levelling-off effect.

Peripheral endurance adaptations are lost more quickly than are the central/transport effects. This feature, coupled with the greater need for specificity in peripheral training, must be contemplated when planning programs of reduced load prior to important contests. Specific peripheral-demanding activities need to be maintained as part of the training load at that time although other forms of training and levels of training stress are reduced in the competitive phase (see Chapter 19).

In comparative studies between continuous and longer, slower interval training, improvements in aerobic power and the level of the anaerobic threshold have been quite similar (Gregory 1979, Robinson and Sucec 1979). Anaerobic threshold, in theory, is best increased by high-intensity interval training, although, in practice, it is effectively increased by long continuous training at levels at or about 1–2 percent below the existing threshold (MacDougall and Sale 1981). Intensive sprint and power training produces more impressive anaerobic benefits than does continuous training (Le Rossignol 1985). Low-power continuous training enhances the oxidation processes that are important in prolonged/endurance efforts. Lower-intensity stimuli also reduce the potential for orthopedic problems unless their duration and frequency is excessive. Low-intensity training is a useful means of strengthening the connective tissue associated with the musculo-skeletal system, a feature that does not result from strength training. By contrast, high-intensity training offers a greater chance of incurring muscle and joint injuries, particularly in activities such as running, where the athlete has to support the body weight.

Endurance exercises that raise the level of lactic acid in the blood to an average of 4 mmol.L^{-1} can be maintained for periods of from 30 to 60 minutes. Such exercise levels train the aerobic capacity. However, exercise intensities that raise lactic acid to a concentration of only 2 mmol.L^{-1} (which is not greatly different from that which exists during rest), do little to improve the functioning of the muscle cells and, at best, serve only to maintain conditioning (*Athletic Performance Review* 1986).

Maximum oxygen uptake improvements that occur through aerobic endurance training usually range from 5 to 25 percent depending on the type and intensity of training and the initial level of fitness of the athlete. In athletes who train all year to maintain a relatively high level of fitness, the potential for improvements in aerobic endurance capacity through further concentrations of heavy training stimuli are relatively small (probably less than 5 percent). While an inactive young man can raise his $\dot{V}O_2$ max from 45 to 55 mL.kg^{-1} through a graduated and intensive endurance training program, he cannot be expected to reach the endurance fitness levels of a champion endurance athlete who might score between 75 and 85 $mL.kg^{-1}.min^{-1}$ in $\dot{V}O_2$ max tests. The champion is genetically favoured with endurance attributes that a lesser-endowed individual may never reach even when fully trained (see Figures 13.2 and 22.2). Thus aspirations to excel in endurance events when an individual is not appropriately endowed with appropriate endurance capacity are not realistic.

Figure 13.2 The Effect of a Two-year Period of Intensive Endurance Training on Maximum Oxygen Uptake in a Normal Individual

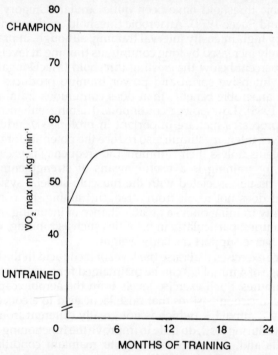

The trained level that is achieved (the 'ceiling effect') is markedly below the characteristic level of a champion endurance athlete.

The $\dot{V}O_2$ max of an active young person is unlikely to improve by more than 15 percent with specific training. The greater proportion of this improvement will occur in the first 12 weeks of intensive endurance training. Further improvements are small and difficult to achieve. After the 'ceiling' endurance capacity is achieved, the athlete must rely on further performance gains to come from increases in mechanical efficiency and techniques, anaerobic energy release, motivation, and tactics.

Methods of Training

There are three basic forms of endurance training: continuous training, fartlek training, and interval training.

The contribution of energy from the aerobic system is greatest in continuous forms of training where lactic acid accumulation is avoided. Major characteristics of the aerobic system are an ability to support extended work; the breaking down of glycogen in the presence of oxygen to produce energy; and the possible use of fats and proteins as auxiliary sources of energy. In pure aerobic work no significant accumulation of lactic acid occurs, and it is less stressful than anaerobic training. A well-trained aerobic system provides three important advantages for athletes: the volume of training that can be tolerated in a session is increased; the recovery from intense exercise within a training session is enhanced; and recovery from general training stress is enhanced.

Fartlek training, a Swedish term which, when translated, means 'speed play', emphasizes aerobic work but also incorporates a number of athlete-determined short anaerobic bursts of speed. Interval training is the most versatile form of training, allowing both aerobic and anaerobic work to occur depending upon the nature of the scheduling of the periods of work and recovery. Volumes of these forms of training produce various forms of endurance adaptation.

☐ Continuous Training

This form of training usually occurs for long periods of time. Continuous activity for longer than 30 minutes usually produces aerobic adaptation at a work rate below the anaerobic threshold. The duration, within reason, should be in excess of the length of the total activity of the competitive performance. An exception to this guideline occurs with marathon events (e.g., road cycling, marathon running, triathlon) where the duration of the competition is of such an extent that were training to be continuously repeated for that time, overuse injuries would almost invariably result in the performer. Another exception would also occur with team games that last for a lengthy period of time (e.g., Australian Rules football, soccer). Continuous training would be employed but for a period less than the normal duration of a game. It should be recalled that the volume of training that is necessary is that which produces maximum adaptation. Volumes in excess of that amount do not produce any further adaptation (see Chapter 4 and Figure 4.6). Too much continuous training can be harmful. Two general subdivisions of continuous training exist.

Low-intensity Continuous Training

This involves easy distance work where, in young adults, the heart rate is kept between 140 and 160 bpm. The blood lactic acid level is kept below 3 mmol.L^{-1}, which is just above resting level (1–2 mmol.L^{-1}). This is a comfortable level of activity that can be maintained for a considerable period of time. It is particularly useful for athletes involved in prolonged endurance activities for it not only develops aerobic adaptation but also strengthens connective tissue in the muscles. It forms the major activity of the basic preparatory phase of training. It is also the principal aerobic training activity for sports that do not have a great energy cost but produce fatigue through prolonged competitive stress (e.g., shooting, archery, golf). Most activities will use this form of training at least at some stage of the annual training cycle.

At very low intensities (heart rate 120–140 bpm), this type of exercise is used as an initial activity for warm-ups, for cooling down after a competition, and recovery from more strenuous forms of training within a training session. At such low intensities no training effects occur.

The effects of low-intensity continuous training are to encourage the oxidation of fat as the fuel for exercise and thus save muscle glycogen; to increase the capacity of the central and peripheral circulatory system; and to gradually strengthen connective tissue (muscle tendons and joint ligaments). Such training also increases an athlete's capacity to perform psychologically demanding sports such as shooting, archery, and sailing. Vigilance, attention, and psychological persistence are improved when aerobic endurance is increased (Rushall 1967).

There are several negative aspects of this type of training. It is very dependent upon the motivation of the athlete. It is hard to control the quantity and quality of the work after the novelty of its performance has worn off. The athlete's feelings have a great influence on the way it is completed. The use of heart rate monitors that signal heart rate ranges are particularly useful for supplying feedback to training athletes about the level of work that they are maintaining. Such devices add to the effective use of this form of training. When this continuous training is undertaken in large quantities over an extended period of time, it de-emphasizes the anaerobic energy system and seriously reduces the ability to produce explosive power (sprinting and jumping). Because of this, it is wise to include some anaerobic training within basic preparatory training so that the capacities of the athlete do not become unbalanced. The final problem with low-intensity continuous training is that its intensity is usually below that required in most endurance activities. Thus specific benefits are lacking. Generally it should not be seen as a form of stimulation for the specific preparatory or pre-competition phases of endurance-based sports. Its use in those phases would primarily involve recovery. However, it would remain as a major form of training in sports which do not have a great physical demand but rely primarily on psychological efforts.

High-intensity Continuous Training

This is a higher quality of aerobic training in which the heart rate is elevated to between 160–180 bpm. Blood lactate concentrations increase to range between 3 and 5 mmol.L^{-1}. Efforts can be sustained at this level from anywhere between 15 and 60 minutes. Since effort levels are increased, it becomes more difficult for athletes to keep a steady level of performance at training. It is usual to observe them undergoing some variations in pace and effort with the result that they periodically produce increased lactic acid levels. They then have to reduce the exercise intensity to remove the excessive lactic acid. Unintentional cycles of efforts and recovery efforts often characterize this form of training. The cycling of work intensities permits an equilibrium to be reached between the rate of lactic acid production by the muscles and its removal from the blood, sometimes referred to as 'anaerobic threshold training'. This type of training is favored by coaches for improving maximum aerobic power, produced by increasing the capacity of both the central and peripheral circulatory systems.

Another name for the most demanding form of this training is 'over-distance training'. It involves greater than race distance or competition duration at an 'all-out' effort level and stimulates aerobic adaptation, with improvements in persistence and mechanical efficiency. However, it is quite fatiguing and so its frequency of use should be carefully planned. It is wise to allow at least 24 and as much as 36 hours for recovery between such training stimuli. Thus attempts to increase the anaerobic threshold of athletes should be planned at most for alternate days keeping in mind that this form of training is particularly hard.

An intense aerobic stimulus produces aerobic adaptation within one week. For a further two weeks gains in aerobic adaptation decrease. Thus, for planning aerobic microcycles, weekly changes in overload stimuli are warranted (Hickson, Bomze, and Hollaszy 1977).

Figure 13.3 illustrates the work intensity zones and ranges of physiological function for both forms of continuous training (see also Table 13.1). The major concern about continuous training is that no lactic acid should accumulate. At its most intense level it approaches and/or equals the anaerobic threshold (90–95 percent of maximum heart rate and 80–90 percent of $\dot{V}O_2$ max). At its lowest intensity, it should not fall below the training threshold to incur a training effect (65–70 percent of maximum heart rate and 50–60 percent of $\dot{V}O_2$ max). The transition from low to high-intensity continuous training occurs at about 80 percent of maximum heart rate and 70–75 percent of $\dot{V}O_2$ max.

Figure 13.3 The Work Intensity Zones for Continuous Training that are Important for Developing Aerobic (Cardiovascular Endurance)

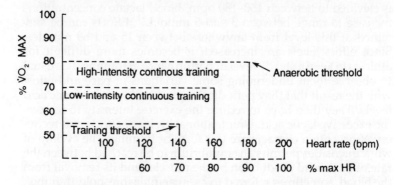

Their relationships to heart rate and $\dot{V}O_2$ max are illustrated. Low-intensity continuous training must exceed the training threshold to produce an endurance adaptation while high-intensity training should mainly hover around, but rarely exceed, the anaerobic threshold.

Table 13.1 Comparison Factors for the Responses to Low and High-intensity Continuous Training

Factor	Low-intensity	High-intensity
Duration	30 min to 3 h	15 min to 1 h
Intensity as percent of maximum performance	70–80%	80–90%
Heart rate		
bpm	140–160	160–180
% max	70–80%	80–90%
% $\dot{V}O_2$ max	55–70 mL.kg^{-1}.min^{-1}	70–80 mL.kg^{-1}.min^{-1}
Blood lactate	< 3 mmol.L^{-1}	3–5 mmol.L^{-1}

The zones for continuous training lie between the threshold for obtaining a cardiovascular training effect and the anaerobic threshold which, if exceeded, results in the accumulation of lactic acid in the blood. Training intensity can be estimated from measurements of pulse rate. After continuous exercise for a period of 10 minutes, the athlete can stop and count the pulse rate for the first 10 seconds. Multiplying the number of beats by 6 will yield the heart rate in beats per minute. It is also useful to have some idea of the athlete's maximum heart rate measured either in a laboratory setting or immediately after a maximum effort at the training site. In a group of young adult athletes, it is not unusual to have maximum heart rates ranging from 185 to 215 bpm. Maximum heart rates decrease with age and in the 50–60 age group rates can fall below 160. A training heart rate of 150 bpm represents a much higher intensity of exercise for an older person with a maximum of 160 than it does for a younger individual with a maximum of 185 bpm. A simpler test of training intensity is the 'talk test'. When exercising below the anaerobic threshold, it is usually possible to talk freely during the activity. However, when lactic acid accumulates, that is, the anaerobic threshold is exceeded, the rate of breathing increases and makes conversation more difficult. Thus when an individual can converse comfortably during exercise it can be assumed that the intensity is below the anaerobic threshold. When conversation is difficult because of the requirement to inhale more frequently and deeply it can be assumed that the anaerobic threshold has been exceeded and that fatigue will occur more rapidly than when talking is easier.

□ Fartlek training

This form of training involves interspersing short bursts of intense/faster work throughout a continuous training activity. It is primarily used as a means of introducing more intensive work. The difference between this activity and pure continuous work is that there is a deliberate attempt to perform at a more intense level which would result in some temporary accumulation of lactic acid. It should be perceived as being harder to do than pure aerobic continuous training. For example, a run may be planned for 45 minutes duration. During that task the athlete might attempt to increase the pace and hold that increase for 1 minute on 6 different occasions. This gives the athlete some control over the training regime while adhering to the objective of increasing the workload for a particular amount of time. It is appropriate to do fartlek training in the latter stages of the basic preparatory phase of the annual training plan as well as in the early stages of the specific preparatory phase. It can also be used for 'recovery', competition phase and transition phase training, warm-up, or as part of training sessions when reduced loads are desirable, such as in an unloading session or microcycle.

Fartlek training provides an entry into doing specific training although it is still, in the main, non-specific in its quality. The intensive work periods introduce the athlete to closer approximations of contest activities. Its adherence is strongly affected by the athlete's feelings so it is somewhat difficult to control the quality and quantity of increased work. Heart rate monitors are useful in this regard. The upper heart rate level signal can be set at the desired level for the intensified work bouts. It then becomes the task of the athlete to keep the signal going for the predetermined period of increased work. By doing that, the quality of the intensified work is guaranteed.

Fartlek training can be both structured or unstructured. Structured activities have clearly defined effort levels, durations, and frequencies. When the appropriate time arises, the effort is initiated (e.g., swim 4,000 meters with one 100-meter swim at 1-minute pace every 400 meters). On the other hand, unstructured fartlek training provides some decision-making for the athlete (e.g., swim 4,000 meters with 10 bursts of 100 meters at 1-minute pace).

□ Interval training

This form of training involves alternating periods of activity and recovery. The advantage of this intermittent training stimulus is that it provides greater amounts of exposure to intensive training without incurring excessive fatigue. Thus it constitutes a method of increasing the repetitions of a particular training stimulus. Since the training response is to develop functional ability when stimulated to do so, the greater number of training units that can be tolerated/experienced in training, the greater will be the training effect. Interval training serves as the main medium for producing specific training effects. It is the principal means for training the oxygen extraction by the muscles that are used specifically for an activity.

Dividing a work distance into units for repetition allows a considerable volume of training to be completed while reducing the amount of fatigue that will occur. For example, it is easier, but nevertheless challenging, to run four 60-second 400-meter runs with 60 seconds as rest intervals between each repetition than it is to run 1,600 meters in 4 minutes (the same 60-second pace) or even two 800-meter runs in 2 minutes each. It is also possible to break tasks into shorter units and then complete each unit at a performance quality that has never been achieved when the task has been done in its entirety. This increased quality of work is the means by which athletes can be trained to perform at a specific level even though this has not been exhibited in a competitive performance. This feature, if used wisely, is the basic procedure for training athletes to exceed previous performance levels. Not only does interval training allow an athlete to work at a greater volume of a particular intensity, it also allows him or her to train harder than is possible in continuous work forms.

The variables that can be manipulated in interval training surround both the work and recovery periods. They are: the duration of work; the intensity of work; the duration of the recovery period; the type of activity done in the recovery period; and the number of repetitions of the work/recovery alternations done in a set. The modification of these variables allows the volume and intensity of training to be prescribed in detail. The specific nature of training effects can be considered to a greater degree of precision in interval training than is possible in fartlek or continuous training.

Interval training can be used to develop both aerobic and anaerobic capacities in varying degrees of emphasis. It also provides the opportunity for developing specific mechanical actions associated with required movement patterns, and psychological factors such as perseverence, mental toughness, and stress tolerance. Volume and work intensity can also be varied to the extent that interval training as a means of developing endurance is appropriate for all stages of training but becomes most important as the specific preparatory phase of training progresses. It is the main form of training for the pre-competition and competition phases.

Interval training is appropriate for events that have considerable anaerobic requirement (e.g, long sprints, middle-distance races, and intermittent team games). The difference between a middle-distance and a sprint event is that in the former the supply of oxygen to the muscles (oxygen intake) is more important than working in the absence of oxygen. The reverse is true for sprint events.

Oxygen consumption is increased when an athlete is subjected to exercise that taxes that capacity to its maximum. On the other hand, athletes who perform anaerobically must train anaerobically. The more time that the athlete spends in an anaerobic state, provided overtraining does not occur, the greater will be the development of anaerobic (muscular) endurance. For the minor parts of endurance events that require the release of anaerobic energy (e.g., finishing bursts) the ability to tolerate working in the presence of lactic acid also needs to be improved. The more frequently lactic acid accumulation occurs, the greater the tolerance for it and the greater the anaerobic capacity will become (up to a limit). The development of anaerobic capacity and high rates of oxygen consumption are best done through interval training, which allows an athlete to be subjected to a large quantity of high-quality work.

The exact prescription of an interval training program will depend on the energy and activity requirements of the sport, the maturation of the athlete, and the training phase. There are three general categories of interval training: long, intermediate, and short.

Long-interval training: This type of training is styled along the lines originally developed in the 1930s by the German coach-scientist team, Gerschler and Reindell. It features work bouts that are primarily aerobic, although anaerobic energy may be brought into play in the latter phase of each repetition. This form of training is appropriate for activities which are predominantly aerobic in nature, for it emphasizes aerobic endurance while also providing some anaerobic endurance training. Long-interval training features the following characteristics:

1. Duration of work	2–5 min
2. Intensity of work	85–90% of best performance standard
3. Duration of recovery period	2–8 min
4. Work–recovery ratio	1 : 1 to 1 : 2
5. Repetitions	3–12

Within each bout of interval work, the effort required to sustain quality performance increases. At the end of each work unit heart rate usually ranges between 180–200 bpm. At the end of the recovery period the heart rate should be in the vicinity of 130–140 bpm. If the work period is extended beyond two minutes, a maximum load is placed on the oxygen transport system and blood lactate concentrations can reach moderate to high levels (6–10 $mmol.L^{-1}$). Because both aerobic and anaerobic energy systems are used, this type of interval training is typical of that employed for middle-distance efforts lasting from 2 to 5 minutes. This makes it an important part of the training menu for 800- and 1,500-meter runners, 200- and 400-meter swimmers, 2,000-meter rowers, and 4,000-meter pursuit cyclists.

Typical examples of long-interval training for a 800/1,500-meter runner would be as follows (note that the dispatch times would be equivalent to the sum of the intensity and recovery periods):

Repetitions	Distance	Intensity	Recovery	Recovery activity
3 ×	1,000 m	2:45 pace	3:15	jogging
3 ×	800 m	2:10 pace	2:20	walk/jog

With the above examples, the work would be primarily aerobic. The first repetition may appear to be easy, but with the incomplete recovery that occurs between each repetition each successive repeat becomes harder. In order to maintain the performance standard for the total set, psychological skills and control will play an increasingly important role. This is a demand that replicates the control demands of a real competitive effort.

Intermediate-interval training. This form of training differs from long-interval work in that the duration of the work period is shortened and the intensity of work increased. The degree to which anaerobic mechanisms are tapped is also increased over the level usually experienced in longer work. Because of that greater anaerobic demand, the work/recovery ratio is also lowered. This form of training is appropriate for training both aerobic and anaerobic endurance. Intermediate intervals feature the following characteristics:

1. Duration of work	30 sec to 2 min
2. Intensity of work	90–95% of best performance standard
3. Duration of recovery period	2–6 min
4. Work–recovery ratio	1 : 2 to 1 : 3
5. Repetitions	3–12

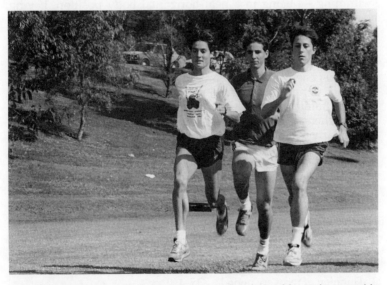

The middle-distance runner requires a mix of aerobic and anaerobic energy and should be exposed to a range of continuous and interval training methods

Heart rates at the end of each bout still remain high (180–200 bpm). The elevated work intensities place a greater load on the lactacid energy pathways than do the longer intervals. Lactic acid concentrations in the blood can exceed 12 mmol.L^{-1}. Because of these high lactate levels, this form of training is sometimes referred to as 'lactic acid tolerance training', where the main adaptations are to increase the capacity to buffer the acid that is produced and to develop a high degree of psychological resistance to, and control over, the discomfort. The exact nature of the work and recovery periods will depend on the sport/event, the individual's capacities, and the phase of training.

Typical examples of intermediate-interval training for a 100/200-meter swimmer are as follows:

Repetitions	Distance	Stroke	Intensity	Recovery	Recovery activity
8 ×	100 m	free	1:05 pace	25 sec	float
12 ×	75 m	free	0:46 pace	24 sec	float

It should be noted that the recovery period for a swimmer is usually much shorter than that for a runner. The characteristics of swimming — being in a near-horizontal body position, having body weight supported, the ease of heat removal in cool water, and the more localized sites of muscle fatigue — promote faster recovery rates than those for running.

Short-interval training: This form of training is specifically designed to generate high levels of muscular power. The duration of the work period is shortened even further than in intermediate-interval training while, with longer work bouts, recovery periods are lengthened. This training is sometimes called 'spurt' training, particularly when used in a running team-game context. It emphasizes anaerobic endurance, particularly the alactacid energy sources when work periods are short, but some aerobic adaptation will also occur. It also allows for very specific training effects to occur as well as for the performance of actions that may exceed the quality that has been exhibited in previous competitions. The characteristics of short-interval training are:

1. Duration of work	5–30 sec
2. Intensity of work	95+% of best performance standard
3. Duration of recovery period	15–150 sec
4. Work–recovery ratio	1 : 3 to 1 : 5
5. Repetitions	5–20

As repetitions are completed, some accumulation of lactic acid (4–6 mmol.L^{-1}) may result from the short intense efforts, but it should not be sufficient to cause extreme discomfort. However, if the duration of each repetition is extended beyond 20 seconds and the intensity is high, a response similar to that experienced in lactic acid tolerance training will occur.

Typical examples of short-interval or spurt training items for a running team-game player are as follows:

Repetitions	Distance	Intensity	Recovery	Recovery activity
5 ×	50 m	100% — 7 sec	23 sec	walk
5 ×	40 m	100% — 6 sec	19 sec	jog
5 ×	30 m	100+%	15 sec	jog

This form of training is the primary means for developing alact-acid energy sources which are required in the first stages of a sustained sprint or middle-distance effort. It is also most appropriate as preparation for stop-and-go action which forms a large part of many team games. The short duration of the recovery period ensures that a high load is maintained on the cardiovascular system, a situation that often occurs in competitive situations.

When training involves an extended and intensive work period, adaptations occur in the provision of energy via glycolytic pathways. However, the necessarily long recovery period lowers the overall load on the cardiovascular system. A comparison of the physiological responses of five active young men first to continuous and then two forms of short-interval training is shown in Table 13.2.

Table 13.2 Average Responses to 20-minute Sessions of Continuous and Interval Training Programs

Training Type	Mean Heart Rate	Blood Lactate
Continuous (90% intensity)	184 bpm	4·7 mmol.L^{-1}
Short interval 1 (90% intensity — 5–15 sec work/recovery ratio)	181 bpm	5·5 mmol.L^{-1}
Short interval 2 (95% intensity — 30–150 sec work/recovery ratio)	150 bpm	8·5 mmol.L^{-1}

The high-intensity continuous training produced a steady state heart rate of 184 bpm which was 20 bpm below the average maximum. A blood lactic acid concentration of 4·7 mmol.L^{-1} indicated some involvement of the lactacid energy pathways during the work. The short sprint training (5 seconds) placed a similar load on the cardiovascular system to continuous training with a moderate energy contribution from glycolytic pathways (blood lactate 5·5 mmol.L^{-1}). The longer, 30-second sprint produced high lactic acid concentrations (8·5 mmol.L^{-1}) but a much lower load on the cardiovascular system (average heart rate 150 bpm). Long recovery periods cause that reduction.

Generally, interval training is completed over designated distances with rest periods being controlled so that recovery between each repetition is not complete. These repetition distances are usually less than the competitive distance but the total distance in the set is greater than the competitive distance. When performing at slower than competition pace or effort (usually a stimulus for developing aerobic endurance), rest intervals are short. However, when the tasks are of competition quality, longer rests are usually planned. Thus the length of the rest periods are inversely related to the intensity of the exercise task.

Variations of interval training. There are many variations and names given to regimens that could be classified as interval training. They all involve different manipulations of training intensity, recovery periods and activity, and the number of repetitions. Some of the more common variations and their appropriate features are:

Repetition training. Units of work are completed at competition quality. Complete recovery is allowed between each repetition, thus, the work/recovery ratio is low. The endurance that is developed through repetition training depends upon the nature of the task, but endurance specific to what is repeated is improved (it may be either aerobic and anaerobic, or both). Specific speed is also trained through this method. This form of training allows controlled quality work to be practised and is appropriate for use in the latter stage of the specific preparatory phase of training and all of the pre-competition phase. This is a good field test protocol for assessing performance improvement. If the quality of each repetition can be increased as training progresses, that is, if the athlete goes faster more often, then it means that the training program is improving performance quality as well as endurance for the task.

Examples of repetition training for swimming are listed below. (Since complete recovery is allowed, the duration of recovery is not stipulated.)

Repetitions	Distance	Stroke	Intensity	Recovery activity
6 ×	200 m	back	2:15 min:sec	easy swim
3 ×	400 m	free	4:15 min:sec	warm-down and rest

Ultra-short interval training. This form of training is based on the principle that sufficiently short intervals of intense work do not produce lactic acid accumulation. It is appropriate for developing alactacid and aerobic endurance and provides the opportunity for specific skill training at competition intensity. It is used for training phases where specific training is important. When this work is alternated with short rest periods, it is possible to complete a large amount of training at competition quality. For example a 1 : 1 work/recovery ratio of periods totalling 20 seconds can be sustained in trained swimmers at 200-meter competition quality for at least 30 minutes. However, when the same work/recovery ratio is maintained but the duration of the task is increased to 1 minute, performance deteriorates quite noticeably in the latter half of the task. Ultra-short intervals do not produce lactic acid accumulation. It is when lactic acid accumulates that fatigue becomes devastating and adequate recovery then takes a markedly greater proportion of time.

Examples of ultra-short training stimuli for swimmers are:

Repetitions	Distance	Stroke	Intensity	Recovery	Recovery activity
20 ×	across pool (20 m)	fly	100 m race pace	20 sec remainder	float
20 ×	across pool (20 m)	back	100 m race pace	20 sec remainder	float

In these examples, the swimmer starts every repetition on a 20-second interval, the rest period being that time remaining from 20 seconds after each effort.

Variable-interval training. There are times when a coach cannot exactly gauge the fatigue state of an athlete. At these times it might be best to allow training to occur with the athlete determining the effort intensity, the assumption being that the selected intensity will be appropriate for the athlete's state of accumulated general fatigue at the time. The athlete's motivation will determine the adherence to this assumption. When prescribing these training units the specification of the repetition intensity and recovery times are omitted, and only the number of repetitions, task, and the total work/rest-time interval are designated. Thus the intensity of the training stimulus is governed by the athlete. Athletes needing recovery or who are still in fatigued states will employ efforts that are not taxing. On the other hand, athletes who feel good have the opportunity to work at even higher intensities than those normally set, although care must be taken that the overzealous athlete does not become injured. The training effect should be that which best serves the needs of the athlete at the particular time.

Some examples of variable-interval training in swimming are:

Repetitions	Distance	Stroke	Work/recovery period	Recovery activity
10 ×	200 m	free	3 min	float
40 ×	50 m	medley	1 min	float

Decreasing-distance interval training. In this progression, the distance to be covered lessens at particular stages in the segment. With each lessened stage there is an increase in the expected intensity of performance. The quality of each effort becomes better than the previous distance segment. Depending upon the nature of the set of repetitions, appropriate endurance qualities will be developed. This form of training is appropriate for the specific preparatory and pre-competition phases.

An example of a decreasing-distance interval set for a female 1,500-meter runner is:

Repetitions	Distance	Intensity	Recovery	Recovery activity
2 ×	800 m	2:35 min:sec	4:25 min:sec	jog and walk
2 ×	600 m	1:55 min:sec	4:05 min:sec	jog and walk
2 ×	400 m	1:10 min:sec	3:50 min:sec	jog and walk
2 ×	200 m	0:32 min:sec	2:28 min:sec	jog and walk

There are numerous other formulations of interval training, some being broken sets, mixed sets, progressive sets, simulators, and pyramids. With the greater variation within a training segment there is a loss of specificity of effect. Most of the innovative or unique forms of interval training are produced to provide variety in a program, that is, they serve more of a motivational function than that of deliberately stimulating the development of a capacity to sustain greater levels of a particular performance. When considering unusual training structures a coach should first determine what physical capacity is being trained and what specific effects on performance will result. If it is not possible to explicitly predict and observe the appropriate training responses of the determined factors then the value of the proposed interval method is questionable.

General Considerations

The value of endurance training comes from the repetition of movements of a particular intensity in an overloaded condition. The level of effort intensity will determine which energy system is being stimulated to increase its functional capacity. Aerobic adaptation occurs in both the central and peripheral domains of the body. Anaerobic lactacid endurance, or muscular endurance, occurs in the periphery or muscles. Alactacid endurance occurs in the peripheral musculature: that is, major developments for all types of endurance occur in the muscles. Training responses in the muscles are specific and do not transfer to any great degree from one activity to another (MacDougall and Sale 1981). These training responses, particularly the extraction of oxygen, are lost more rapidly than are effects on the central circulatory transportation of oxygen. Thus specific training is the primary essential feature of effective endurance training. It needs to be considered right up to and during the period of competitions. Departures from specific endurance training will cause rapid deteriorations in peripheral adaptations.

The three general forms of endurance training described above have different formats of execution and largely different effects, although interval training can be devised to achieve almost any form of endurance adaptation. Interval endurance training is more taxing than continuous or fartlek training, since it is harder for participants and will require more motivation in the athlete to persist over long periods of time. This means that the scheduling of the different forms of training must be seriously considered. Continuous and fartlek training at easy intensities can be programmed twice a day. Moderate continuous and fartlek training work should be scheduled daily and when of high intensities, on alternate days. Moderate interval training should be scheduled every 36 hours, while hard interval training stimuli usually require 2 full days for recovery.

The severity of the endurance training program stimuli will affect the scheduling of the session load. Considerations of those loads lead to sequences such as hard, easy, moderate, easy, hard, easy, easy, hard, etc., rather than expecting as much work as possible from athletes at every training session. The variation in session load intensity is one of the ways that recovery from fatigue can be accommodated and controlled. Recovery is as important as work. Good training programs will feature varied session loads to allow both stimulation and regeneration (training effects) to occur.

The programming of endurance training is difficult when more than one athlete is considered. With group training, the principle of individuality is usually compromised. It is difficult to gauge the various endurance capacities of a number of athletes and then accommodate them with an exact training program when they all train on only one program. Group training programs obscure individual adaptation capacities. Fox, Bartels, Klinzing, and Ragg

(1977) trained two groups of untrained athletes. The first used sprint training (19 high-intensity/high-power runs) and the second used longer (lower-power) runs (7 × 2 minutes duration) on a treadmill, 3 times per week. Each was continued to produce the same heart rate levels at the end of the work (175–180 bpm) and at the end of recovery (120–140 bpm). Each group improved the same in aerobic and anaerobic endurance measures. It was concluded that both forms of training produced similar effects. However, it is likely that individual capacities and response patterns are obscured in group training studies and programs. If groups have to be tolerated, then it is best to provide a variety of stimuli for all endurance features. With that approach, some of the athletes will always be accommodated some of the time by the training stimuli. It makes no sense to expect to maximize the training of individuals when they are trained in group programs.

Most sports requiring sustained levels of effort require aerobic and anaerobic endurance training. The degree to which each needs to be stimulated depends upon the sport. Thus training sessions will include mixing different forms of endurance training. The order in which training stimuli are presented is important. Anaerobic training should occur before aerobic training in a session. Chapter 18 describes in detail the ordering of training session items.

Table 13.3 presents a summary of the various general forms of endurance training.

Table 13.3 A Comparison of Features of Several Intensities of Continuous, Fartlek, and Interval Training Modes

Feature	Characteristic
Endurance Capacity Trained	
Low-intensity continuous	aerobic
High-intensity continuous	aerobic, some lactacid
Low-intensity fartlek	aerobic
High-intensity fartlek	aerobic, some lactacid
Long-interval	aerobic, some lactacid
Intermediate-interval	lactacid, some aerobic
Short-interval	alactacid, aerobic
Frequency of Use	
Low-intensity continuous	twice per day
High-intensity continuous	once per 24–36 hours
Low-intensity fartlek	twice per day
High-intensity fartlek	once per day
Long-interval	once per 36 hours
Intermediate-interval	once per 48 hours
Short-interval	once per 36–48 hours

Lactic Acid Levels Achieved

Low-intensity continuous	< 3 mmol.L^{-1}
High-intensity continuous	3–5 mmol.L^{-1}
Low-intensity fartlek	2–3 mmol.L^{-1}
High-intensity fartlek	3–6 mmol.L^{-1}
Long-interval	6–10 mmol.L^{-1}
Intermediate-interval	> 10 mmol.L^{-1}
Short-interval	4–6 mmol.L^{-1}

Recovery time

Low-intensity continuous	8 hours
High-intensity continuous	24–36 hours
Low-intensity fartlek	24 hours
High-intensity fartlek	36–48 hours
Long-interval	36 hours
Intermediate-interval	48 hours
Short-interval	36–48 hours

Load on Athlete

Low-intensity continuous	light
High-intensity continuous	moderate to high
Low-intensity fartlek	light
High-intensity fartlek	moderate to high
Long-interval	moderate to high
Intermediate-interval	high
Short-interval	moderate

Appropriate Training Phases for Use

Low-intensity continuous	basic preparatory
High-intensity continuous	basic preparatory, early specific preparatory
Low-intensity fartlek	basic preparatory, early specific preparatory, transition
High-intensity fartlek	specific preparatory, competition
Long-interval	basic preparatory, specific preparatory
Intermediate-interval	specific preparatory, pre-competition, competition
Short-interval	specific preparatory, pre-competition, competition

Factors Trained

Low-intensity continuous	physiology
High-intensity continuous	physiology, psychology
Low-intensity fartlek	physiology, psychology, some biomechanics
High-intensity fartlek	physiology, biomechanics, psychology
Long-interval	physiology, biomechanics, psychology
Intermediate-interval	physiology, biomechanics, psychology
Short-interval	physiology, biomechanics, psychology

14
Strength Training

The principal object of strength training is to increase the force that can be exerted in a sporting performance. There are also other objectives such as injury rehabilitation and muscular definition and development. Strength is an important ingredient of sports such as weight-lifting, power-lifting, and body-building. Its value for many other sports is revered by many but is not well understood. It is the purpose of this chapter to clarify the current status of strength training for sports.

There are three major forms of muscle contractions that differentiate types of training:

1. *Isotonic exercises* traditionally involve an absolute external resistance and employ two phases of action: an eccentric contraction involving the lengthening of the muscle as part of the preparation to produce force and a concentric contraction which is the productive exertion that is developed through a shortening of the muscle. Both concentric and eccentric contractions are involved in many movements, for example, lowering a weight (eccentric) after it has been lifted (concentric), and the foot strike in running (eccentric) followed by push-off (concentric). Most sporting activities involving large amounts of strength employ isotonic forms of exertion.

2. *Isometric exercises* involve exerting effort against a stationary resistance. This is also termed a static contraction. It has some relevance to sports where maintaining a posture is of importance, for example, the stance in shooting and archery,

the crucifix in gymnastics, and many pushing activities in contact sports where little movement is achieved (e.g., the scrum in rugby).

3. *Isokinetic exercises* involve a constant movement speed while exerting a variable force. This form of contraction has few counterparts in sporting movements but is commonly used in strength testing and training programs.

Because there are three different types of contraction, there is the possibility that they may be mixed in some actions. For example, to initiate a pushing movement in a rugby scrum, an isometric contraction that increases in force could occur until the resistance of the other scrum is overcome. From then on, a variety of isotonic contractions which develop forward propulsion, produced mainly by the legs but directed by the alignment of the body, cause the scrum to move forward. Similar situations arise in many combative sports where one athlete attempts to overcome the resistance provided by another individual. When analyzing the strength needs of a sport the biomechanical force components need to be carefully determined for all elements of an action, not just the obvious movement features.

There are a number of strength terms which are commonly associated with sport:

1. *General strength*, the strength of the whole muscular system estimated from a combination of measurements of the strength of major muscle groups.

2. *Specific strength*, the strength of the primary muscles involved in a particular action (usually measured by isolating the large muscle groups and measuring maximum strength in each).

3. *Maximum strength*, the highest force exerted during a single voluntary contraction of a particular action, also referred to as 'absolute strength' or one repetition maximum (1 RM).

The physiological requirements and movement patterns of a sport and a particular individual will dictate which facet of strength is important for training.

Physiological Responses to Strength Training

☐ Neural Adaptations

Rapid increases in strength develop during the first two to eight weeks of training (Fleck and Kraemer 1988c, Thorstensson, Hulten, von Doblen, and Karlsson 1976). These marked improvements occur without any increase in muscle size. Strength training effects first occur at the neuromuscular level. This means that the first response to strength training is a harnessing of existing capacities and resources. Training a group of muscles in a particular exercise will increase strength in that exercise but will not generalize to any appreciable degree to another exercise involving the same group of muscles (Sale and MacDougall 1981). The neural adaptations that occur are very specific. There are four responses that produce strength increases without any anatomical (morphological) changes: neural adaptations appear first and improve technique; the firing rate of motor units increases; additional motor units in the muscle are recruited; and the synchronization of the motor units is improved. It also has been suggested that inhibiting the self-protective mechanisms of the body (golgi tendon organs) allows for a more forceful contraction (Ikai and Steinhaus 1961). Morphological adaptations occur after neural adaptations are exhausted (Bosco, Rusko, and Hirvonen 1984, Fleck and Kraemer 1988c, Moritani and de Vries 1979). The major factor for the practitioner to understand is that the initial response to strength training is one of skill acquisition. Morphological adaptations only occur after skill levels have been developed.

□ Hypertrophy or Hyperplasia?

After eight weeks of training increases in muscle size may become noticeable. Size changes may be due to either or both of two processes. Hypertrophy occurs when a muscle's cross-sectional area is enlarged due to an increase in the size and number of actin and myosin filaments and the addition of sarcomeres within the fibers (Fleck and Kraemer 1987). In hyperplasia, muscle fibers split due to the damage a muscle experiences when stimulated excessively. However, this phenomenon has only been observed conclusively in animals. The doubters about the role of hyperplasia contributing to muscle size enlargement are in the majority. Hypertrophy results in an increased total amount of connective tissue (ligaments and tendons) so that this tissue keeps pace with the developing muscle tissue (Fleck and Kraemer 1988b).

Training with low volume heavy loads results in greater hypertrophy of fast-twitch fibers than occurs with high-volume lower loads. Conversely, high-volume low-load stimuli result in greater hypertrophy of slow-twitch fibers. This supports the fact that muscle fiber recruitment is dependent on muscle tension. High tension recruits fast-twitch fibers while lower tensions recruit slow-twitch fibers. Thus the training stimulus will determine the site of hypertrophy.

☐ Cellular Adaptations

There are three reactions at the cellular level that could occur with strength training:

1. *Mitochondrial density:* Muscle size increases through strength training are not accompanied by a similar increase in the number of mitochondria. This is probably due to the anaerobic nature of resistance training which provides little stimulus for using oxygen as a source of energy.
2. *Capillarization:* There appears to be a differential response in the number of capillaries in muscles depending upon the type of training. Fleck and Kraemer (1988b: 111) speculate that in a typical body-building session (heavy resistance at moderate to high intensity, with high volume and short rest periods), there is an increase in the total number of capillaries but no change in capillary density. This is the result of an accompanying increase in fiber cross-sectional area. On the other hand, with power and Olympic lifters (heavy resistance training at high intensity and low volume, with long rest periods), hypertrophy occurs with no change in the number of capillaries per fiber. This results in decreased capillary density.
3. *Intracellular fuel stores:* Anaerobic energy stores (ATP, CP, glycogen) are increased by as much as 66 percent through resistance training (MacDougall, Ward, Sale, and Sutton 1977). However, the availability of substrate glycogen does not seem to be a limiting factor in strength performance.

☐ Muscular Endurance

High repetitions of moderate loads increase the ability of a muscle to exert force for a sustained period of time. Apart from alterations in movement efficiency, the force of movements also increases. This translates into fewer fibers being necessary to sustain a certain workload. Consequently the time to exhaustion is extended (Hickson, Rosenkoetter, and Brown 1980). Training stimuli which adapt the slow-twitch fibers do not increase strength; they only produce increased muscular or aerobic endurance.

☐ Cardiovascular Adaptations

There is considerable debate as to whether weight training produces cardiovascular gains. The controversy is confounded because of the different effects of types of training programs. At one extreme there are circuit training formats (moderate repetitions, low resistances, short rests, several total sets) which produce slow-twitch fiber adaptations. The aerobic endurance gains from such programs are small and less than could be achieved by training specifically for aerobic adaptation in an activity (e.g., running, swimming, cycling). The load of resistance training is such that heart rates are much higher for a given level of VO_2 max than in endurance training, so caution should be used when individuals with cardiovascular problems train to voluntary fatigue. Also, the elevated heart rate is likely to produce an overestimation of the energy expenditure of weight-training exercise.

Muscular strength and aerobic endurance are poorly correlated. Hypertrophy without a proportional increase in muscle oxidative capacity might actually be viewed as being harmful to the performance of an endurance athlete, particularly in activities such as running where body weight has to be supported (MacDougall, Sale, Moroz, Elder, Sutton, and Howard 1979). Assuming that mitochondrial volume density reflects the oxidative potential of the muscle it would seem that not only does heavy resistance training fail to enhance the endurance characteristics of skeletal muscle, it may even be harmful to endurance performance by decreasing oxidative potential per total muscle mass (MacDougall *et al.* 1979).

The reverse is also proposed as being true, aerobic training interfering with the development of maximum strength, the training responses being incompatible (Poliquin 1985). When both characteristics need to be trained, macrocycles need to be alternated to emphasize each capacity. With regard to this programming strategy Poliquin warns that *mixed training gives mixed results.*

A further confounding factor in the strength–endurance comparison is the nature and fiber composition of the trained muscle itself. The long head of the triceps is a predominantly fast-twitch muscle whereas the vastus lateralis is considerably more heterogeneous in fiber composition. Thus the response tendency of these two muscles will be different depending upon the training stimulus. The triceps will react noticeably to strength training but unimpressively to endurance work. The vastus lateralis will respond to both forms of training. The practitioner must consider the muscles being trained to determine the potential for training improvements.

Modifying Variables in Strength Training

□ Speed of Development

Strength is a capacity that can be gained quickly. Asfour, Ayoub, and Mital (1984) found that 70 percent of the gains in strength occurred in the first 10 sessions of a weight training program. Over the next 20 sessions, the gains were less than 30 percent of the original strength values. They concluded that the development of correct technique was the main factor that contributed to this gain. Hickson *et al.* (1980) also recorded rapid strength gains. Strength increased 19 percent after 3 weeks, 27 percent after 6 weeks, and 38 percent after 10 weeks. The initial rapid gains can be encouraging and motivational for athletes. However, as gains then become less obvious adherence to a continuing program of strength training may become a problem because of diminishing returns.

The speed of development of strength could mislead coaches. It resides in increases in the skill of doing the specific exercises of the training program. It should not be concluded that such strength improvements will transfer to a sporting action. The strength improvements are neuromuscular and specific to the exact exercise being performed. Since there is no anatomical change one should not expect any performance change in another exercise. This is a difficulty that must be confronted by adherents of intensive strength training programs for sports.

Like all physiological capacities, there is a ceiling level of strength development. There is also a level at which the attainment of further training effects is not a worthwhile pursuit. For most sports where strength is not the primary capacity for performance, a certain amount of strength assists performance. Above that level, the extra capacity is not taxed or used. Whether or not that excessive level has been achieved can be determined in the following manner: combine resistance and specific-sport training together; measure improvements in both areas; and cease strength training while still monitoring strength and specific-sport performances. If there is no performance regression in the sport but there is in specific-strength measures, then it might be concluded that the strength gains were not specific determinants of the sporting performances. What this suggests is that there is the possibility that strength training may be very useful for bringing weak athletes to a level of strength that is appropriate for their sport. Any further strength gains might then be unnecessary. The following illustrates this point (Derriman 1989: 30):

> And on the institute's [Australian Institute of Sport's] courts, biomechanists have been using radar guns to measure the velocity of tennis serves in a study of how strong players need to be. What they found is that if you build up a player's strength you will increase the speed of the player's serve — but only up to a point. Beyond that point, further increases in strength make no difference. The important thing for coaches, therefore, is knowing when that point has been reached. Darren Cahill is one player who seemed to benefit from this research.

While he was at the institute his serving speed rose from about 120 km/h to about 150 km/h, largely through a build-up of strength.

The above principle might not be applicable to all activities. In some sports (e.g., soccer, rugby, cricket) the frequency of occurrence of a particular action may not be sufficient to stimulate even strength maintenance. However, even though the rate of occurrence is low, the isolated cases when such actions are needed are very important. Thus extra strength training for these actions needs to be followed to achieve a level of strength that is above that which is supported purely through participation in the sport.

□ Loss of Strength

Once strength has been developed for certain exercises, it may only be important to maintain this, rather than continuing to attempt to develop it further. Programs of strength maintenance can be conducted less frequently than those aimed at producing strength change (see Chapter 4). Stimulus intensity is a more important factor than training frequency in maintenance training for strength. The practical implication for this is that muscular strength can be maintained over a relatively long period, such as during the precompetitive and competitive phases, by performing as little as one intense training session per week (Graves, Pollock, Leggett, Braith, Carpenter, and Bishop 1988). This means that strength capacity can be retained as a competition period approaches even though the time allocated to strength training is greatly reduced.

□ Technique

The technique used in a resistance exercise will determine strength gains. Adherence to a specific technique will produce specific improvements in a very short period of time. If techniques are varied, then improvements will be slowed because of the dissipation of training stimuli over a greater variety of neuromuscular patterns. This accounts for simple movements improving rapidly and complex movements taking longer. However, the more restricted a technique and/or the simpler a movement, the less transfer there will be of strength gains to a sporting action. A failure to understand the mechanics of strength exercises has led many coaches to prescribe wrong training exercises (Poliquin 1985).

A dilemma arises for the coach and athlete. If one uses a device or piece of equipment that severely restricts the range and locus of movement, then the benefit of such an activity will be negligible for sports performance. However, since modern sport facilities commonly invest large sums in movement-limiting equipment, such as leg- and bench-press machines, the value of the investment for potential effect on performance has to be questioned. It is probable that other forms of specific sport training, such as concentrating high-intensity repetitions of actual actions, are a better means of developing strength than relying on artificial actions and devices to promote a change.

☐ Speed of Movement

The magnitude of the resistance used in strength training will dictate the speed of the movement employed to execute one repetition as well as the number of repetitions that can be completed without a necessary rest. Low-speed, high-resistance exercises produce strength increases only in slow-speed movements. High-speed, lower-resistance exercises produce strength effects in both high- and low-speed movements, although the low-speed benefits are not as great as those developed by low-speed exercises (Moffroid and Whipple 1970). This means that for activities where speed of movement is a notable feature, quickly executed resistance exercises would have more general value in terms of training effects than would those exercises which are performed with slow movements. This suggests that strength exercises should at least be performed at the speed of contraction of the sporting activity for any potential benefit to occur.

There is another confounding factor involving the speed with which an activity is performed. As the velocity of contraction increases, the force that can be developed decreases, despite maximum effort. This means that when faster movements are employed in an activity absolute strength has a lesser influence on performance. It is possible to have excess strength developed for a sport, because the actions of the sport do not allow that excess to be tapped. For example, in a 100-meter sprint, strength is an important factor at the start, particularly in the first few strides when the body mass is accelerated from a stationary position. Once in full sprinting stride, strength is less important. Speed of movement becomes a critical determinant (Sale 1975). Thus a concentration on strength training in activities that do not require great amounts of such training may be a waste of time. Strength only needs to be developed to a level that is moderately in excess of that which is required in a sporting performance.

Sale and MacDougall (1981) suggested that strength training should be limited to the speed of the sport action. The specific-training effect that results from strength work is related to the controlling function of the brain rather than to the energizing capacity of muscle fibers. Muscle growth is related to the amount of tension produced in the muscle by the training stimulus. Slow-velocity training may be necessary to stimulate maximum adaptation within the muscle. On the other hand, low resistances and high repetitions do not produce hypertrophy and only stimulate a restricted number of muscle fibers. Thus it may be best to combine activities of varying velocities to produce added training effects. Fast movements might be used to train the nervous system, and slow movements to train the greatest number of fibers. This supports the usual practice of athletes engaging in strength training with high resistances and lower speeds before power training with lower resistances and higher movement speeds.

□ Resistance Magnitude

The brief maximum contractions associated with heavy-resistance training require a very high rate of energy production which can be met only by the muscle's high-energy phosphate reserves and, to a lesser extent, glycolysis. An increase in the total content of the high-energy phosphate stores as a result of high-resistance training would not be expected to affect the maximum rate of power output from a muscle. It would increase the total energy from this source and thus prolong the duration of sustaining strength output. On the other hand, repeated low-resistance contractions develop significant increases in the capacity of muscle to oxidize pyruvate and fatty acids as a result of both increased mitochondrial number and size (MacDougall, Ward, Sale, and Sutton 1977).

The implication of this is that low-resistance, high-repetition training produces aerobic changes that might be achieved better by specifically doing the activity itself. Strength training with a high resistance produces changes in stored energy sources for maximum power output. No change in performance speed or rate should be expected. Therefore strength training may be useful only for strength and power activities rather than ones involving substantial endurance qualities.

□ Contraction Type

The manner in which muscles contract determines the type of changes that occur. For example, muscles exert more force when contracting eccentrically than when performing concentrically. Eccentric contractions can be three times as forceful as concentric ones. There may be an advantage to doing eccentric training because it stimulates a greater number of muscle fibers in the contraction. Eccentric contractions are used in plyometric or 'rebound' training which activates the stretch-shortening cycle and embellishes the force of contraction (see Chapter 15). The state of knowledge on eccentric training is far from complete. Eccentric contractions are involved in most sporting movements. Eccentric training is likely to be most effective where muscles are compelled to exert high magnitudes of eccentric force (e.g., running, jumping, bounding, tumbling) where lowering the body weight is resisted.

It is known that the transfer of training effects from one form of contraction training to another form is very low. Pipes (1978) compared training effects on the same exercise using universal (isotonic contraction) and Nautilus (isokinetic contraction) equipment. A strength improvement of 25 percent on a universal machine only transferred to a 10 percent improvement on a Nautilus device using the same movement. Indeed, the effects of strength training are so exact that for any transfer to occur from the training activity to the sporting activity, the type of contraction must be the same. Thus isotonic contractions may be the most useful for training since they are the most common form of contraction in sports. On the other hand, isokinetic contractions rarely occur in the sporting world and thus would appear to have limited value for sport training. Poliquin (1985) advised against using isokinetic exercises and equipment for power sports which involve an element of velocity change or acceleration. While all forms of muscular contraction appear to have some value for the rehabilitation of muscles after injury, it must be emphasized that rehabilitation is different from sports training.

Specificity of Strength Training

Strength training in one exercise will increase strength in that exercise but not in another, even though the same muscle groups might be involved. Thorstensson and Karlsson (1974) reported that a much greater improvement in leg-squat strength than isometric leg-press strength was obtained as a result of leg-squat training. The muscular strength adaptations gained through squatting only partially transferred to the leg-press action. Thorstensson *et al.* (1976) showed that isometric training of the quadriceps muscles at 90° on a leg-extension exercise resulted in an increase in strength at that angle but not at 60° or 30°. The load is carried in a different manner by the muscles in the thigh when they function at different knee angles. Even a change in posture can affect the specificity of strength training. Rasch and Morehouse (1957) reported that a training program that increased elbow flexor strength in the standing position had less effect on the same action when in the supine position. Thus alterations in exercise from one position to another will drastically reduce the transfer potential of strength gains. These studies demonstrate the specificity of the movement exercise that is used in training.

The type of contraction used in strength training determines the specific effects which are derived. Specific contractions produce specific neural adaptations (Sale and MacDougall 1981). For specific training effects to occur and transfer from strength training, the action used should simulate that of the sport activity. Such a simulation may be difficult to produce unless the exercise is that of the sport itself (Costill *et al.* 1985). There are attempts to dissect a sporting activity and train using exercises that only partially simulate the total action. An example of the reasoning for this approach is as follows (Konstanty 1989: 15):

> An offensive lineman in American football must possess exceptional muscle strength and power in the legs, as he drives forward from a three-point stance. Great upper-body and arm strength is also needed. Attempting to simulate the movement patterns of an offensive lineman through strength training exercises may be next to impossible. The blocking sled found on most practice fields may be used to help improve leg strength. The strength training environment could enable a lineman to simulate the force of contraction by performing exercises at a higher velocity and in an explosive manner (e.g., controlled high-velocity leg squats or presses) . . . Though the movement pattern is not replicated, the neural mechanisms may be trained to respond to quick, powerful movements. The quick, forceful contractions experienced in the weight room may enhance performance on the football field.

The value of this form of training has not been adequately demonstrated. It proposes the use of specific exercises to enhance a gross, integrated, and variable action. The benefits from specific weight exercises do not transfer well, if at all, to sporting actions. There is no guarantee that the velocities, types of contraction, and movement patterns of strength training will be the same as those occurring in the various situations that arise when blocking. The argument rests on the assumption that the characteristics trained in a series of simple exercises focusing on strength and speed will carry over into another integrated movement. The principle of movement specificity indicates that such an assumption is not likely to be correct. The principle of specificity is so pervasive that reasoning of the type given above should be interpreted with caution and some scepticism.

A training zone exists in developing strength that will produce the best returns. Any training in which the resistance is less than 60 percent of maximum will not stimulate strength increases. It will enhance muscular endurance if the activity is repeated enough to produce significant fatigue. It is typically asserted that sports which involve a large number of submaximal contractions (e.g, swimming, basketball, cross-country skiing) should incorporate strength exercises of 8 to 10 repetitions at 75–80 percent of maximum. Though the contractile force of the muscles in the sport is smaller, the athlete is concerned with maintaining a level of muscle endurance. The recruitment of fibers towards the end of a maximum endurance set involves a similar mechanism to that in a single maximum effort. Hence the benefits gained from strength and muscular endurance programs can be quite similar. The implication of such thinking is clear. Strength training exercises that produce a 'similar' type of fatigue to that experienced in an original action might transfer to that action. However, such a transfer has not been demonstrated and until it has *coaches are advised to avoid such an assumption when devising strength training for low to moderate strength activities*. Rutherford, Greig, Sargeant, and Jones (1986) trained the quadriceps muscles of men and women on a leg-extension machine for 12 weeks (4 × 6 repetitions, three times per week). Males increased their maximum strength by 20 percent while women only improved 3 percent. There was no change in maximum power output on a cycle ergometer. The strength improvements did not transfer to the cycling activity although leg extension was emphasized in both actions.

A similar argument is made by the proponents of supplementary strength training (Konstanty 1989: 16):

> For sports involving a few maximal contractions, a strength training program should incorporate the performance of 1 to 3 repetitions at 90–100 percent of maximum. Athletes in sports such as weight lifting, power lifting, football, and some field events should benefit most from a low-repetition, high-resistance program. The athletes would maximize the contractile force of the muscles involved in the strength exercises. Hypertrophy and increases in joint tissue would also be stimulated. Tissue damage (strains and tears) would also be minimized.

Whether or not these benefits transfer to the actual sporting environment and activity is debatable. The preponderance of evidence suggests that they would not. The overriding factor to be considered about the transfer of training effects has to do with neural patterns. Such patterns are particularly specific and do not transfer in whole or in part. Thus *if strength gains are due primarily to neural patterns, one should not expect transfer to occur*.

In terms of the specificity of strength training, four conclusions can be drawn:

1. Strength training activities which are not related in movement pattern (technique), movement speed (velocity), contraction type, or contraction force are useless for enhancing specific-sport performances. They may be of benefit for sport injury prevention or rehabilitation or for building muscle mass that can be incorporated into a movement.

2. The smaller the group of muscles used in strength training activities, the lower is the potential for transfer of training effects to sporting activities.
3. The more restricted/localized the strength training activity, the lower is the potential for transfer of training effects to sporting activities.
4. Because of the restricted nature of any transfer effects the benefits to be expected from general strength training programs have to be realized as being relatively insignificant or trivial.

☐ Cross-training

The concept of cross-training implies that the development of physical capacities in one activity will transfer ('cross over to') another (e.g., the benefits of bench-pressing will carry over to shot-putting). This has already been argued as being a false assertion in Chapter 6. It is surprising that many proponents of cross-training admit that there is no evidence to support this contention but still promote its use. In strength training, cross-training has perhaps its most fervent advocates. Essentially, there are two opposing positions:

1. *Specific effects:* Strength training exercises should simulate the sport movement as closely as possible in terms of movement pattern, velocity, contraction type, and contraction force. Each departure from these simulation requirements lessens the amount of transfer of strength training effects to a target activity.
2. *General effects:* Strength training exercises need only train the muscle groups without much concern for specificity. The cross-training position contends that it is only necessary to train muscle groups (multilateral training, biomotor development) for a large proportion of training time. The gains that are made in such training can then be 'educated' into sports actions. Thus the benefits of general strength training are supposedly 'transferred' or 'converted' into specific sporting performances after a period of specialized training.

Bompa (1986) advocated the educating strength gains viewpoint. In planning strength training programs he stipulated 5 developmental phases:

1. the build-up phase, where supplementary strength training is gradually introduced to athletes
2. the maximum strength phase, where intense exercising and overloads are experienced

3. the conversion phase, where specific-strength gains are re-educated into sporting actions
4. the maintenance phase, which retains strength improvements through enacting reduced frequencies of intense training
5. the cessation phase, which occurs prior to the commencement of a period of important competitions.

Sale and MacDougall (1981) evaluated the two opposing viewpoints. They concluded that strength-training effects were specific and did not transfer in any appreciable degree to other activities. There was no evidence to support the 're-education' or cross-training theory for strength gains.

There is much that needs to be discovered and understood about the benefits and limits of strength training. It is the position of these authors that the specificity principle governs strength training to a similar limiting degree as it does with other physical capacities.

One hypothetical way in which strength benefits may be incorporated into specific physical activities might be as follows:

Develop strength improvements/changes prior to commencing technique training. This might best be achieved as an emphasis of off-season or transition-phase training. It could be contended that alterations in physical capacities, particularly strength in the muscle groups that are used in a particular sport, are best done at this time when little, if any, sport-specific techniques are pursued. This overcomes the problem of skill learning being disrupted by non-specific and heavily loaded movement patterns.

Once the specific preparatory training phase commences and sport-specific intense techniques are 'relearned' or altered to reflect technical improvements, these alterations should include the new strength capacities and structural changes which have been achieved in the previous training phases. This is where strength changes might be 'converted' into a technique. The reasoning behind this assertion is that strength in sports is primarily a neuromuscular adaptation: that is, a neural pattern is established using the body's resources and capacities at the time of learning. Thus, with the relearning of techniques in each annual plan, it is possible to incorporate strength-change benefits which have occurred prior to the learning experience.

Once the neural patterns for an action are established for a period of continuous specific training, they will not be altered and will continue to use the level of physical capacities that existed during their development. Any new capacity changes, particularly strength, will not be incorporated into technical efficiency. The body will continue to employ the capacities and movement patterns that it originally developed. Unless there is a drastic change in the technique pattern followed by sufficient practice repetitions to allow the new technique to develop a greater conditioned strength than the original pattern, and assuming the changes incorporate the new strength gains, there will be no carry-over of in-season strength training gains to sporting activities. Once neural organizations of the body's capacities are developed into a technique, any further changes in strength will not be used by these established techniques. That is why training effects are specific. Strength gains made after techniques have been established will not be incorporated into sports performances.

The above reasoning proposes that it may be possible to transfer strength training benefits into sporting activities. These benefits should be developed before specific and intense technique training occurs if they are to be 'educated' into the activities. Training programs aimed at changing strength capacity, should not be done in concert with or after techniques have been developed. They should be completed prior to the commencement of technique work. The only beneficial in-season strength training would appear to be of a maintenance nature.

The arguments presented above are purely speculative. They indicate that the timing of strength training gains could be the important factor in governing any transfer of benefits. However, with regard to current practices, the direct transfer of general strength training effects to many sporting activities is, at best, of minimum to trivial value.

Despite this rather negative general picture for strength training, there are obvious values for its use in high-resistance strength sports; correcting physical weaknesses and deficiencies in practicing athletes; and rehabilitation programs. If the conjecture of these authors about the timing of strength training in relation to the learning or relearning of skills is also true then it could also be a beneficial form of training. The following section discusses strength training programs.

Programming Variables in Strength Training

The stimulus for an increase in muscle strength is a tension in a muscle fiber that surpasses the stimulus threshold. When the fastest and most effective increase in strength is desired, the greatest training stimulus should be applied, that is, an athlete must exert the muscle with maximum tension. The force of a muscle during isometric contraction is always larger than that of the concentric phase of an isotonic action. Thus isometric training may be a valuable adjunct to isotonic training for stimulating the greatest strength increases (Stegeman 1981).

In physically active people who are not athletically trained, muscles of the body which are often used (for example, forearm flexors and extensors) are already at a high level of their final strength capacity — as much as 75–80 percent (Stegeman 1981). Other muscle groups may have a level that is much lower than their capacity following training. This means that expected improvements should be determined by the initial level of the strength of the muscle groups to be trained.

Final strength is dependent upon the specific effects of the training stimulus. It is unlikely that many of the specific training effects will be used in other actions. Thus the specialized effects of strength work need to be considered when planning a training program.

The time in which strength is gained is of primary importance relative to how fast these gains will be lost. Strength which is gained rapidly is lost faster than strength which is gained slowly (Stegeman 1981). Thus the intended uses of strength gains will determine how training is programmed, implemented, and altered from change to maintenance orientations.

□ Isometric Strength Training

Although the effects of isometric training are specific, it would seem to be valuable for training the stabilizing and postural muscle groups in the trunk, shoulders, and spine.

An isometric exercise is performed with force being applied against a stationary resistance. Bompa (1986) indicated the following considerations for programming isometric training:

1. The level of exertion should exceed 70 percent of one's maximum.
2. It should be used mainly with mature athletes who have a good history of strength training.
3. Overload increases are achieved by increasing the number of repetitions, not the effort levels.
4. Each contraction should last from 6 to 12 seconds, with a total of up to 90 seconds per muscle group per session.
5. Rest intervals should be from 60 to 90 seconds and should employ recovery exercises such as stretching or light aerobic work.
6. Alternating isometric exercises with isotonic exercises will assist recovery and the development of training effects.
7. One should consider doing intermediary contractions where the action is stopped and resisted at several stages across a range of motion.

The last feature listed is important. It may be a method of stimulating maximum adaptation in the motor units of a muscle group. When it is combined with isotonic training it may produce the most desirable effects. It may even be more effective than a combination of low-repetition high-resistance and moderate-repetition moderate-resistance isotonic exercises. Again, this is pure speculation and needs to be evaluated through appropriate research.

□ Isotonic Training

There are several terms that are associated with isotonic strength training that are used to describe programming options. *Intensity* is described in two ways, the actual amount of resistance lifted per repetition in a training exercise, or a percentage of maximum strength. *Volume* is the number of exercise repetitions performed in one continuous exercise set. *Repetitions maximum (RM)* refers to completing the volume of an exercise with maximum effort. Therefore, 10 RM is the maximum load that can be lifted ten times. The maximum strength in one effort is 1 RM. *Number of sets* refers to how many times a training stimulus set is repeated in a session. *Frequency* indicates how often training stimuli are repeated, usually during a week. *Recovery duration* indicates the time period to be used for recovery. *Recovery activities* are performed during recovery periods to stimulate accelerated recovery from the specific fatigue of an exercise.

Training overloads can be altered through increasing the resistance, decreasing the recovery interval, and increasing the number of repetitions. Only by increasing the resistance will strength magnitudes be increased. Decreasing the recovery interval and increasing the number of repetitions are the means by which muscular endurance is stimulated. Thus, to become stronger, an athlete has to experience step-like increases in absolute resistances.

The number of sets of repetitions normally ranges from one to three when strength training stimuli are first introduced. This allows for habituation and reduces the soreness that could result from overworking while in an untrained state. When the stage of adaptation for the stimulus has been entered the number of sets should increase to between 3 and 6 (Fleck and Kraemer 1988a). Performing multiple sets of an exercise induces greater developments and faster increases in strength and muscular endurance gains than do single sets (Atha 1981, McDonagh and Davies 1984).

A major factor in strength training is the number of repetitions. Fleck and Kraemer (1988a) suggest the following:

1. Six or less repetitions seem to be most effective for increasing strength and power.

2. Training with heavy loads and as few as 2 repetitions produces smaller gains than more moderate loads of 4 to 6 repetitions (low repetition work volumes are not as high as those attained with greater repetitions).
3. As the number of repetitions increases beyond 6, the strength training effect is progressively lost, while muscular endurance increases. Strength is not noticeably stimulated beyond 20 repetitions.
4. The inclusion of maximum voluntary contractions at some point in the training session will enhance the likelihood of strength gains.

The frequency with which strength training sessions are programmed depends upon the trained state of the individual. In early adaptive phases, the frequency may be as low as twice per week to allow for complete recovery of the soreness and stiffness that may result. If muscle soreness remains after a previous session then the frequency of training intensity is probably too great. A program that aims at steady strength increases should be planned for every other day. As individuals adapt to training they can tolerate greater frequencies. These will be determined by the overload stress, the type of strength work, and the recovery capacities of the individual. Residual fatigue (general and local) from resistance training must be considered when programming extensive strength training or combined training programs. High-volume low-intensity training that requires a large total energy expenditure is associated with chronic fatigue to a much greater extent than is lower-volume higher-intensity training (Scala, McMillan, Blessing, Rozenek, and Stone 1987). High total workload training sessions require longer recovery periods than do those of moderate stress.

Heavy resistance work causes muscle phosphagen to be depleted. Sufficient recovery time should be allowed for its replenishment. Short and inadequate recovery periods (normally less than one minute) contribute to the accumulation of lactic acid in the blood. If that occurs, the length of the training period will be determined by how fast lactic acid accumulates. It is argued in Chapter 18 that strength training is best completed without increases in lactic acid.

The agonist–antagonist balance of the musculature is a matter of controversy. It is possible that strength/power imbalances between sets of muscles might contribute to an increased susceptibility to joint and soft-tissue injury (Fleck and Kraemer 1988a).

Proper form/technique should always be maintained during a resistance-training exercise. If a movement is altered, then muscles will be used that are not intended to be stressed by the exercise.

This reduces the possible training effect on the targeted muscles. Effective training only occurs when the intended muscles are used by employing correct movement patterns. Improper execution also increases the possibility of injury.

It is generally advocated that for moderate resistances, one should breathe in during the effort phase and out during the relaxation phase. However, this changes with heavy resistances and high effort levels. The breath should be held during the effort phase (the resulting high intra-abdominal and intra-thoracic pressures may help support the spine and stabilize the trunk) and expired once the effort is completed. Whatever inspiration–expiration pattern is adopted, breathing should be rhythmical for the exercise set.

The selection of exercises is a critical consideration. Resistance equipment can involve body weight, elastic bands and cords, a partner's resistance, medicine balls, simulation machines, fixed resistances, dumbells, pulleys, and various manufactured apparatuses (e.g., Nautilus, Universal). The exercises should adhere to the principle of specificity. The use of free-weights usually requires more sophisticated and complex techniques than those needed for machines. They also allow movement in all three planes whereas machines usually direct actions in only one. Free-weights using whole body activities (e.g., squat, clean and jerk, bent-over rowing) and involved movement activities (e.g., pulleys, medicine balls) are more akin to performing sport actions than are the particularly restricted or simpler machine determined actions. There is likely to be a greater amount of transfer to sport movements from more complicated free-weight exercises than simpler machine exercises. They are considered to be a better choice for sport training than are resistance machines (Fleck and Kraemer 1988a).

Steps in Sequencing an Isotonic Strength Training Session

The decisions that need to be made when developing strength should encompass those factors which best stimulate its development.

Strength training is scheduled within a training session after all learning, speed, and power work has been completed. If activities associated with these factors have been enacted, it is most likely that the body will be sufficiently warmed to start strength training. However, it is advisable to always precede a strength activity with some stretching that employs the muscles that will be exercised. The use of general and specific stretching between sets also accelerates the rate of recovery. If strength training activity has not been preceded by a warm-up, it will be necessary to complete one. Such a warm-up should at first be general with the main objective being to raise the central core temperature to a state where a light sweat is evidenced all over the body. Then a general stretching routine employing all major muscle groups, as well as the muscles to be used in training session, should be completed. Strength training activities should combine specific stimuli for training effects and stretching exercises for active recovery.

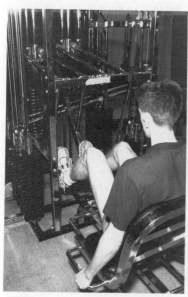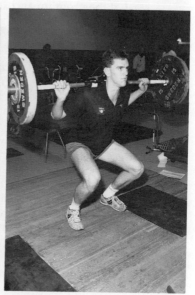

There is likely to be a greater transfer of sports movements from more complicated free-weight exercises such as squats and the clean and jerk than from simpler machine exercises such as the leg press and knee extension

The programming of strength training should follow the steps outlined in Chapters 18 and 19. The major decisions that have to be made are as follows:

1. Determine the objectives of the strength/resistance training program.
2. Develop the program for the appropriate training phases.
3. Plan the transition from general to specific exercise content across the training phases.
4. Decide the number of repetitions to be used to achieve the desired capacity development (at one extreme pure strength, in the middle a strength and muscular endurance effect, and at the other extreme a muscular endurance effect).

5. Decide the range of loads to be used for each individual.
6. Select the exercises for the program objectives.
7. Test maximum strength for each exercise, the capacities developed by each exercise, and the carry-over of training effects to the sport.
8. Take appropriate anthropometrical measurements at the start of the program and at the end of each macrocycle.

Kraemer and Fleck (1988) suggested an exercise prescription model for strength training, which is summarized below:

1. *Assess the needs of the participant.* The health and fitness of the athlete will modify program needs. The starting level of fitness has a dramatic effect on the improvement capabilities of a participant. The higher the initial strength level of the athlete the slower and less obvious will be strength improvements. In a group where the strength of participants varies considerably, differing improvement rates could become a source of motivational and exercise adherence problems. The capacities for strength gains is also related to each athlete's genetic potential. Those with the greater number of fast-twitch motor units in muscles are likely to perform better and show greater improvements on strength exercises than do individuals endowed with more slow-twitch fibers (Dons *et al.* 1979).
2. *Establish program objectives.* The objectives that are formulated will determine the nature of the exercises that are used. Five different areas that require different exercise prescriptions are strength development and/or maintenance, muscle hypertrophy, changes in body composition (decrease body fat), muscular endurance, and power.
3. *Determine session training variables.* These incorporate the stimulus qualities which will be employed to achieve specific effects. Not all programs that are labelled 'strength' produce the same effects.

The choice of exercises should be based on an analysis of the muscles and joint angles to be trained. Every time the posture of exercising, the range of movement, and the rate of execution changes, the potential training effect is altered. Thus exercises must adhere as perfectly as possible to a particular form otherwise their value will be lost to unintended effects gained through technique alterations. The degree to which an exercise mimics the qualities of a sporting action governs the amount of transfer that will occur. 'For many sports this requires a wide variety of exercises for muscle groups that contribute in different ways to athletic performance'

(Kraemer and Fleck 1988: 71). The principle of specificity should be heeded when selecting exercises. Non-specific exercises will produce non-significant effects for a specific sport.

The order of the exercises requires planning. Usually large muscle groups are worked before small groups. It is customary to alternate the muscle groups to be trained, for example, legs, arms, and then trunk before doing the next arms exercise. However, the recent and growing popularity of pre-exhaustion exercises, where muscles are deliberately fatigued before the next exercise, appears to be threatening this traditional approach. The benefits of this tactic have not been adequately researched and coaches should be wary of its use. On the surface it seems to have a number of potentially negative effects: it increases the level of fatigue which would then necessitate greater periods of recovery to achieve training effects; it smacks of the advocacy that 'if some work is beneficial then a lot more work should be better', an approach which has not served athletes well in the past; and excessive fatigue does not enhance the level of training effects over those which are optimally stimulated (the extra work producing no extra gain and also increasing the chances of muscle soreness and injury).

The resistances to be used should be based upon the capabilities of each athlete. They should facilitate the execution of sufficient repetitions to achieve the specific training objective. The number of repetitions that are performed should be of high intensity. Thus the resistance chosen should be that which requires a maximum effort for the number of repetitions prescribed. These will govern the type of training effect. General guidelines for determining what number of repetitions are appropriate are as follows:

1. 3–8 RM produces primarily strength gains.
2. 9–15 RM produces both strength and muscular endurance gains (mixed effects), each predominating at either extreme.
3. 15–20 RM produces primarily muscular endurance with strength effects diminishing as the repetitions increase.
4. greater than 20 RM trains only muscular endurance.

It can be seen from these that as the number of repetitions increases, strength gains diminish.

The length of recovery periods modifies training effects. Shortening recovery periods increases the amount of lactic acid that accumulates in the muscles. In turn, this reduces the volume of work that can be achieved. Short-recovery intervals are used by bodybuilders for definition and size but are not appropriate for the development of maximum strength. It would seem that coaches would be advised to provide recovery periods that err on the side of length. Between-exercise activities, particularly stretching, massage, and posture alterations, will accelerate the rate of recovery.

The number of sets is the last determination for session programming: 1–3 sets is recommended for beginners since they cannot handle large amounts of work. As the state of training improves, the number of sets should increase, to a maximum of between 3 and 6. The actual number which is selected will be influenced by the ability of the athlete to maintain the form and rate of the exercise and the capacity to recover between sets. Multiple sets of strength exercises produce greater gains than do single-set programs.

□ Circuit Training

Circuit training consists of performing a repeated series of exercises according to some schedule. The exercises usually focus on resistance training, but often include activities to develop other physical capacities. Circuit training has good organizational qualities for it allows a relatively large number of athletes to train within the same time period on the same activities when equipment is limited.

Since circuits (a series) of exercises are completed and then repeated a number of times, the activity supports two good features of training. First, within a circuit, activities are alternated which allow recovery from one exercise while completing another. Second, the repetition of circuits provides a greater number of opportunities to develop beneficial effects of fatigue followed by recovery. The programming of exercises to promote these two features is necessary to gain the best results from this form of training.

Circuit training was once touted as a procedure that could result in all manner of physical benefits, including muscular strength, power, and endurance, as well as flexibility and aerobic endurance. Research has shown that some of these benefits were inflated. It is the nature of the exercises and how they are performed that governs the benefits that are derived from this form of training. When flexibility exercises are included in a circuit there is likely to be some improvement in flexibility. Similarly, when power actions are included power will likely be improved. Although circuit training was originally designed as a strength development procedure the inclusion of various activities that stimulate other physical capacities has led to it being a more general program of exercising. When a circuit deliberately focuses on strength by following correct procedures for its development, it can be used for strength training. However, for each activity that attempts to work another physical capacity, the potential for maximum strength benefits is diminished by a corresponding amount.

Circuit training can be used to develop muscular endurance, possibly some strength (if the repetitions are low enough and the resistance high enough), and is often mixed with flexibility and free-standing power and agility activities. There have been claims that circuit training also increases aerobic endurance. Those claims have diminished recently in light of research evidence. While doing circuits, heart rates are usually within a range that suggests an adequate workload for aerobic adaptation. However, these cardio-vascular responses are not accompanied by sufficient elevation of oxygen uptake and so one should not expect much aerobic benefit from circuit training (Hempel and Wells 1985, Hurley, Seals, Ehsani, Carter, Dalskey, Hagberg, and Holloszy 1983). Even when a circuit is expressly designed for cardiovascular fitness (lighter loads of 40–60 percent RM, rest periods less than 30 sec, 12–15 reps) one should not expect changes in aerobic power that exceed 5–8 percent (Fleck and Kraemer 1988a, Gettman and Pollock 1981). It has even been suggested that focused strength training may be harmful to endurance performance because of decreased oxidative potential per total muscle mass (MacDougall *et al.* 1979). At its best circuit training provides only marginal benefits to cardiovascular fitness (Hempel and Wells 1985, Fleck and Kraemer 1988b). Train-ing with high repetitions produces minor aerobic changes that can be achieved better and more quickly by doing exercises that are properly prescribed for endurance work in the activity itself (MacDougall *et al.* 1977).

It is recommended that circuit training be used to focus on muscular strength and endurance, and, to a lesser extent, flexibility development. If fatigue or blood lactates are high, then increases in speed and power will be difficult to attain. Generally, the benefits from circuit training will be mixed because it includes mixed activities for different physical capacities. While it may be an ideal method for developing general fitness when accompanied by pure speed and power training methods as well as other forms of endurance training, it has no value for specialized sports move-ments because of its mixed and non-specific effects.

There are some clearly justified uses for circuit training. Under-standing that a circuit should be designed to match these capacities which are appropriate for a particular sport, its greatest value would seem to be for the basic preparatory and transition phases of training, where multilateral training benefits are sought. There are some sports which need a variety of physical capacities devel-oped, have actions that require forceful movements, and often place a performer in unusual positions. Contact sports frequently require athletes to experience and cope with physical demands for which they have not specifically trained. Wrestling, Australian

Rules football, and American football are good examples of sports where the combinations of physical stress that arise during their competitions are particularly varied and often infrequent. For such sports, circuit training may be an expedient form of beneficial conditioning. Its general training effects may produce an overall physically trained state that would better prepare the body to cope with unexpected events than would restricted specific training effects. For contact sports, it is suggested that circuit training may be engaged in through the specific preparatory and pre-competition phases of training because of the general fitness that it produces.

Circuit training has some other values which support its use. It is motivational in that it provides standards (time on task, number of repetitions) for the athlete. Thus it may be an ideal activity for training outside scheduled practice periods as well as at practice training. When performed in groups, the fact that all athletes are striving for similar standards of performance (hopefully groupings would account for the individuality principle), suggest it as a possible team-building activity emphasizing a work ethic of unity.

A coach will have to carefully consider when to employ circuit training, if at all. Its use as a vehicle for general fitness training in the early phases of an annual plan is justifiable. From then on it should only be used when it can stimulate specific physical capacities that are appropriate for the athlete and sport in a particular phase of training. On the other hand, its general effects can be applicable to sports which have varied and general demands on physical capacities. This is usually the case in contact sports.

□ Programming Circuits

It is recommended that circuits be designed to focus on strength and muscular endurance development. Exercise circuits require a certain number of decisions to be made before they are implemented. These include: the capacities to be trained; the exercises to be performed; the number of repetitions for each exercise; exercises (if any) to be completed in the recovery period (flexibility activities are most appropriate); the number of circuits to be repeated; and the time to be spent on each exercise/recovery phase at each station.

The most difficult feature to determine in circuit training design is the work-to-recovery ratio. In group situations, there will be considerable variation in the time that it will take for each individual to complete a particular number of repetitions of each exercise. Thus if time is used as the basis for moving from one exercise to the next (e.g., if one minute is allotted for the number of exercise repetitions and recovery to take place), there will be different work: recovery ratios within a team or group because of the various completion times for the exercise component between individuals at each station. Despite that drawback, a possible benefit is that work intensities for each exercise can be moderated by the athlete to produce more appropriate training stimuli in much the same way that occurs in variable interval training (see Chapter 13). It is recommended that the coach plan sufficient time at each exercise station for work and recovery to occur rather than specifically designating recovery times, which will in any case need to be varied for each individual.

The manner in which the training loads are progressively increased for a circuit exercise is dictated by the best method for the physical capacity that is being trained. However, there is an overall fatigue that is produced by a circuit. Repeated exposures to this can be used as a method for increasing the capacity of an athlete to perform with intensity in fatigued states. The possible programming parameters for increasing the overall strain of a circuit training program are:

1. increase the number of repetitions for each exercise while still maintaining the same time for each activity
2. decrease the time for each activity while maintaining the same number of repetitions
3. increase the number of circuits
4. change the resistances of each exercise

A general circuit which has been used with Australian football players is shown in Table 14.1. The exercises are illustrated in Figure 14.1 — 5 stations require weights; 3 barbells or sets of dumbells at each station can cater to the range of body weights existing within a team. The circuit shown employs fixed loads and allows 50 seconds for each exercise (the completion of three circuits takes 25 minutes). Three levels of intensity are described. When level A can be completed comfortably in the allotted time period, then the athlete progresses to the next level of difficulty. If an individual loading for the exercises is required, then the athlete can be tested on each activity for maximum performance in 1 minute. The circuit exercise loading then would be 75 percent of the maximum score. Usually with activities such as skipping and bench-stepping a 2-minute test is conducted and 50 percent of that performance is the 1-minute load for the circuit. Bench-stepping can also be increased in loading by raising the height of the bench, sit-ups can be done on an inclined board, and weights can be increased.

Table 14.1 A General Training Circuit for Australian Rules Footballers

Exercise	Apparatus	Circuit		
		A	B	C
1. Skipping	Rope	80	100	120
2. Clean and Press	Barbell — 20% body weight	10	15	20
3. Half-squats	Barbell — 50% body weight	10	15	20
4. Press-ups	None	20	25	30
5. Bench-stepping	45 cm bench	30	40	50
6. Arm-curls	Barbell — 20% body weight	10	15	20
7. Burpees	None	10	15	20
8. Upright Rowing	Barbell — 20% body weight	10	15	20
9. Bench Jumps	Dumbells — 10% body weight (total), 35 cm bench	10	15	20
10. Sit-ups	None	20	25	30

Exercises can be tailored according to the capabilities of those for whom they are designed. For example, press-ups can be done with the knees supported on the floor, sit-ups with hands on the abdomen, and the bench height and barbell/dumbell weights reduced from those indicated in Table 14.1. These exercises can also be made more difficult.

Considerations for Planning Strength Training

The success of any training is determined by the coaching decisions that are made. A number of factors need to be contemplated when planning strength training in an annual plan.

The number and type of exercises for strength training is modified by the level of performance of the athlete, the specific needs of the sport, the age of the athlete, and the phase of training. What is incorporated into a strength training program should be governed by the implications of this book. Strength is merely one physical capacity that requires stimulation, overload, recovery, and appropriate programming. For example, Chapter 20 indicates that young athletes should be exposed to a wide variety of exercises, while élite athletes should emphasize sport-specific activities. This is also true for strength programming. A wide variety of strength training stimuli, exercises, resistance apparatuses, and overload types should be constructed to produce a general strength fitness. It would be incorrect to specialize too early when attempting to train strength because later specializations are best built upon a sound basis of general capacity.

Figure 14.1 Examples of General Circuit Training Exercises for Australian Rules Footballers

(continued overleaf)

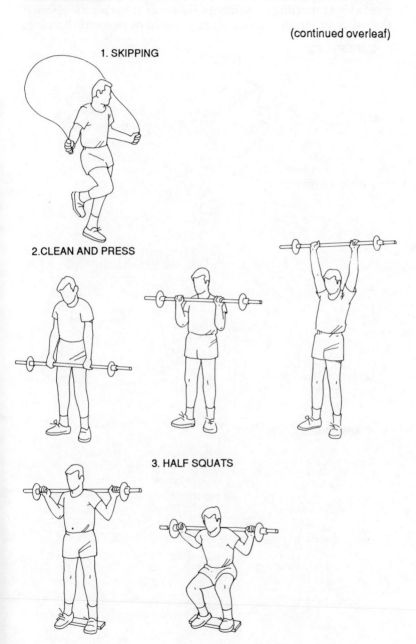

A decision has to be made as to which type of strength training is best. It would seem that isotonic exercises are those which are most akin to sporting movements. However, it has been suggested that when isotonic exercises are augmented by isometric training,

4. PRESS-UPS

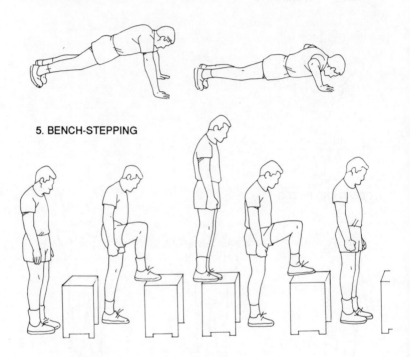

5. BENCH-STEPPING

6. ARM CURLS

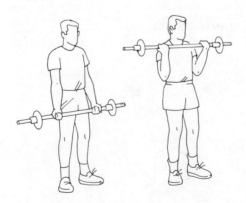

results may be even better (Jackson, Jackson, Hnatek, and West 1985). Impressive strength gains were demonstrated when isotonic activities were supplemented with isometric exercises that focused on the most difficult part of the exercise (the 'sticking-point'). A

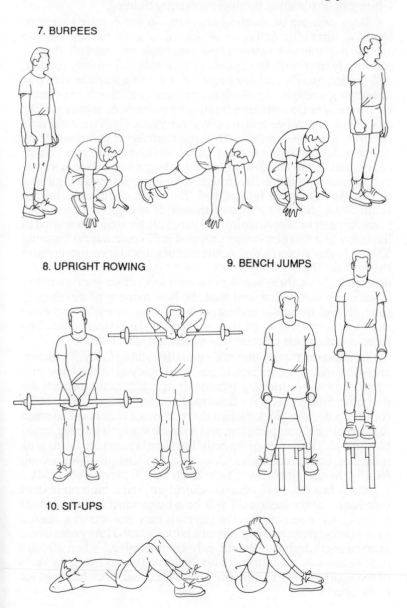

7. BURPEES

8. UPRIGHT ROWING   9. BENCH JUMPS

10. SIT-UPS

program employing full-range movements could be enhanced by using isometrics in this fashion. The implication of this combination seems to make sense but further research needs to be conducted to determine whether it is of any further value than that which can be obtained by single-modality training.

A large number of sporting activities do not require excessive levels of strength. Activities which have a substantial aerobic energy requirement warrant less emphasis on strength than is commonly asserted. The sports of running, swimming, rowing, and cycling usually employ augmented training sessions aimed at developing strength. As much as one-quarter to one-third of training time is spent in resistance training by swimmers, using a variety of exercise machines and in-water activities. Such an emphasis would seem to be excessive. The important factor that needs to be developed for activities of this type is muscular endurance. Costill, Sharp, and Troup (1980) assessed the relationship between swimming speeds and the ability to exert force in a simulated swimming action. An anaerobic fatigue test (muscular endurance) lasting about 50 seconds best indicated the use of strength in swimming. Some 80 percent of swimming 100 yards (91 meters) was related to the test, while that percentage dropped to 50 percent for swimming 500 yards (457 meters), that is, the role of muscular endurance and strength declined as the performance distance increased. It was determined that there was a minimum level of strength required to sprint in swimming and that the best manner of developing strength and muscular endurance was to repeat maximum exercises that duplicate as closely as possible the skills needed. The recommended best exercise was maximum sprint swims.

It would seem that augmented strength training for cyclic, endurance-dominated sports would best be employed in the basic preparatory phase of training where non-specific training effects are desirable. Strength is not a dominant performance capacity, but it could be a deciding factor when the margins of victory are so small in international competitions, and so some strength training could be justified. The nature of the activities should focus on developing muscular endurance rather than absolute strength. This would require the use of relatively light loads (40–50 percent of 1 RM), a relatively fast rate of rhythmical execution, and a high number of repetitions. Since lactic acid will be a by-product of this form of training, some recovery in the intervals between sets in a session as well as between training sessions is important. Heavy resistance, pure-strength training should only be entertained when athletes have below-adequate strength for the correct execution of the skills of the sport. Excessive strength levels are usually not required for cyclic sports.

For court and field games which require maximum efforts and speed, some resistance training could be of value. What was indicated by Costill *et al.* (1980) for swimming would also appear to be true for these activities. Maximum efforts aimed at performing as fast and vigorously as possible would be the most appropriate form of resistance training during the specific preparatory, pre-competitive, and competitive phases of training. Augmented resistance training should be employed in the basic preparatory training phase. The speed of the exercises should be fast. The resistance should be the maximum that can be handled without slowing the speed of execution. Since the employment of any strength gains would be associated with speed development, the intervals between sets of exercises should allow total recovery to occur. If lactic acid is allowed to accumulate it will interfere with the movement speed.

For the two classes of activities discussed above, it would be wrong to complete too many repetitions in a workout. If more exercises are needed, the number of workouts should increase, not the length of the training session (Poliquin 1985).

The planning of resistance and strength training programs should follow the guidelines of sound programming. The application of overloads should be 'periodized' into stepped increases, with the end of each step employing a session of reduced stimulus intensity. Variations in exercise stimulation are needed to make optimum gains in strength and power. Thus a general feature of programming will be to employ a variety of tasks to achieve the same training objective (Fleck and Kraemer 1988).

Because of the limited transfer of training effects, strength training is, in many cases, only remotely related to performance improvements in non-strength-dominated sports. However, even small gains in strength may be sufficient to produce the minor performance improvements that are critical for success in élite competitions. Specific regimens aimed at developing strength would seem to be important for élite athletes. Other performance improvement factors are more important for youthful and maturing athletes. Thus, as a general principle, strength and resistance programs should be general for developing athletes, but should become more specific as the level of athlete achievement rises. It would be wrong for a coach to employ specific-strength training as a means of performance improvement in a young athlete. The short-term gains would compromise possible long-term improvements (see Chapter 20).

As the training of an élite athlete progresses, only specific-strength exercises should remain at the end of the pre-competitive training phase. It is debatable whether strength training should be used in the competitive phase. If it is, the focus should be on maintenance, not development.

Final Considerations

Augmented strength and resistance training is not the ultimate form of training to develop sport strength. In some circumstances it may contribute to the basis of performance by increasing the strength of the muscles that control the dynamic posture of large muscle groups, particularly the spine, trunk, and shoulders, and provide an element of a multilateral base that could be included in new performance developments.

The ability to use strength is inversely proportional to the speed of the performance action. Very fast activities do not need high levels of strength while slow activities do. In some sports it may be necessary to develop strength for relatively slow movements (e.g, starting from the blocks in a sprint race) but not for other aspects of the activity (e.g, running as fast as possible in the sprint phase of the race). Thus strength training would seem to be of greater value for slower forms of movement even within a sport.

The value of the time that is dedicated to augmented strength training sessions has to be reconciled with the amount of time that is spent in training for the sport. There is the possibility that strength training could be overemphasized to the point where it interferes with the performance gains that can be expected from other training forms. If the residual fatigue from a resistance training session carries over to actual training, then the learning of skills and the development of capacities such as speed, power, and aerobic endurance may be hindered. If the time spent is such that specific-sport training is reduced to accommodate it, then performance improvements will be lessened because of the reduction in the volume of specific training. This leads to the recommendation that *augmented strength or resistance training should only be employed when it is not possible to entertain further sport-specific training.* A coach should not sacrifice an opportunity to practice on the football field or in a swimming pool in order to complete a strength-training session.

When strength gains lessen (that is, when a ceiling level of development is approached) and performances still improve, the need for strength training becomes one of maintenance. The training time released through a maintenance program should be employed for more beneficial sport-specific training.

Although research shows that physiological changes occur with resistance training, one has to ask if these changes can be used effectively and beneficially in sports. Because of the specific effects that are produced by strength training exercises, the benefits to be gained for many sports are minimal. Popular coaching practices seem to overemphasize strength training and its importance for performance improvements. A moderation of that emphasis is warranted. Many programming decisions for strength and resistance training appear to be driven by belief rather than by an understanding of scientific knowledge.

15
Power and Speed Training

Power is usually described as a function of both the force (strength) and speed of movement. One could assert that any movement is a power movement, for all movements entail some strength and speed. However, when an action is very fast and seems to require relatively little effort it is usually classified as a speed movement. On the other hand, when an action seems to need considerable effort it is a power movement. The two concepts are, however, interrelated. The basic difference between a power event and a sustained sprint event is that in a power event the athlete never reaches his or her maximum energy capacity. Further, the difference between a sprint event and a middle-distance event is that in a sprint anaerobic energy release is more important than oxygen consumption, whereas in the middle-distance event the opposite is true (Bompa 1986).

The performance of power or speed activities is dependent on their interrelationship. Every activity has a desirable speed of performance that is accompanied by a maximum level of useable strength. Thus for power and speed actions there are very specific combinations or balances of speed and strength.

Power and speed movements are purely learned actions. Their improvement is primarily determined by a neural reorganization of existing physical structures and attributes. Bobbert, Van Ingen Schenau, and Huijing (1985) concluded that the adaptations associated with improvements in explosive power are subtle, and are heavily dependent on connective tissue dynamics and neural inputs. Grabe and Widule (1988) determined that much of the training effect from explosive power training is due to the motor learning of the skill associated with the activity. As was indicated in the previous chapter on strength, neuromuscular patterning as an adaptive response is very specific. Power and speed training should be as specific as possible to a sport. In fact the actual activities of the sport would seem to be the best training exercises for the development of both speed and power.

To illustrate the potency of neuromuscular patterning for determining power performances, Grabe and Widule's (1988) study will be recounted. They examined the differences in technique of Olympic-type weight-lifters of varying performance levels. The better performers exhibited a more economical acceleration of the bar, accomplished by generating the upward momentum of the jerk phase of the clean-and-jerk with a shorter duration (faster) motion and by reducing the depth of the squat and the length of time spent braking in the counter-movement. The better performers also had a greater economy of work for a given weight as they reduced the distance travelled by the bar by dropping lower for the catch and eliminating unnecessary horizontal motion of the bar. This description implies that subtle changes in technique can account for relatively large changes in the performance of power events and that technique is the major determinant of power. Bobbert et al. (1985) also concluded that technique is a major factor in power training when they suggested that in addition to training the appropriate muscle groups at high forces and velocities, the specific joint kinematics should be duplicated as well.

Several studies have been conducted to assess the development and evaluate the potential of testing for power (Bedi, Cresswell, Engel, and Nicol 1987, Berg, Miller, and Stephens 1986, Mayhew, Schwegler, and Piper 1986, Tharp, Johnson, and Thorland 1984). A synthesis of these works led these authors to contend that the results of various testing methods of explosive power cannot be applied across sport groups and many of the tests may be significantly influenced by factors other than explosiveness. Close attention needs to be paid to the validity of power tests. While some sports certainly involve vertical jumping (e.g, volleyball, basketball) and short running sprints, the relevance of stair climbing, cycle sprints, and ball-throwing tests of muscle power must be carefully evaluated in relation to the movements involved in the sport.

Training for power and speed would seem to be relatively simple. The activity itself should form the basis of the form of movement, the technique should be as economical as possible, and given the restrictions of this, the action should be as intense as possible. However, a dilemma arises for the coach training for power and speed. If these types of action use existing capacities (the trained states of fast and slow-twitch fibers) then it would seem to be best to have these in the best state of training possible before they are coordinated into a powerful or speedy action. Training for power and speed is far from optimum if the muscle fibers are not physically adapted for strength and muscular endurance. Before power and speed training of a specific nature is entertained, there needs to be considerable multilateral training of strength and muscular and aerobic endurance achieved. These enhanced physical attributes will then be employed as the power and speed activities are 'learned'. There are a number of general training implications that can be drawn from this:

1. Multilateral strength and muscular and aerobic endurance should be maintained to a relatively high degree in the transition phase of training and then emphasized more in the basic preparatory phase than power or speed training.
2. Late in the basic preparatory phase of training, multilateral power and speed activities should be developed.
3. In the middle of the specific preparatory phase, specific technique power and speed training should be commenced. It is advisable to continue with specific strength and muscular endurance training while specific power and speed are developed. This will maintain the physical status of the muscle fibers.
4. The specific training of power and speed, with particular relevance to sport technique (Brown *et al.* 1986) and the maintenance of its supportive strength and muscular endurance activities, should continue through the pre-competition and competition phases of training (only being reduced during a peaking macrocycle).

Essentially, the concept underlying power and speed training is the same. Trained muscle fibers are coordinated through a learning process to function in an economically improved manner. The level of that improvement is determined by the mechanical efficiency of movements. Thus the technique that is taught, the physical status of the muscles, and the opportunities for learning and performance refinement will determine the success of training for power and speed. Factors which dictate how training should be prescribed are:

1. Lactic acid production should not be encouraged by each set of repetitions or exercise. Adequate recovery should occur between trials.
2. The highest possible intensity of an exercise should be the aim. Anything less than a maximum effort will train different neuromuscular patterns. If these are conducted in

sufficient volume, there will be poor, and even negative, transfer to maximum efforts.

3. Given the above two factors, the volume of training should be as high as possible. The time spent at training doing power and speed work of a specific nature will determine the improvement that is possible.

4. Power and speed work at a training session should be scheduled early so that no residual fatigue or lactic acid will interfere with its development (see Chapter 18).

It would seem that the best form of power and speed training, once the prerequisite physical states of the muscles have been attained, is maximum effort at a particular skill. Any training other than a maximum effort should be considered to be counter-productive. There are many activities that are proposed as being power and speed activities but their effects have to be verified.

Power Training

In sports where high resistances need to be overcome the power generated is largely dependent on the amount of force that can be exerted. Strength is an important factor in accelerating heavy objects or the body weight (e.g., rugby-scrummaging, shot-putting, sprint-starting, weight-lifting). When light resistances are encountered the speed factor dominates and great strength is not required. This is the case in baseball-pitching, football-kicking, and javelin-throwing. The generation of muscular power is dependent on the coordination of both the fibers within muscles and groups of muscles. The relationships between force, speed, and power are shown in Figure 15.1. Large forces cannot be exerted at high speeds, that is, sports that require fast movements do not need unusually high levels of strength in their athletes. Peak power is generated at that speed which allows a force in the 30 to 40 percent of maximum force range. The nature of an activity should be considered before assigning resistances that enable athletes to work at specific points on the force–velocity curve. Sports requiring athletes to overcome high resistances quickly would do power training towards the lower end of the force–velocity curve while those requiring faster movements would work closer to the higher end of this curve.

Since power training involves moving resistances quickly, a training program should include rotary movements, rather than just those in one plane, and a balance between prime-mover and antagonist muscle activity. Power training should only be initiated after a sound preparatory program of muscular endurance and strength training. That will allow established strength to be coordinated into movements and will decrease the likelihood of injury. Specific power training should also be planned to coincide with the initiation of skill development so that continual refinements of performance can be made to include power gains. Training activities usually involve 15–20 repetitions of an exercise with the resistance being between 30 and 50 percent of 1 RM. Power gains will not be made if the exercise technique does not stress maximum speed in each repetition.

Figure 15.1 A Stylized Curve Illustrating the Relationships between Force, Speed (Velocity), and Power

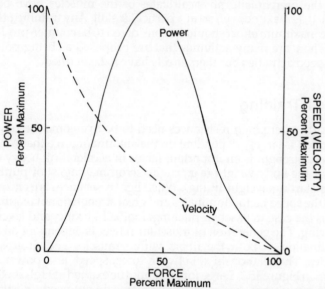

There are three major features of this graph: when speed is very high the percent of maximum force that can be exerted is very low; when maximum forces are to be exerted the speed of movement should be very slow; and maximum power (the best combination of force and speed) is achieved at that speed which uses 30–40 percent of maximum force. These relationships have obvious implications for the emphases of training items that are planned for power and speed development.

Plyometrics

One of the most popular activities for developing power is plyometric training. It attempts to use the weight of the body itself or pieces of equipment to increase the stimulus of training. Plyometric exercises use the force of gravity to increase stored elastic energy in muscles during the eccentric contraction (preparatory phase) of an action. Some of that stored energy is then released in the concentric contraction (release phase) which immediately follows. This extra stored energy facilitates an elevated performance. Plyometric exercises are used to train the eccentric aspect of muscle action (Wilt 1975). There are a variety of forms of this type of training ('rebounding', 'bounding', 'depth-jumping'). The major ingredients of these exercises are:

1. the elevation of the centre of gravity of the body so that when it drops to the ground, the added force of gravity creates a greater than normal amount of stored energy in the musculature
2. contact with the ground and movement direction change
3. the projection of the body either vertically, horizontally, or some combination of the two
4. the performance of the exercise in a smooth, integrated fashion in which there are no obvious decelerations or pauses

There are two major components developed with plyometric exercises. The first is the athlete's neuromuscular reaction during the 'amortization' phase. This occurs for the time that the athlete is in contact with the ground. The shorter this phase, the greater the athlete's neuromuscular reaction to the ground contact stimulus. The implication here is that with the greater stimulus during the preparatory phase of a jump, greater power will result. The second component is the amount of elastic strength the athlete possesses. Elastic strength relates to those properties of muscle-tendon tissue which allow it to be stretched rapidly, thereby increasing internal muscular tension (stored energy), and subsequently facilitating a rapid forceful shortening of the muscle (Chu 1984).

Wilt (1975) described why plyometrics should work in sports:

1. Maximum tension develops when active muscle is stretched quickly. Thus, when the speed of an exercise is increased by the force of gravity, it produces a faster eccentric contraction and muscle stretching in the preparatory phase of the action. This results in a better concentric contraction being produced in the ensuing movement.
2. The rate of stretch in the eccentric contraction phase of a movement is more important than the magnitude of the stretch. This means that fast stretching is achieved by doing a fast preparatory movement in the exercise.
3. The increased forces in an exercise that result from using gravity to its maximum effect will produce greater levels of training overload and therefore, as a result of training, will produce eventually greater levels of performance.

To illustrate the above point, it is predicted that jump-squat training (where the feet leave the ground as a result of rapid eccentric and explosive concentric contractions in the leg and hip muscles) will eventually produce more powerful movements than will squat training (where the feet always remain on the ground during the exercise). *It is the speed component of this form of exercise that is important* (Brown, Mayhew, and Boleach 1986). Slow exercises, such as when one does very heavy squatting, do not produce training effects for fast movements.

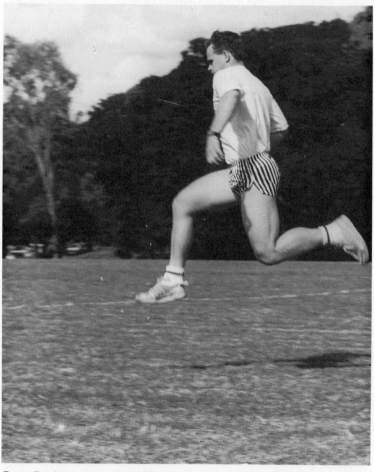

Bounding is a commonly used plyometric exercise in which the contraction force of the muscle is increased by stretching it forcefully when the body is lowered

To illustrate the features of plyometric exercises, the majority of this section will use the vertical jump as the example activity. It is an action where the contributions of different body segments act on the centre of gravity of the whole body. The vertical jump is an accepted test for determining leg-power in athletes (Pyke 1980).

The basis for using plyometrics as a training method lies in the elasticity of the muscles. Bosco and Komi (1979) compared vertical jumps for a static, a semi-squat, an erect counter-movement jump position, and a depth-jump. The pre-stretching of the muscle involved in the counter-movement and depth-jumps caused storage of elastic energy in the muscles which resulted in better levels of performance. The depth-jump produced the best performance. This was explained as being caused by the mechanical work that developed through a spring-like behavior in which restitution of elastic energy played an important role. Asmussen and Bonde-Petersen (1974) also demonstrated the ability of muscles to store elastic energy for later use. They also concluded that there is an optimum height for depth-jumping. Heights which are low do not produce maximum stimulation while excessively high heights exceed the individual's capacity to use the forces generated. However, Bedi et al. (1987) did not find any significant difference between depth-jumps of various heights. It was shown that trained jumpers (e.g., volleyball players) performed significantly better at all heights than did non-jumpers. The determination of the height for depth-jumping should be made by finding the drop-height which produces the best resultant jump. As performance improves, the height should be increased gradually. As a rule of thumb, the height of the drop should match the height of the rebound.

Research on vertical-jump training has produced mixed results. When isometric and isotonic resistance programs were used for improving quadriceps strength, strength changes were noted but no change in vertical jumping occurred (McKethan and Mayhew 1974). This suggested that the strength training regimen did not transfer to the power of vertical-jumping. However, Blattner and Noble (1979) compared isokinetic (3 × 10 maximum speed leg-presses), plyometric (3 × 10 jumps from 0·86 meters), and control groups on vertical-jumps. Both training groups improved but were not significantly different. This suggests that plyometrics was an effective, but not the only, method for improving vertical-jumping.

Strength training combined with almost any kind of jumping can be an effective training regimen. They also suggested that plyometric depth-jumps are useful for athletes who are doing no other jumping, but the activity adds nothing extra to that which was obtained from 'normal practice', where a good deal of maximum-jumping occurs.

Brown *et al.* (1986) compared plyometric with no plyometric training in basketball players during a competitive season. They concluded that the superior performance of the plyometric group was derived from 57 percent jumping skill and 43 percent strength gains. The plyometric training appeared to enhance the coordination of the arms (a learned factor) with strength development in the legs even though the sport itself supported reasonable jumping ability while not inducing maximum jumping potential.

For vertical jumping it appears that depth-jumping has a considerable degree of transfer of training effect. However, there is a suggestion that maximum jumping in sports such as volleyball will also produce similar improvements. It would seem that the common factor between the two possibilities for training is that the *jumps must be maximally executed*. Anything less, such as most of the jumping that occurs in basketball, will not effect an improvement. Additionally, weight-training, other than maximally explosive efforts of an isotonic type, will also have little value for effecting the power involved in a vertical-jump. The research seems to suggest that depth-jump training is valuable for non-jumping athletes to produce greater vertical-jumping capacity. A generalization from that contention is that explosive and plyometric activities are the types best suited to producing power in physical performance.

☐ Training with Plyometrics

The essential feature of plyometric training is that it aims to employ a faster rate of preparatory action (the eccentric contraction phase) of a movement followed by a maximum-effort release (concentric contraction phase). Some external force is added to the preparatory action; for example, gravity in depth-jumps. However, there are a variety of methods and pieces of equipment that can produce a faster movement than that which occurs doing a normal exercise. For arm extension power, explosive press-ups that allow a hand-clap to be executed at the end of the arm-extension movement will produce a more power-oriented activity than that which occurs in straight press-ups when the hands do not leave the ground. Similarly, a military press with a bar release at the full extension position (so that the bar is caught on the way down) should produce power for arm extension activities in an upright posture. These are two examples of modifying standard exercises to produce more power and speed in their execution which also develops greater eccentric contractions in the preparatory phase.

The tossing and catching of medicine balls increases the eccentric loading of muscles in the upper body. Using various pieces of gymnastic equipment as well as performing stunts that require the weight to be taken on the hands also appear to use the principles of plyometric exercise. For leg work, depth-jumping from varying heights is one of the most common exercises (particularly for long, triple, and high-jumpers). Sets of continuous maximum bounds for distance are popular activities amongst the top skiers of the world. Double-leg bounding over obstacles is another action that is frequently suggested. However, bounding loses its potential benefit if the exertion is not maximum (i.e., if athletes clear obstacles by manipulating their legs and trunk rather than by projecting the centre of gravity in a maximum fashion). The essential feature of plyometric training is that *athletes have to seek the opportunity to produce the greatest force possible by incurring the greatest load possible.* Half-hearted plyometric exercises will be of little value.

The loads that can be incurred in plyometric work are very severe. This is one activity where injuries are possible and the coach must be extremely cautious in the way it is programmed. Light workouts should be planned in the early stages, with increments of overload being too small rather than too large and being introduced in a step-like fashion. Thus, maximum plyometric work should only be employed when a thorough conditioning and developmental program has been completed. A sample progression of activities in a developmental program for leg power is:

Stage 1	Repetition hops (single- and double-leg)
	Repetition steps
	Lateral hops and steps
Stage 2	Same exercises for Stage 1 but introduce greater depth and extension in movements
Stage 3	Repetition hops over low obstacles (adds a vertical component)
	Repetition hops on and off benches
	Combination hops and steps for distance (single- and double-leg)
Stage 4	Depth-jumping
	Elevated take-off:
	— rebound
	— horizontal (forward)
	— vertical (upward)
	— combinations of the above

The determinant of the depth for a jump or any plyometric activity is that the height of the drop should match the height of the rebound. Similarly, for medicine ball work, the distance from which a ball is caught should not exceed the distance of the return throw executed in the same action. It is important to understand that the preparatory and release phases of plyometric exercises are performed as one coordinated movement. Any break in the natural rhythm of the action will negate its intended benefits.

At the start of a depth-jumping program the bench height should be no more than 30 centimeters but can be progressively elevated to 80 centimeters or more over the course of a training program. As a general rule, depth-jumping should only be introduced after several weeks of horizontal bounding exercises. Heel cups should be used and the drills done on soft surfaces, such as mats or grass, to protect the lower limbs. The knees should not be flexed beyond 90° during the preparatory phase of the action.

General plyometric exercises appear to be a good form of activity for multilateral power training in the basic preparatory phase. If they can be made more specific they should be continued into the specific preparatory and pre-competition training phases. Some multilateral work should be performed to maintain the capacities developed in the basic preparatory phase.

Extra-load Training

This form of training uses weight added to the body to increase the effort required to perform 'normal' activity. The additional weight can be situated on the extremities, as with wrist and ankle weights, or centrally on the body. There was considerable research on the value of wrist and ankle weights (i.e., low resistances) for improving performance in the 1960s. The belief behind this training procedure was that the extra load would make the athlete work harder (possibly more powerfully), which would result in better performances. After reviewing the research literature Rushall (1970) reported that these devices did not improve performance. Adjustments to technique to handle the 'minor' loads might produce negative training effects because of the subtle alteration to refined neuromuscular movement patterns. Extremity weights have the potential to be more damaging than beneficial. Indeed, there have been commercial attempts in tennis to use heavier racquets and balls, in baseball to use lighter balls, and in running to use ankle weights, but they have not been widely accepted. It is a common response of élite athletes to dislike factors which alter a 'grooved', relatively successful pattern and feeling of movement. This can also be the problem when weighted pulley systems are used to simulate throwing, kicking, or pulling movements. If the movements are similar, but not quite 'right', they run the risk of being rejected by the athlete. Extra-load resistances that are used on the extremities have not been shown to be of value for training.

A positive effect of wearing a weighted vest (7–8 percent of body weight) was reported by Bosco *et al*. (1984). The subjects for both experimental and control groups were sprinters who were no longer improving. Vests were worn all day except in skill acquisition training. After three weeks the controls had no performance or test variable changes. The experimental group improved in the 15-second continuous jumping test and the drop-jump test. This meant that the power in these activities had been improved and the force–velocity curve shifted to the right. Anatomical measures were not altered but the mechanical power was clearly enhanced by the extra-load conditioning. This desirable outcome needs to be replicated before it is advocated as being a training principle. However, a case can be made for considering its effectiveness. The vest might act to 'centralize' the extra-load where it may not be disruptive to the 'feeling' of an action. Since an athlete can work with a usual technique, but in a harder manner, there is a potential for improvement through overload, in much the same way that plyometric exercises further overload an exercise. It would seem that the continual wearing of significantly weighted vests with a view to improving power in power and speed sports has potentially beneficial effects.

Extra-load training might influence performance in a positive sense if the load is centrally placed on the athlete's torso. It is not beneficial when it is applied to the extremities. The continual wearing of a vest has the potential for multilateral benefits as well as specific training benefits. To preserve the integrity of neuromuscular skill patterns, the vests should not be worn during exact skill learning or practice but should be alternated with these activities within a training program.

Speed Training

Speed work involves an emphasis on completing an activity in the shortest time possible. The amount of strength that can be employed while moving fast will determine how much power (speed × strength) is applied. The development of speed is subject to all the factors that surround effective learning. Apart from the physical activities that are used to stage speed training, the psychological factors of feedback and attentional focus are paramount to achieving results. For pure speed training, the exercise should be limited to avoid any development of lactic acid, with sufficient recovery allowed between repetitions. Speed training should terminate when technique changes due to fatigue (*Coaching Review* 1985).

The following discussion of speed development will be restricted to sprint running so that one topic can be explored fully. The coach will have to take the general principles which are discussed and adapt them to a particular sport. Non-scientific journal articles on sprinting and jumping cover a wide range of training regimes including the use of quite unusual devices. Arakelyan, Raitsin, Manzhuev, and Brazhnik (1985) described attaching a harness system to a sprinter and then applying various loads to the thighs by means of weights and elastic bands while the athlete sprinted. This suggestion may seem to be innovative but one must suspect that it will alter the basic kinematic properties of sprinting (e.g., support and flight times, stride length, rhythm, stride rate). Such an alteration will not facilitate the practice and refinement of the correct neuromuscular pattern that would occur in non-restrained sprinting. The use of such devices would violate the principle of specificity and may be harmful if employed in any phase of training other than the basic preparatory one.

Running on a downhill grade has been suggested (Yakimovich 1986). The benefit of such an activity would be determined by the similarity of techniques used in flat and downhill running. The more dissimilar they are, the less value the activity would have. A practical determinant of similarity in sprinting techniques is the amount of stiffness and fatigue that results from the new technique. Thus if an athlete has been training exclusively on the track and then attempts some downhill speed work, the subjective reports of the severity of stiffness and soreness after 24 hours or a night's sleep will indicate how dissimilar the activities are. The maximum downhill slope that can be used to produce increased running speeds is $-2°$. Slopes greater than $-2°$ will alter technique in a non-productive fashion. A potentially beneficial training procedure is to perform as much training as possible with a following wind. Reductions in wind resistance could facilitate supra-maximal sprinting.

A popular tendency in sprint training is to use a program of varied activities. This smacks of a multilateral approach and has the potential to be excessively time-consuming, produce harmful fatigue, and distract the athlete from more beneficial activities. Derbaba and Petrov (1984) recommended a comprehensive program of sprint, flexibility, plyometric, jumping, and weight training to improve performance for long and triple jumping. When multiactivity programs are provided it is not possible to determine which activities are and are not influential for producing a performance change. The suggestions of the Soviet writers are representative of the lack of consistency found between the training methods for sprint training.

One factor that has not been researched thoroughly is that of reduced resistance training. Karvonen, Peltola, and Saarela (1986) compared altitude (1,850 meters) training with sea-level training in Finnish national-level sprinters during final preparations for a main competition. Reduced air and gravity resistances at altitude increased speed and explosive strength. Altitude training is popularly considered as an environment that might be beneficial to endurance runners (see Chapter 9). This benefit is questionable. However, it has not been popularly advocated for sprint and power events for which it might be better suited.

□ Effects of Speed Training

The physiological effects of speed training have not been studied in the same detail as those of endurance training. However, some features have been established:

Muscle fiber changes: Increases occur in the size of fast-twitch muscle fibers, the total phosphagen content of muscle, and the concentration of enzymes responsible for splitting glycogen to lactic acid (with sustained-sprint training) and breaking down high-energy phosphates. These improvements closely relate to increases in alactacid and lactacid anaerobic energy capacities.

Anaerobic power: Improvements in both the strength and speed of contraction of the muscles are commonly observed. This has been displayed through improvements in anaerobic power and speed.

Aerobic power: Only small increases in $\dot{V}O_2$ max have been induced by traditional sprint training. However, there are likely to be significant effects achieved through ultra-short training. When brief bursts of activity are interspersed with short recovery periods, the cardio-respiratory system is taxed. When longer sprinting distances are used for training, there usually is insufficient volume of work to stimulate significant aerobic adaptation. However, the magnitude of this change relates to the level of aerobic fitness of the individual and is probably non-existent in a trained athlete undergoing specialised sprint training.

Neuromuscular considerations: External manifestations of improved mechanics, such as increased stride length, movement-cycle rate, and range of joint movements (e.g., height of knee lift in running) have been shown to result from sprint programs. The neuromuscular events responsible for a large and smooth expression of force appear to be of considerable importance but, as yet, have not been well studied. However, it seems logical to suggest that these mechanisms are enhanced by sprint training.

☐ Programming Speed Training

A challenge for programming speed training is how to get the sporting activity to be performed at a speed which exceeds that of the contest activity. Sufficient repetitions of such supra-maximal activities could be used to train the body to move faster than normal, that is, the supra-speed neuromuscular patterning has to become strong enough to supplant a slower established pattern. Consequently, activities have to be devised that will produce super-speed in sport-specific actions. Since speed is a neural organization activity, non-specific speed training will have insignificant to no transfer to a specific-sport action.

The basic requirements of speed training for any activity are those that underlie strength and power training: the technique, the nature of the muscular work, the speed of movement, and the intensity of the activity should be the same as those desired for the competitive performance. The major task is to stimulate enhanced performance speeds and then train the athlete to produce them for the duration of the competition. Improvements in sprinting skill can be achieved by attending to the training emphases of skill, fitness, and psychology.

☐ Skill

Sprinting speed is a product of action length (stride) and rate (turnover, striding tempo). The optimum length and rate of movement results from a complex and synchronized series of neuro-muscular events that are designed to suit both the physical characteristics of the individual and the specific nature of the task. An increase in either or both length and rate of action will produce greater speed of movement. In sprint running, there are two phases of the task which are worthy of attention.

1. *Acceleration.* The initiation of movement from a stationary position requires a strength component which rapidly diminishes in importance as the runner accelerates to maximum speed. The characteristics of a running technique to produce acceleration are a forward lean, an exaggerated foot strike rate, and quick, short arm actions which minimize rotary movements. Attention to teaching these features and their gradual alteration through the transition stage to full-speed running is necessary.

2. *Full-speed running.* The maintenance of full-speed running is facilitated by a technique which demonstrates a high knee lift which produces a resultant longer ground contact and leg-drive action; a foot placement being on the toes or ball of the foot which effectively lengthens the limb and im-

proves the mechanical efficiency of the leg muscles; an upright, relaxed posture (unnecessary tension will inhibit moving in the fastest manner possible); and a full-arm action in which the movement is directly backwards and forwards from the shoulder, with elbows close to the side, also contributing to the length of the stride.

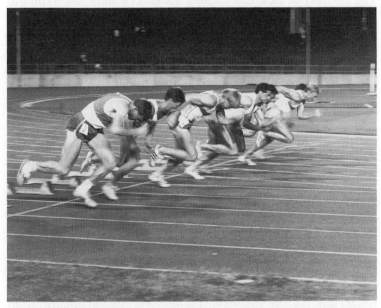

The ability to accelerate quickly is vital in sprinting events and in many team sports. An acceleration training program must include practice of specific techniques associated with body position and arm and leg action

The coach should concentrate on eliminating faults in technique and develop appropriate changes at slower speeds before progressing to faster ones. Fatigued states should be avoided when attempting to correct faults. For activities where running speed is incorporated with directional alterations, drills involving lateral movements, reversals (e.g., shuttle runs), and changes in body position (e.g., lying or kneeling to running) are important ingredients of an acceleration and agility skill training program. Reaction drills involving the practice of fast responses to common stimuli such as sound, light, or movement are also useful in this context.

The techniques used in speed activities offer the greatest avenue for speed improvement. Fitness developments are limited, and psychological factors enhance performance only to the limits of mechanical and fitness attributes.

☐ Fitness

It is not possible for an athlete to maintain maximum speed for the duration of a 100-meter or longer running event. Thus fitness training should aim at developing the greatest capacity to extend the length of time that maximum running speed can be maintained. The intensity of all sprint training activities should be maximum, since anything less should not be expected to contribute to improvements in either speed or acceleration.

The most appropriate form of sprint training would appear to be ultra-short interval training (see Chapter 13). The repetition of shorter-than- race distances is programmed. The duration of the training task should be such that no lactic acid is accumulated, and the primary source of fuel is the alactacid energy system. Since the capacity to develop this energy source is restricted, sprinting improvements resulting from fitness are quite limited. However, ultra-short training can be used as a program activity to alter fitness as well as a stage for altering and practicing sprinting technique.

In some sports (e.g., swimming, rowing) the work/recovery ratio can be as little as 1 : 1, but in sprint running the ratio is likely to be higher. One reason for that elevation is the need to accelerate and decelerate after each burst of super-speed running. Those two features consume considerable amounts of energy and so have to be factored into the work/recovery ratio. The response of each individual to the demands of the exercise and the energy cost of each repetition will determine the work/recovery cycle of each repetition. For sprints of 25–40 meters which include acceleration from a stationary position, the rest period is likely to range from 30 to 45 seconds. As the distance increases and lactic acid starts to be produced, the duration of the recovery will begin to extend markedly. The coach has to *develop training stimuli which produce the greatest volume of repetitions of super-speed running while minimizing the occurrence of harmful fatigue.* This will usually require the allocation of a much longer than normal training session for speed work, a greater proportion of which will be spent in recovery and returning to the area in which the sprint is to be performed after deceleration has occurred. The recovery period should also include activity (flexibility exercises and constant movement) so that the total body remains warm and functional. This will accelerate recovery and diminish the possibility of injury due to cooling. This is important and is often neglected by coaches, particularly those who believe that only 'hard' work, that is, the development of fatigued states, is the secret to success. It is also important to schedule speed work as the first physical capacity to be developed in the training session so that no residual or accumulated fatigue from training the other capacities occurs. This is contradictory to the practices of sports such as rowing, swimming, and many team games where speed work is normally entertained at the end of practice sessions. Since speed development is a neural adaptation it is important to provide as many trials as possible using the exact neuromuscular pattern of the intended competitive performance.

The general fitness of the body is also important for speed work. For example, a major technique factor is being able to produce a stable central torso against which forces can be applied. If the body posture cannot be maintained, alterations and movements will absorb some of the energy that is produced (i.e., it acts like a shock absorber). It is necessary that the greatest proportion of the sum of all developed forces be applied to moving the body. Consequently, a general fitness that can support the technique features of speed work is needed. Strength, power, and flexibility training are necessary supplementary training considerations that should be continued throughout both change and maintenance stages of training.

The selection of the most appropriate fitness training depends on the individual athlete. If strength or stride length problems are diagnosed, the amount of uphill work facilitating an increase in muscle strength and power and stride length should exceed that undertaken downhill or on the flat (possibly by as much as a ratio of 2 : 1). On the other hand, if a limitation in stride rate acts as a barrier to speed gain, it is probably more desirable to do more downhill and flat running that aids movement speed than uphill work. Attention to the details of technique and fitness training for speed development is of paramount importance.

Speed-oriented fitness training should only be implemented when athletes are well conditioned. The intensity of the efforts is such that injuries are possible. It is important that the warm-ups be extensive and specific to the activities that will be performed. Attention should also be paid to maintaining a warmed and prepared state during recovery periods in the training program.

There are various forms of interval training for sprinting that should be considered for programming.

Ultra-short interval sprint training for running: This training form should be the most commonly programmed for it offers both alactacid energy and technique improvement. Guidelines for this form of training are:

1. Duration of work	3–6 sec
2. Intensity of work	100% (maximum) +
3. Duration of recovery	30–45 sec
4. Repetitions	until performance starts to deteriorate
5. Energy system	alactacid (ATP–CP)

Examples of ultra-short repetition for running for a male high-school sprinter would be:

Repetitions	Distance	Intensity	Work/recovery period	Recovery activity
15 ×	30 m	100%+	30 sec	stretch/walk
10 ×	40 m	100%+	60 sec	stretch/jog

Short interval sprint training for running:

1. Duration of work		6–15 sec
2. Intensity of work		100%
3. Duration of recovery		1–2 min
4. Repetitions		until inadequate recovery or performance deteriorates
5. Energy system		alactacid with some lactacid when longer intervals are used

Examples of short-interval training items for a female college sprinter are:

Repetitions	Distance	Intensity	Work/recovery period	Recovery activity
10 ×	60 m	95%+	90 sec	stretch/walk
5 ×	75 m	95–100%+	2 min	walk/stretch

Sustained-sprint training for running: The ability to sustain speed and tolerate elevated levels of lactic acid in the muscles is particularly important in events lasting between 20 and 60 seconds, but it can also play a role in efforts that take considerably less time. Because the work period is prolonged and the effort intense, the anaerobic release of energy by the process of glycogen splitting to lactic acid predominates. A minor portion of the energy will be derived from aerobic processes. This training is extremely strenuous and should be included in the latter stages of the practice session but before pure aerobic work is entertained. It should form part of the preparation for events such as the 400-meter run and, for that matter, any event where a sustained sprint is required (e.g., towards the end of a middle-distance effort). Sustained sprinting should only be incorporated after a substantial aerobic base has been established (i.e., the latter stage of the specific preparatory phase). Using an interval format, the factors involved in sustained-sprint training are:

1. Duration of work	20–45 sec
2. Intensity of work	95% (as fast and relaxed as possible)
3. Duration of recovery	3–5 min
4. Repetitions	5–10
5. Energy systems	alactacid, lactacid, and some aerobic in longer intervals

An example of sustained-sprint training for a national-caliber male runner would be:

Repetitions	Distance	Intensity	Work/recovery period	Recovery activity
7 ×	200 m	90–95%	3½ min	walk/jog
5 ×	300 m	> 90%	5 min	walk/jog

An alternative form of programming for sustained sprinting is to complete two-thirds of the competition distance at racing speed before permitting a recovery period. Hence, a 400-meter runner might do a series of 250-meter efforts at 400-meter racing pace. Lactic acid would gradually increase throughout a series of 6–8 repetitions and would be close to maximum at the end of the training bout.

Summary

Both power and speed training require attention to two necessary factors: the technique of the training activity needs to be specific to the sport (the best suggestion is to do the sporting activity itself), and each repetition must be performed with maximum velocity. Minor departures from these two specifications will greatly reduce the value of any activity for the development of either useful power or speed. The best interpretation for both speed and power training is that what is practiced is learned. The adaptations that occur through power and speed training, because neither is done to fatigue, are neuromuscular patterns. Thus athletes will improve in the manner in which they practice. Anything less than exact practice will not result in desired outcomes.

Attention should be paid to when specific power and speed training is instituted in an annual plan. The trained states of strength and muscular endurance will determine the energy capacities that exist during exercise trials. A sound aerobic base will permit an increase in the quantity of power and speed training that can be performed. Specific power and speed training should only be initiated when the more fundamental physical capacities that govern the nature of these types of responses are in a relatively high state of training.

16
Flexibility Training

Flexibility is an important characteristic for human performance because it governs the range of movement that is used in a technique and the length of the movement over which forces can be generated. It relates to the range of movement around a joint. It has beneficial effects in terms of the reduction of injuries and the promotion of muscle relaxation. Stretching exercises are used to train flexibility and as part of the specific warm-up for an activity.

Flexibility is specific to each joint (Fleishman 1964, Harris 1969), differs between each athletic group (Song 1979), and is specialized between individuals and sports. The combination of the needs of each athlete, the activities in which they engage, and the state of training, are individual and need to be determined by flexibility testing before developing a training program. The flexibility needs of sports vary considerably. Some activities, such as gymnastics, figure skating, and diving, require the greatest range of flexibility to be developed and maintained for adequate performance. Team games do not usually require extreme flexibility except when a joint is forced beyond normal range of movement. Thus, there is a need to maintain considerable flexibility although it will be used relatively infrequently. For endurance sports, flexibility work can be used as a restoration process. Stretching of the Achilles tendon and calf muscle after a distance running workout facilitates recovery in that muscle and reduces soreness.

Joint mobility is restricted by bony and fleshy masses that block movement in the end position and by the skin, muscles, tendons, ligaments, and capsules that act as ties and which are put on stretch in the limiting position. The shape of bones, the elasticity of liga-

273

ments and muscles, the strength of the antagonist muscles, and the effort of movement also determine the maximum range of movement. A variety of external factors also affect flexibility: heat treatment (Grobaker and Stull 1975), preliminary exercise, short-wave diathermy (Asmussen and Boje 1945), hot showers (Carlile 1956), muscle soreness, tolerance for pain, ability to relax, and room temperature (Scott and French 1959). These factors could cause day-to-day variations in flexibility in athletes and need to be considered prior to exercising. Frequent physical activity also produces an adapted level of flexibility in the appropriate joints. Specific physical activities, such as weight-training and calisthenics (Denk 1971, de Vries 1962), dance (Campbell 1944), yoga (Meyers 1971), basketball (Turner 1977), and ice-hockey (Chevrier 1981) produce changes in flexibility as a result of participation. Each sport appears to generate a range of flexibility that suits the majority of activities that are performed. This means that conscientious training and participation in a sport will eventually produce an habituated level of flexibility that will meet *most of the usual demands* of a sport. However, extra flexibility training will be necessary to accommodate unusual circumstances when limbs are forced beyond a natural participation-developed range (see Injury Prevention, below).

Research on flexibility has yielded mixed and contradictory results. Some have shown flexibility to help an athlete's performance while others have found no such benefits (Chevrier 1981). Those that support the claim would acknowledge that a lack of flexibility would be a severe setback. Travers (1973) stated that poor flexibility has three consequences: it is impossible to perform skills properly, there is an increased risk of muscle injury; and there will be a loss of power in the range of movement. Cureton (1941) suggested that flexibility exercises, if employed in sufficient dosages, may condition muscles, tendons, ligaments, and bones to a greater tensile strength and elasticity. On the other hand, excessive flexibility may cause problems because adequate stability cannot be provided, for example, the shoulder in the rugby scrum (Cureton 1941, Davis, Logan, and McKinney 1961). Generally, the effects of a lack of flexibility on performance are confined to opinions rather than research.

Flexibility Methods

There are several training methods each purporting to enable the athlete to achieve a number of benefits. One needs to discern which is the most effective and efficient in terms of achieving for the performer the greatest range of flexibility in the shortest time with the most enduring effects. There is little information, either from the laboratory or the field, concerning the relative merits of different flexibility training methods or the relevance of them for the practitioner (Holt 1973). Clarke (1975), after an extensive review of the literature, suggested three factors that influence flexibility development, notably types of exercise, warm-up, and the length of time that the effects of flexibility stimulation last. Clarke (1976) stressed that exercises must be based on principles of joint dynamics, fulfill their objectives, and be within the physical capabilities of the athlete performing the exercises. Slow-active stretching (SAS) (Jacobs 1976), Proprioceptive neuromuscular facilitation stretching (PNF) (Holt 1973), and the traditional ballistic or bounce stretching (de Vries 1974) are three methods that have received support for use in sports.

□ PNF Stretching

The PNF method is based on the neurophysiological principle of proprioceptive neuromuscular facilitation and developed from the work of Kabat (1952). It involves the muscles being placed in a relaxed and lengthened position. The attainment of that position is usually assisted by light pressure from a partner or an external force. After that, an isometric contraction of the antagonist muscle group is performed against an immovable resistance. This is repeated until the scope of movement cannot be increased without pain. The reason that PNF works is that it uses the physiological principle that a contracted muscle returns to a lengthened state upon relaxing. With isometric contraction, the muscle is longer after the contraction than before. Each repeated isometric contraction increases the lengthened state of the muscle group and subsequently, the range of movement about the joint improves. Holt, Travis, and Okita (1970) compared a subtle variation of the PNF method with fast (ballistic) and slow-passive stretching. Under well-controlled conditions the PNF method was shown to produce the greatest effect on flexibility. Tanigawa (1972) compared a method which was basically similar to the PNF procedure with passive mobilization. The former produced greater and faster improvements in flexibility. Pyke (1980) advocated PNF as the best stretching procedure for sports and pointed out that these exercises promote both flexibility and muscular strength. Since there is a learning stage for both the athlete and partner when using this technique, exercises should be performed with less than maximum effort until both parties become accustomed to the procedures and are confident that no injury will result. The steps for PNF stretching are:

1. After a substantial warm-up, the athlete and partner assume
    the position for the exercise (Figure 16.1 illustrates a number
    of PNF exercise positions).

Figure 16.1 Examples of PNF Stretching Exercises

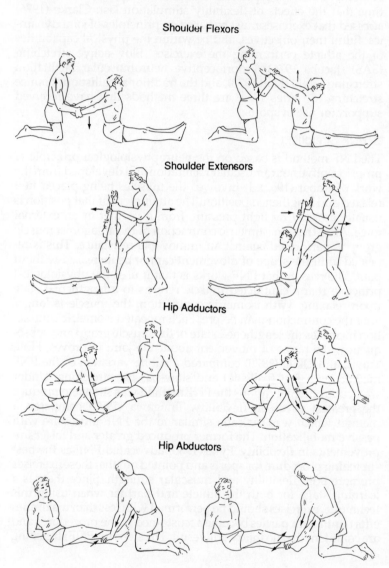

Shoulder Flexors

Shoulder Extensors

Hip Adductors

Hip Abductors

Knee Flexors

Knee Extensors

Ankle Extensors

Ankle Flexors

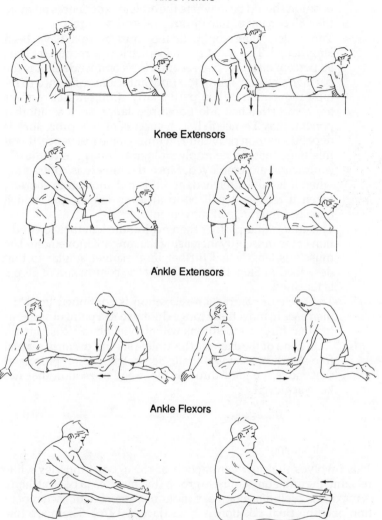

For a more complete presentation the reader is referred to the publication by Holt (1973).

2. The athlete relaxes the muscles that are to be stretched and the partner applies pressure so that the relaxed muscles are *slowly and carefully* lengthened. That lengthening is actively assisted by the athlete trying to attain the position. Ex-

plosive forcing should be avoided. The extent of the forced position should be to where the athlete experiences no more than 80 percent of maximum pain or discomfort.

3.   The athlete then contracts the muscles that have been lengthened. This must be an isometric contraction (at least 90 percent effort for 5–6 seconds is recommended). It is the partner's responsibility to apply sufficient resistance to inhibit movement. When particularly strong muscle groups are being stretched additional resistance, such as another person, may be needed. The success of this procedure is dependent upon providing an immovable resistance. It is at this stage that the neurophysiological principles of muscle contraction are employed. Since the muscle is contracting when it is fully stretched, and it is not allowed to shorten, when it relaxes it will be in an even longer state which increases the range of movement.

4.   The athlete and partner then exploit the lengthened condition of the muscle by increasing the range of movement. The muscle is lengthened further in a manner similar to that described in Step 2 and the isometric contraction of Step 3 is repeated.

5.   The cycle of contraction-relaxation is continued until the increases in movement range diminish to a point of suggesting that further repetitions will not yield beneficial gains.

6.   At the end of the exercise the athlete should perform several free-standing exercises (ballistic stretching is appropriate) that move the joint through the range of motion that has been achieved.

□ SAS Stretching

This involves the slow contraction of the agonist muscles while relaxing the antagonist muscle group (the muscles to be stretched). A maximum voluntary range of motion is attained for each repetition and the final position is held (Jacobs 1976). There are few studies that have reported on the SAS method. The procedure for SAS stretching is:

1.   After a significant warm-up the athlete assumes a position for stretching the muscle group that is targeted (see Figure 16.2 for examples of starting positions).

2.   The athlete then slowly and cautiously moves the appropriate body part to stretch the muscle as much as possible. The extent of the movement is that which can be voluntarily

Figure 16.2 Examples of SAS Stretching Exercises

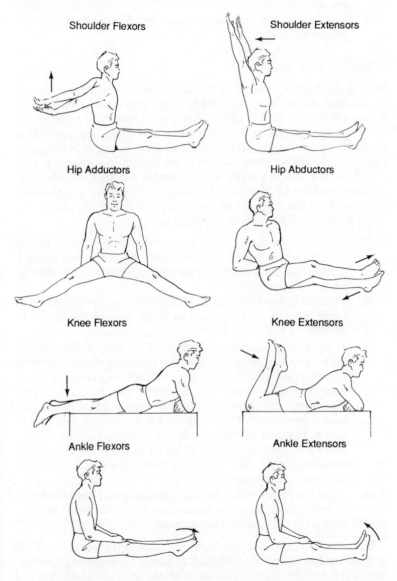

Shoulder Flexors

Shoulder Extensors

Hip Adductors

Hip Abductors

Knee Flexors

Knee Extensors

Ankle Flexors

Ankle Extensors

maintained for ten seconds. It is important that no additional force be added to that which is purely generated by the agonist muscles.

3. The athlete relaxes and reassumes the starting position.

4. Step 2 is repeated and should result in an increased range of movement.
5. The cycles are continued until beneficial effects are no longer achieved.

☐ Ballistic stretching

This is the common method of stretching. It requires the use of rhythmical actions to apply force to lengthen a muscle. Weber and Kraus (1949) concluded that ballistic stretching was superior to forms of slow-active and slow-passive stretching. However, this method has received a number of criticisms for it can injure muscles (particularly with tearing) and it often results in soreness if executed improperly. As well, when muscles are stiff and the first actions produce some pain, tenseness in the athlete can develop which delays the progress of increasing the range of movement. The procedure of ballistic stretching is:

1. The body should be very warm with an obviously raised core and muscle temperature before this technique is used. It is best used after either of the other two forms of stretching have been performed.
2. The athlete uses some form of controlled and relatively light force (usually body weight or some part of the body) to generate a force to 'stretch' the muscle group.
3. A slow soft bounce is performed to stretch the relaxed target-muscle group. The speed of the bounce increases with each repetition but never becomes severe enough to be a near-maximum force. The degree of pain associated with the bounce should never exceed 80 percent of the maximum tolerable amount. It has been shown that if the bounce is too severe in terms of the pain that is generated, an avoidance and protective response will occur in the muscle to guard against injury. This will actually reduce the degree of stretch reached by the muscle.
4. Light but comfortable bouncing is continued until the range of movement ceases to increase and the athlete is comfortable with moving to that extreme.

Both the PNF and SAS methods are sound in theory. The PNF procedure has been substantiated as being superior to more traditional flexibility training methods (Holt 1973). The SAS method was evaluated against the PNF method and was found to be only marginally less effective (Chevrier 1981, Turner 1977). The principal difference between the two methods of training is that the PNF technique involves two phasic contractions and the use of an immobile resistance for each trial whereas SAS involves only one contraction procedure for each repetition.

Considerations for Flexibility Training

□ Warm-up

Since warm muscles stretch more easily it is advisable to precede each bout of stretching with a general activity that elevates the muscle and central core temperature of the body. The degree of warming that is beneficial is that which produces light sweating on the forehead and the back of the hands. This requirement contradicts the common practice of stretching being the first activity that is undertaken by athletes in warming-up for a training session or competition. It is usual to see swimmers enter onto a pool deck and commence stretching without having done any previous activity. Runners find a place near a track and start to stretch their hamstrings, ankles, and other joints. We advocate that an athlete does not stretch when the body is at a resting temperature. Stretching produces its best effects and is safest after an activity that raises body temperature.

The use of passive warm-up is not frequently considered but it does have the benefits of raising the core temperature of the body in place of exercise. Carlile (1956) showed that as little as ten minutes of hot-showering warms the body to a level that facilitates performance. Similarly, the wearing of sufficient clothing to trap body heat and create a micro-climate which would lead to a raised body temperature is another option. When it is not possible to do general activities, such as jogging, cycling, and total-body calisthenics, these methods should be considered as possible ways to prepare the body for a full stretching or flexibility training routine.

□ Habituation

When an athlete participates seriously in a sport, that sport develops flexibility in participants of sufficient ranges to meet its most common demands. Turner (1977) found that after six weeks of playing basketball, flexibility improved significantly in a control group that did no particular stretching program. Both PNF and SAS stretching programs improved flexibility to a great degree but a large proportion of those gains were lost within two weeks of cessation. The PNF and SAS athletes did not regress, but stopped at the level that was stimulated by the activities of basketball.

Some sports require greater ranges of movements (e.g., gymnastics, a contact sport such as ice-hockey). After a while, the flexibility of athletes habituates at very extreme ranges such that stretching work serves only a warm-up function, that is, the athletes cannot improve their flexibility any further. Chevrier (1981) trained collegiate male ice-hockey players to use both PNF and SAS procedures. He found that the training did not increase flexibility over that which already existed. The ranges of movement caused by a pre-scrimmage warm-up were not maintained during the scrimmage, where two-thirds of the time was spent sitting on benches. However, upon completion of the scrimmage and its warm-down routine, flexibility once again was at pre-scrimmage levels. An interesting finding of the study was that flexibility was not retained during the simulated competition. It appears that the bench-sitting was sufficient to allow players to partially 'tighten-up'. It could be suggested that during an ice-hockey game, and other games where time is spent on the interchange bench (e.g, basketball, rugby league and Australian football), stretching while off the playing arena should be performed to stop the loss of movement range. This activity might decrease the susceptibility of players to injury during the contest. There is also the implication that for athletes who develop a good range of flexibility because of their participation in a sport, the main role of flexibility and stretching is that of warming-up.

Some coaches might conclude that the activity itself is sufficient for training flexibility. It should be remembered that it takes considerable time for the habituation to take place. During that time it is advisable to perform stretching routines as an injury prevention procedure and to accelerate the attainment of habituated flexibility.

☐ Frequency

Flexibility is gained and lost quickly. Studies on retention have generally shown that the effects gained from serious flexibility training, over and above that which is habituated from participation, are lost within one to two weeks (Chevrier 1981, Turner 1977), although isolated studies and claims contend that the effects last much longer (Holt 1973, McCue 1953). This means that flexibility training programs have to be continued through all phases of training. With other physical capacities it is possible to reduce the amount of training by one third once maintenance training is instituted. However, for flexibility work that reduction is not advisable. Some of the effects of stretching are lost within a few hours, particularly when inactivity and cooling occur. Within 24 hours a major portion of the benefits are lost. When flexibility training is incorporated into a specific warm-up it serves a dual function and therefore does not become a burdensome task. It is the recommendation of these authors that flexibility training be a daily activity that is performed the whole year, irrespective of the training phase or sporting season.

□ Injury Prevention

Even though frequently occurring activities in a sport produce a general range of movement that accommodates them there are still instances when external forces may cause joints to exceed their normal range of movement. This is particularly the case in contact sports. Such distortions often lead to injury. Consequently, the use of a deliberate stretching routine that covers particularly vulnerable joints (e.g., ankles, knees, hips, and shoulders) should be part of training, warm-ups, and performed at appropriate opportunities during the contest (particularly at half-time, the end of regulation periods, or when there are excessive delays or time-outs).

There is one class of event where the intensity of the competitive effort is such that injuries could occur. In 50-meter and 100-meter sprints, all throwing events, and indeed, sports where extreme bursts of speed and effort are required, there is a tendency for muscle pulls and tears to frequently occur. It is recommended that in such sports, stretching of the agonist and antagonist muscle groups that control the actions which produce these excessive forces be a frequent activity during the pre-competition and, where appropriate, in the competition period. Bleier and O'Neil (1975: 159) offered the following anecdotal assessment of stretching and injury prevention:

> Paul was also a fine gymnastics coach, which is how he developed a unique set of stretching exercises for the legs and back. When he introduced them to the Steelers [Pittsburgh Steelers] our number of muscle pulls and serious leg injuries was cut by more than half.

It would seem that a greater use of stretching exercises at breaks within a competition might be an advisable activity for injury prevention. As well, such activity, because of its nature, will also accelerate recovery at these times. The institution of stretching as a recovery activity within a competition is worthy of consideration and assessment.

□ Sequencing

There are three types of stretching that could be used for beneficial gains. Each should only be used after a general warm-up that has raised body temperature. SAS and PNF methods should be used to first stretch the muscles and for flexibility training. Ballistic stretching should then be used to maintain the temporary gains derived from the other two methods. It is important that ballistic work be included in the warm-up for it is the form of stretching to which muscles are subjected in a sporting activity. The use of ballistic stretching as being the only form of stretching is less than desirable. It is not as effective for producing changes in flexibility as the other two methods.

Conclusion

Flexibility training and warm-up stretching can be performed as a single practice segment so that two benefits are produced. The PNF and SAS methods are the most useful stretching procedures and need to be taught and incorporated into the training program. Being the most temporary of the physical fitness capacities, stretching work needs to be a daily activity performed independently of the training phases and competitions. Stretching exercises also are useful to stimulate recovery as part of an active-recovery routine. It is recommended that the frequency and volume of use of stretching exercises be increased over that which is commonly evidenced in the training and competitions of most sports.

17
Team-sport Training

The majority of team sports require a variety of physical capacities to be developed. Since most require individual and team skills and frequent competitions over extended time periods, a number of compromising decisions have to made when programming training. Participants need to experience a balance of emphases that will produce the best competitive performances. It is not possible to discuss every sport, competitive schedule, and level of competition in one text. This chapter will focus primarily on college or semi-professional activities (e.g., soccer, Australian football, rugby, basketball) which have weekly competitions and players who divide their time between work/college and the sport. For the sake of consistency, the large majority of examples used will be for Australian football, a game that requires a mix of fitness components such as endurance, speed, power, and flexibility.

In team games it is necessary to constantly emphasize the development of individual and team skills. However, such development will largely be dependent upon the provision of energy as a result of the athlete's physiological capacities. Competitive performances, performance improvements, and the capability of an athlete to endure an extended period of competition will be influenced by the physical training of all the necessary capacities for the game.

Functional Fitness

A knowledge of the physiology of the sport is important for a coach. It provides information that will allow effective planning, monitoring, and analysis of training and conditioning programs.

The functional fitness required to meet the demands of the sport, testing to assess players' levels of preparation, and the extent to which training objectives are being met by a program need to be considered.

A successful player must develop all the physical capacities which are essential to cope with the physical demands of the game. For example, Australian football is a running sport that necessitates covering distances of up to twenty kilometers at varying intensities in games. While this requires *endurance*, much of the distance covered is in short bursts of high intensity sprinting alternating with short recovery periods. Players also require *speed* and *agility* to accelerate quickly, change direction, recover from loss of balance, and to twist and turn in maneuvering actions. They also need *power* to jump and dive for ball possession and to spoil the efforts of opponents as well as kicking and passing the ball long distances. *Strength* is required for execution of body skills and when contact is made with other players and the ground. *Flexibility* is important for performing with maximum efficiency and avoiding injuries. An Australian Rules football player needs to be trained in all the major fitness elements.

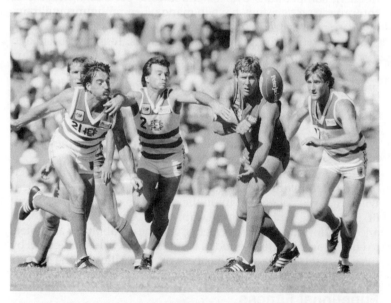

Australian Rules football is a running sport that requires a number of components of fitness: endurance, speed, agility, jumping power, strength and flexibility. As with many team games, fitness programming is very complex and must give attention to each factor

It is possible to train various fitness capacities and improve them in isolation. These include pure running, strength training, and agility activities. However, in adherence to the principle of specificity, as the competitive season approaches it is necessary to develop physical fitness in such a manner that the fitness is functionally appropriate for the sport. Functional fitness will allow a player to effectively meet the demands of the game. The major determinants of functional training is that it be as game-like as possible, and of sufficient repetition and loading to cause training effects to occur. Thus, training programs should not consist of a number of unrelated activities, but rather should be of activities which combine to develop fitness components and skills at the same time, especially during the competitive season.

The most specific types of functional training are interval running which reflects the type, duration and intensity of game-running, and interval skill-drills that add the use of equipment in the development of skills. Skill practice activities should be conducted in such a manner that small group and team plays are facilitated, that is, talking, thinking, positional responsibilities, and anticipatory actions are encouraged. Table 17.1 indicates a general assessment of the demands Australian football makes on the energy systems, muscular qualities, and skills. The hypothetical figures will have to be adjusted to accommodate the individual physical qualities of each player and the different demands of particular positions. Coaches should make their own estimates of the fitness and skill demands of their sport (see Chapters 11 and 12) and use them to determine the objectives of and prescriptions for training programs.

Table 17.1 Estimates of Fitness and Skill Demands of Australian Football

Energy Systems	20%	Muscular Fitness	20%	Skills	60%
Aerobic	50%	General strength	15%	Individual skills	20%
Anaerobic	50%	General muscular endurance	25%	Small-group skills	30%
		Specific power	50%	Team plays	50%
		Flexibility	10%		

Source: Woodman and Pyke 1990

Phases of Team-game Training

Team games are usually seasonal, with a three- to four-month preparation period followed by an extended competition period of as much as six months. The remaining time is off-season and should be considered as a transition period between the competitive season and the next preparation phase. The Australian football year could be considered as consisting of the following phases:

Phase	Professional Clubs	Amateur Clubs
Transition (Pre-November)	8 weeks	18 weeks
Basic preparatory (November–December)	6 weeks	3 weeks
Specific preparatory (January–March)	12 weeks	5 weeks
Competition (March-September)	26 weeks	26 weeks

☐ Transition Phase (Off-season Training)

Off-season training is aimed at physiological and psychological recovery from the demands of the preceding season's training and competition. It also includes an evaluation of the previous season and the planning of the next year's training. As a general principle, players should maintain endurance fitness and control their body weight. The activities of this phase should not necessarily involve the sport. Each player should aim to enter the new season with the level of conditioning in all the important physical components a step higher than existed at the commencement of the previous season. This is one of the main purposes of multi-year planning, involving, in particular, the following of defined activities in the transition phase. Allowances have to be made for individual differences, especially for older players and players recovering from injury when determining what training is to be done.

The transition phase is also the most suitable time for undertaking specialised programs aimed at overcoming diagnosed weaknesses in body structure, fitness, and skill. Individualised training programs such as strength training, speed development, and skill improvement can be undertaken at this time. However, participation in such activities should not be of an intensity that will interfere with total recovery from the previous season's stresses. Restoration through non-specific activity should be emphasized as much as development through sport-related training. If one were to err in one direction, it would be to provide too much respite rather than too little. However, the most important objective of transition phase activity is not to allow detraining of the physical capacities that are important for the sport. Thus multilateral training through a variety of activities that challenge those capacities should be scheduled. For example, football players should aim at running ten-kilometer or half-marathon recreational races, participate in beach or track sprinting, play basketball or soccer, and generally get involved in activities that stimulate the maintenance of a reasonable degree of fitness. This will allow the next season to be initiated with a considerable degree of general fitness. These associated activities should not be competitively demanding.

☐ Basic Preparatory Phase

The aim of this phase is to build a solid foundation of fitness and basic skills for the more specific work that will follow. It can be accommodated satisfactorily over a 6- to 12-week period. It is used to progressively condition the energy systems appropriate to the sport as well as practise basic skills. The coach should also use this time to develop the elements of team play using activities that will develop effective cohesion between team members.

Early microcycles should involve high-volume training, each increase in overload being planned in a step-like fashion. Workout demands should vary from low to moderate intensities so that high volumes of training can be accommodated.

For Australian football the program should follow a sequence of continuous, fartlek, longer-slower interval training (15–120 seconds of work, 45–360 seconds of recovery), shorter-faster interval training (5–15 seconds of work, 15–45 seconds of recovery), and interval skill drills. A mixture of these training methods with additional strength, speed, and flexibility work can be continued into the specific preparatory phase and on into the competition phase. The main objective should be to establish a base upon which later more specialized training can be built. The volume of work is progressively increased to the end of this training phase.

☐ Specific Preparatory Phase

The main objective of the specific preparatory phase is the development of specific performance capacities and new levels of skill. In the early stages, the volume of training continues to increase although the content becomes more sport-specific. One-third of the way through the phase the physiological emphasis should be evenly divided between volume and intensity. From then on intensity should increase gradually as the volume of training remains constant or is slightly reduced.

As the phase progresses an increasing emphasis should be placed on skill and strategy practices which continue into the competition phase. The Australian football activities associated with the two preparatory phases of training in the pre-season period are illustrated in Figure 17.1. A 90-minute training session could be divided into six sections as illustrated in Figure 17.2.

Figure 17.1 A Guide for the Basic Preparatory and Specific Preparatory Phases of Training for Multi-capacity Team Games

	WEEKS										
Lower Grades	1	2		3		4		5	6		
Higher Grades	1	2	3	4	5	6	7	8	9	10	11	12

TRAINING					
Endurance and Sprint Running	Continuous	Fartlek	Longer Slower Intervals	Shorter, Faster Intervals interval Skill Drills Sprint Training	
Muscular Endurance, Strength, Power	General Muscular Endurance		General Strength		Specific Strength and Power
	Circuit Training				
Flexibility	Flexibility Work				
Skill	Individual Skills			Group Skills and Team Plays	

When any training plans are implemented, the transition from one phase to the next is not as clear or definitive as theory would suggest. Good implementation will make such transitions transparent to the participants. This is because the times of achievement of training objectives differ and the needs of players should be adjusted to their rates of progress. Thus, even though two preparatory phases are planned, their obvious differences are evident at the start of the basic and the end of the specific periods. In between there are less-than-exact characteristics of both. To illustrate this when implementing training phases, the following is a 9-week pre-season training plan of a leading Australian football team:

Three weeks of 5 sessions per week
Monday, Wednesday, and Friday — approximately 30 minutes each on circuit training, running, and skills
Tuesday and Thursday — players meet at venues for 45 minutes of distance or fartlek running; injured or 'sore' players may need hydrotherapy sessions (running in water, swimming) rather than running

Figure 17.2 Suggested Activity Allocations for a 90-minute Practice Session

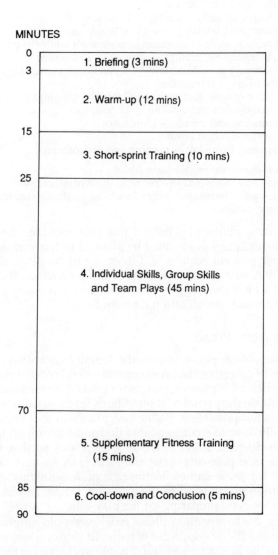

The order of the activities is important but the duration of each type of activity can be altered to suit the specific needs of the team and sport.

Three weeks leading up to practice games
    Monday, Wednesday, and Friday — continue with circuit training,
        skills and running being combined into skill drills using footballs,
        each drill appropriate to the game, and each 90-minute session
        following a basic format:
    • warm-up and stretching — 15 minutes
    • lane work (starting slowly) — 10 minutes
    • partner work — one team in possession while the other applies
        'pressure' but minimizes contact — 20 minutes
    • recovery period of 'slow' skill practice (e.g., marking against a
        partner) — 10 minutes
    • three-quarter ball or mad ball (intense running) — 15 minutes
    • two-on-two and tackling — 15 minutes
    • running and circuit — 15 minutes
    • warm-down at leisure
    Tuesday and Thursday — running and hydrotherapy

Three weeks during the practice game period
    Monday and Wednesday — running and hydrotherapy
    Tuesday and Thursday — normal training gradually emphasizing
        game qualities

The training philosophy behind this plan includes that players
who are genuinely 'sore' must be allowed to recover; that senior
and older players require less intensity of training, since they
generally have a good knowledge of game demands and pride in
keeping a high level of general fitness; and that injury avoidance
is an important consideration for training.

☐ Competition Phase

The competition phase covers the lengthy competition period.
Chapter 19 describes the pre-competition and competition phases
as being desirable planning stages for peaked performances. However, because the period of competitions for most team sports is so
long, it is not possible to define two phases of that kind. What is
essentially done to accommodate a demanding competition schedule is to disguise shifts in training emphases so that when the
end-of-season play-offs occur, the team is in the very best shape
possible for these games. In the case of Australian football, the
competition phase handles the extensive league games and then
starts to focus on preparing for the play-offs.

During the competition phase coaches should emphasize skill
practice and the development of game strategies while working to
maintain the fitness levels in all capacities achieved in the previous
phase of training. The primary mode of maintenance conditioning
is the employment of repetitive skill practices and small games that
require intensive effort. Because of the demands of competing, high

intensity training is necessary to compensate for the reduced frequency and volume of training.

Conditioning and skill activities should be mixed and balanced throughout all training phases, as should periodic testing of physical capacities (a diminution in a capacity could account for a deterioration in play). Figure 17.3 illustrates two different macrocycles of training, each stressing a different form. When physical conditioning is emphasized, the objectives of skill work are maintenance and consolidation. When skills are emphasized, condition is maintained. Skill practices are generally low in intensity while conditioning is of high intensity. The use of interval skill drills and grid practices can produce high-intensity training which also has a conditioning effect. The illustrated alternating pattern of 4-week emphases, first on a particular capacity and then having a break from it, is aimed at producing a better level of adaptation and improvement in that capacity. This cyclic planning of macrocycles throughout the competition phase is important because it adheres to the following principles of training:

1. It allows the development of specific performance aspects to occur in a step-like fashion.
2. The accommodation of periods of maintenance training allows athletes to experience stages where stress for that aspect of the sport is gradually reduced (psychological fatigue is therefore avoided).
3. It avoids the spectre of mixed training which will produce mixed results.
4. The alternating emphases make training more dynamic.

Examples of common variations in the types of microcycles that could be used during the competition phase are listed below.

Team A
Sunday	Free recovery day
Monday	Running and circuits
Tuesday	90–100 minutes of intense competition simulation
Wednesday	Optional
Thursday	60–75 minutes of individual and team skills
Friday	Free
Saturday	Game

Team B
Sunday	Free recovery day
Monday	Light training session — alternative activities (running, swimming, court games)
Tuesday	No organized training
Wednesday	High-volume training session

Thursday	No organized training
Friday	Short, intense session aimed at sharpening skills and team play
Saturday	Game

Figure 17.3 Two Hypothetical Macrocycles Illustrating a Typical Pattern of Changing Volume and Intensity while the Total Training Stress Increases from Week 1 to 3 in Each

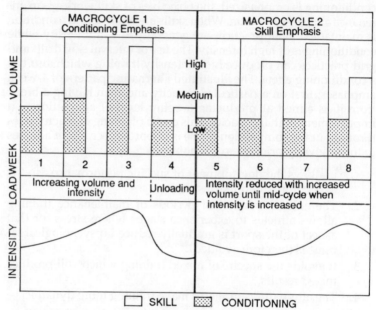

The fourth weeks are unloading microcycles that allow for adaptation and recovery to fully occur. These macrocycles are also appropriate for a phase where physical states are still be altered, that is, undergoing change training (*Source:* Woodman and Pyke 1990).

Some teams follow a Monday-Wednesday-Friday system regardless of the actual match day. This has the advantages of being systematic and providing rest days after the game and Monday and Wednesday training. Others follow a pattern of organized training on Tuesday-Wednesday-Thursday nights. Players usually undertake a light run or other recovery activity on Monday nights. This arrangement allows for good recovery after even the most stressful games. This sequencing is particularly beneficial to older players with almost three days of recovery between the game and the next hard training session.

An improvement on this programming would be to add recovery activities directly after the game and on Sunday. In some players this can promote faster recovery which would allow more training to occur during each week. Attention to injuries should be provided immediately after a contest so that healing can be promoted in the fastest fashion.

Training loads usually increase throughout the preparatory phases, are reduced in the early competition phase, build again during the middle of the phase, ease again, and then follow a final build-up through the latter stage of the phase leading up to the play-offs (see Figure 17.4). Endurance, speed, strength, power, flexibility, and skill are all important factors in team game performance. This variety of factors, along with the requirements of individual players and the need to prepare for weekly contests, increases the complexity of planning for team games when compared with that of individual sports.

A planned systematic approach to training is just as feasible and workable in team games as in any sport, and it allows the coach to develop a purposeful plan and strategy. Training programs based on sound principles can be implemented and modified according to periodic needs. Chapter 19 of this text discusses the phases of training in an annual plan in more detail than has been covered here.

Macrocycles

The structure of each macrocycle will depend on the objectives of the training phase. However, the integrity of periodization must be maintained for the phase, that is, step-like increases in overload for several microcycles followed by an unloading microcycle. It is the nature of the training stimuli and their associated overloads that changes the content of each macrocycle (see Chapter 18).

Usually, a preparatory phase macrocycle emphasizes step-like overload increases through volume increments. At the end of the specific preparatory phase changes in intensity supplant further changes in volume. In the competition phase, training intensity is often emphasized over volume. The training intensity of each macrocycle is organised in a wave-like pattern with the load peaks increasing throughout each training phase (see Figure 17.4). The cyclicity of workloads is meant to allow athletes to have the opportunity to fully recover and to guard against overtraining. Volumes and intensities change through low, medium, and high levels throughout each macrocycle. High volume is usually matched by low intensity, while higher and maximum intensities are usually accompanied by correspondingly lower volumes.

Figure 17.4 A Sample Annual Training Plan for a Professional Australian Rules Football Team

MONTHS	OCT.	NOV.	DEC.	JAN.	FEB.	MAR.	APR.	MAY	JUN.	JUL.	AUG.	SEP.
COMPETITIONS												Play-offs
PERIODIZATION	Transition	Basic Preparatory		Specific Preparatory		Competition						
MACROCYCLES		Conditioning General Basic			Specific Basic				Unloading		Taper	Peak
ENDURANCE		Aerobic Capacity	Maximum Aerobic Power		Anaerobic Alactic Capacity			Anaerobic Alactic Capacity and Power			Maintenance	
STRENGTH		General	Maximum		Power			Maintenance				
FLEXIBILITY			Develop					Maintenance				
SPEED			Running					Movement				
TECHNIQUE (SKILL)		Maintain Basic Remedial		Improve Basic	Aquire Variants	Acquire Advanced		Maintain and Develop Rhythm and Coordination	Consolidate and Synchronize			
TACTICS (TEAM PLAYS)		Maintain Elementary										
PSYCHOLOGY	Assessment and Individual Program Development			Specific Mental Skills		Competition & Motivation Development			Positive		Specific Play-offs Preparation	
% TRAINING TIME CONDITIONING		70	60	50	40	30	20	20	20	20	30	20
SKILL		30	40	30	30	40	40	40	40	30	20	20
TACTICAL				20	30	30	40	40	40	50	50	60
TRAINING LOAD 100% / 80% / 60%												

KEY: —— Volume   --- Intensity   ■ Grand Final   ▰ Final   ⊠ League Games   ▨ Pre-season Games

Source: Woodman and Pyke 1990

Microcycles

A 7-day microcycle accommodates weekly competitions. However, with modern scheduling in Australian football, games are sometimes irregularly spaced. The time period between games can range from 3 to 9 days, with an occasional longer period occurring for representative games and special events.

The structure of a microcycle will depend upon the number of training sessions and competitions each week. Junior teams may only be able to train twice as a group whereas more senior teams may train 3–4 times weekly or even daily. Professional athletes should be expected to train as often as necessary. Group work should be scheduled into available team training times whereas individual work could be planned outside practice time. A restricted number of training sessions will compromise desirable training schedules. However, it is still good coaching to include variations in the training load by altering the intensity, volume, and activities of team practices. Recovery should still be considered to be an important variable even though practices may not occur with the desired frequency. The variations in session loads will be determined by the macrocycle and training phase objectives.

Even in professional sports, the problem of fitting in enough training still confronts the coaching staff. An emerging trend seems to be that of scheduling two practices per day, each with a very different objective. Since fatigue interferes with learning, morning training sessions focus mainly on the learning and repetition of skills without damaging fatigue being incurred. The later session focuses on overloading the athlete through specific and general training activities. Since performance improvement is directly related to the number of correctly executed skill trials (Ashy, Landin, and Lee 1988), it would seem that constructing training circumstances which allow an increased number of skill-learning opportunities to occur is a step in the right direction. The common practice of trying to incorporate large amounts of skill improvement and the stimulation and maintenance of various physical capacities into a few training sessions may not be the most efficient method for training team game athletes. This alternative procedure should not be confused with training twice a day where noticeable fatigue is incurred at both sessions. The concept of separate skill training and physical training sessions allows adequate recovery and beneficial skill development conditions to coexist.

A typical, but not necessarily the most efficient, training microcycle is illustrated in Figure 17.5.

Figure 17.5 A Typical Microcycle for a Sport with Important Weekend Competitions

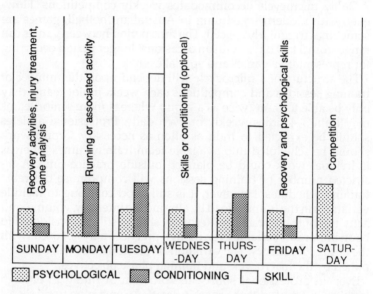

Sport-specific skill development, physical conditioning, and mental skills training are accommodated. Some activities are scheduled for both Sunday and Friday, but their nature will not interfere with recovery. The frequent but low volume conditioning activities are flexibility activities, a capacity that is best trained on a daily basis. Psychological work is also part of the total training plan.

Monitoring the Training Load

Training periodization is necessary because of limits to the body's ability to adjust to heavy training loads and particularly stressful competitions. Recovery should be of as much concern to the coach as is overload. Attempts to sustain heavy training loads and/or peak form will cause overtraining and a corresponding deterioration in performance.

Overtraining in team games can be caused by many factors, such as:

1.　too many 'important' competitions which produce physiological and psychological fatigue
2.　sudden increases in the amount of training (this often occurs when in the light of a team's poor performance the coach

makes a panic decision and assumes that the performance was due to 'not being fit enough' and drastically increases the volume and/or intensity of training)

3. a long period of sustained high-intensity training and competitions

The mix of competitions and training is particularly stressful on most athletes, particularly when their positions as starters or members of the first team is constantly under threat. The stress of uncertainty caused by that situation makes each contest more complex and fatiguing for the player. This should be remembered by coaches and compensated for in the training loads, schedules, and game roles of each individual. This more complicated source of fatigue affects individuals in different ways. 'Sensitive' athletes break down faster under psychological stress of the nature that surrounds team games than do less sensitive ones. Thus performance slumps could occur at different intervals and be caused by differing amounts of psychological and physical fatigue. Physiological testing of essential performance capacities to determine if poor performances are caused by reduced physical capacities should be conducted at the end of each unloading microcycle. The regular use of self-report stress analyses (see Chapter 8) to determine declining psychological states should occur. Skill deteriorations are best monitored by the skill 'experts' who are involved with coaching. These three evaluation sources should cover most of the reasons for performance reversals.

With extended competition schedules and after approximately 12–16 weeks of intensive one-session-per-day training, the body will cease to respond favourably and changes must be made to the training programs. After 8–12 weeks in the competition phase the training load should be reduced for as much as 2–3 weeks. That reduction can be as much as conducting only one or two formal training sessions per week and allowing adequate rest to occur preferably through engaging in unrelated activities. Activity must be continued although the workload is markedly reduced. A noticeable decrease in activity could produce lethargic athletes.

The basic principles of periodisation apply to contact team games as much as to individual sports, the major difference being the need to win enough regular season games to qualify for the play-offs which is the key time for players to reach their 'peak performance potential'. The ability to sustain a high level of performance from week to week is important. The closer a team can consistently perform to its peak the better but the risk of overtrained or 'burnt-out' players increases when this is attempted, and a team of jaded or fatigued players will not perform well. Accommodations for recovery and reduced training/competition loads need to be planned even during the competition phase.

Peaking

Peaking so that the best possible performance can be achieved at a particular time is a complex process. It becomes even more complicated when a large number of very different individuals has to achieve that state at the same time.

Effective peaking involves not only a long-term build-up of physical conditioning, psychological skill development, and technical and tactical improvement, but also a tapering of sport demands to ensure maximum recovery and overcompensation at the time of important competition. Factors such as nutrition, rest, and a reduction in stressors outside sport also play an important part in peaking. For peaked performances to occur, the majority of factors that influence game performances have to be considered to be in a better-than-normal state by the athlete (see Chapter 8). Coaching decisions are going to directly affect the ability of team members to achieve peaked states for serious competitions.

Peaked states are easier to achieve in individual sports where only one or perhaps two peaks are attempted each year. Peaking is only possible for a short period of from 10–14 days and is usually followed by a decrease in performance. Under special conditions it may be possible to maintain a peaked state for a slightly longer period (see Chapter 4). In team game situations it is only useful to bring a team to a peak for finals.

Although peaking every week is not possible, it is important to try to maintain a consistently high level of performance throughout the season and avoid dramatic performance peaks and troughs. Performance consistency will usually carry a team through to making play-offs. To produce this consistency and the necessary number of victories, performance can be maintained by the appropriate manipulation of training volume, intensity, and activity selection. It can be facilitated by having moderate to heavy workouts early in the week, heavy mid-week sessions, and lighter sessions closer to game day. In a repetitive and arduous competitive season, the emphasis on skill enhancement and development should remain consistently high, with the physiological demands of training being moderated to allow training intensities to vary. During the season, consistent execution of high quality drills is usually the major factor that determines if a team does or does not qualify for the play-offs.

The implementation of a correct peaking program can mean the difference between winning and not winning a championship.

Tapering training to ensure a peak for finals means dropping the volume of training while maintaining and possibly increasing the quality of work (see Figure 17.4). What is most important is to ensure that there is full recovery between training sessions and before games. Reducing or tapering the training load lowers the level of fatigue, increases the efficiency of movement and the capacity to prolong effort, as well as increasing the ability to develop greater strength and power. Poor monitoring and control of training can be a cause of a team peaking at the wrong time or not at all.

Peaking usually involves two aspects: reaching and sustaining or improving top form, and organizing a specific preparation for peaking. The high-intensity training and competitive stress required to reach and stabilise top performance is fatiguing both physically and psychologically. The period of this special training to achieve this can only be maintained for six to eight weeks. This means that a particular 'peaking' macrocycle will need to be constructed for the latter stage of the competition phase of training. This special period may have some of the characteristics of the pre-competition phase of training that is described in Chapter 19.

When top performance is reached, it can be maintained by reducing the total workload to allow the body to reach maximum skill efficiency and physical capacity. For Australian football this approach should occur in the four weeks leading up to the finals, with a specific peak-maintenance phase being used during the finals. The maintenance of a peak is primarily determined by performing with high performance quality at training and being allowed to recovery fully between training sessions (residual fatigue is not allowed to depreciate the standard of training performances). A general approach which could be adopted for a finals series in Australian football is as follows:

1st week:	Recovery and low-intensity but high-quality training.
2nd week:	Start the week with high-volume and low-intensity training and then gradually reverse the balance of the two as the week progresses.
3rd week:	High-intensity, low-volume training if the team qualifies for the Grand Final; otherwise, as for the fourth week if playing in the Preliminary Final.
4th week:	Grand Final Week — very specific high-quality training, low volume but intensity varied to permit adequate stimulation of all physical capacities. Recovery must be complete with rest and diet at optimum levels.

These training manipulations will be dependent to some degree on the route through the play-offs. It is important to realize that at this stage it is too late to improve fitness or to develop new techniques. Skill precision and amplitude as well as increasing the degree of confidence that the athletes have in their training should be the objectives of training sessions. Training stimuli of sufficient quality and intensity should be experienced to maintain the highest possible levels of fitness capacities.

There is often a temptation to introduce a new training item or emphasis in the name of variety or novelty (to serve a 'motivational' purpose). For example, the sudden introduction of an aerobics session or new stretching exercises, in which players do exercises to which they are not accustomed, might leave them sore for a few days when they least need it. This occurrence should be avoided.

The peaking process is largely psychological. Athletes must be prepared for all manner of unusual events and increased levels of attention and expectations. The preparation for serious competitions of this nature is in itself a special topic and requires specific skills, training, and procedures (Rushall 1979c). However, the correct stimulation of physical capacities, a perception of increasing skill proficiency, and the general impression of feeling better than normal in most aspects of life are crucial features that can be directly enhanced by the coaching decisions that are made.

Specialized Training Methods

☐ Acceleration/agility Sprint Training

The ability to accelerate quickly is often the key to gaining possession of a ball in a team game. Stopping and changing direction are also the key components of eluding opponents and defensive maneuvers. It is common to find players who can sprint fast once they have started but can neither accelerate nor change direction quickly. The fastest runner over 100 meters may not be the fastest over 10 meters or in an agility sprint over 10 seconds. Improvement in the ability to accelerate and decelerate quickly can be made by attending to each of the three basic factors in team-game performance — skill, fitness, and psychology.

1. *Skill.* The main points to emphasize in a straight sprint are forward lean to accelerate, backward lean to decelerate; frequent foot strike; and short quick arm actions to minimize rotary movements. Attention to these aspects of technique assist in overcoming acceleration problems associated with over-striding and remaining upright. Drills involving lateral movements, reversals (as in shuttle runs), and body position changes (assuming lying or kneeling positions as

starts for short bursts of running) are important ingredients of an agility and skill training program. It must be remembered that these are skill learning activities and that as many repetitions as possible should be completed but *only in the absence of fatigue.*

2.   *Fitness.* Maximum efforts are required before acceleration improvements can be expected. Sprints of 5–8 seconds interspersed with recovery periods of 30–60 seconds are recommended (ultra-short interval training is a desirable form of programming). General upper and lower body strength training could be a useful supplement to sprint training particularly if the athlete is not particularly strong. Bounding or depth-jumping (plyometric training) is valuable in that it activates the stretch-shortening cycle of the specific muscle groups involved in accelerating. However, the strenuous nature of these activities can produce muscle soreness and injuries if overdone.

Fitness could also be stimulated by a number of activities that add variety to training and may enhance the capacity being trained by the focused attention that they demand. Speed-resisted running involves adding weights to the body (e.g., weighted vests); towing weights (e.g, sled or log); sprinting in a harness against mechanical devices; running uphill; and sprinting up sand dunes. All can be considered to develop muscle power, a very important ingredient for acceleration. Speed-assisted running down slight slopes (2°) or with a following wind provides a supra-maximal stimulus that could enhance sprinting speed. However, the actual value of these forms of activity needs to be determined through research because each of them theoretically violates the principle of specificity. It is recommended that these activities should be performed in the basic preparatory phase of training with a view to 'transferring' their 'benefits' through more specific activities.

These forms of training should only be implemented when players are conditioned well. Since they employ maximum efforts they should be gradually introduced across a number of microcycles in step-like increments. They should be implemented in the absence of fatigue and occur early in the training session after both a general and specific warm-up (see Chapter 18).

3.   *Psychology.* Improvements in speed and agility come primarily from learned factors. Physical activities provide the channel through which learning to use existing capacities in more efficient ways occurs. Feedback about the quality of performances is essential for changes to happen. Thus it is important for measures to be provided frequently for each

repetition of an exercise that is used for training. The replication of game situations will increase a participant's ability to read cues earlier and more accurately. The speed of decision making, which directly affects response time, is dependent on the number of experiences that an athlete has with a particular setting and with executing the appropriate response. Speed of recognition and anticipation of situations can improve the effectiveness of a response. This means that even though capacities are trained through particular activities, unless these capacities are then practiced in real life or simulated situations it is unlikely that any noticeable benefit will occur in games. The quality of game simulations that are practiced at training will determine the extent to which speed and agility can be improved in a competitive sport setting.

□ Flexibility

Stretching exercises are an important part of team sports. They help to increase the range of motion at the joints and hence aid certain aspects of performance (e.g., kicking, sprinting) and also assist in the prevention of injuries. For maximum benefits exercises should be performed early in the workout following a substantial and effective warm-up. Stretching should be periodically repeated throughout training and during competitions to avoid the loss of flexibility that occurs through disuse.

Static, PNF, and ballistic stretching all have some role to play in the warm-up routine. Static and/or PNF stretching should precede ballistic stretching. Arguments have been advanced against ballistic stretching being the first form of stretching to be used (see Chapter 16).

□ Endurance through interval skill drills

The development of aerobic and anaerobic endurance can be effectively achieved when repetitions of sport specific drills are programmed. These are termed 'interval drills' and are an important part of team game training. A common situation is to present a group of three or four players with a task that takes about 10 seconds to complete. Three other groups then take the next three 10-second periods to do the same exercise. The result is that the groups are working on a 1 : 3 work/recovery ratio within the confines of a skill practice. The work periods should be kept to less than 15 seconds otherwise accumulated lactic acid will start to interfere with the quality of execution. This efficient use of energy sources allows a high intensity of effort to be continued for 10–15 minutes without fatigue interrupting the transfer of skill learning process. The use of interval skill drills should not be abused. They are appropriate for practising learned skills. They are not the stage for introducing new skills or skill elements. Learning should be conducted under certain conditions that lead to the best learning response. Once the action to be learned has been performed relatively consistently in a 'learning environment' it should be practiced in circumstances that better resemble game situations — one of the roles of skill drills. Purely learned skills can be transferred to conditions that simulate game demands. The best use of skill drills occurs at a particular time in the sequence of activities for a training session (see Chapter 18).

Interval skill drills can also be developed to practice effective patterns of play in team games while still stimulating physiological adaptation. The creative coach should pay careful attention to the number of players in each sub-group and to the specific responsibilities of each player. The objectives of play pattern drills should be to:

1. assign players to positions and responsibilities that are similar to those experienced in a game
2. position the players in such a way that the ball can be moved forward in a coordinated manner
3. utilize the energy sources that are used predominantly in the game

The skills of a team game can be practiced separately. For example, each of the four sections of a field hockey playing area can be used to practice a different skill, within the interval training format. During a period of 5–10 minutes, four players in each quadrant can work on drills which involve, for example, trapping and shooting, trapping and pushing, tackling and intercepting, and dribbling. At the conclusion of this period the groups change activities until all skills have been completed. The 'grid' system of organization leaves the coach free to identify and remedy problems rather than simply supervise a practice session. This system is being used in many team sports and, because players are well organized, it optimizes the use of training time and effort.

The same principles of interval skill drills can be applied to racquet sports. Tennis players can be involved, in turn, in a sequence of shots most likely to be encountered in a game. Five balls can be fed to different parts of the court so that the player hits a forehand drive, backhand drive, forehand approach shot, volley, and smash in that order. The player then retrieves the balls and replaces them in the supply bucket. Six players can be involved in the drill which provides skill practice and energy utilization that is appropriate for tennis. A series of interval skill drills for squash have been described by Elliott *et al.* (1980).

Interval skill drills may have to be supplemented with some shorter, faster interval sprint training completed outside the confines of skill practice. This is because the commitment to skill often inhibits the team game player from running at top speed and hence the energy systems involved do not get fully taxed.

There is often a tendency for a coach to want to achieve too much through the use of skill drills. From a physiological perspective, they may be too limiting to stimulate adequately all the physical capacities that are needed for a sport, particularly those required for body and ground contact. The value of interval skill drills can also be overestimated. For example, when the performance level during an exercise starts to deteriorate noticeably, the resulting effect is not beneficial. If fatigue is of sufficient magnitude to interfere with specific performance levels, then the correct neuromuscular patterns of the skills are not being practiced and training effects are doubtful. The major effect of continuing the deteriorating repetitions may be learning to cope with fatigue, something that will not enhance performance. Thus the sequencing, alternation, repetition, and termination of the drills are critical programming decisions for the coach.

The training for team games that require multiple physical capacities is complicated. Each capacity should be developed as effectively as possible with adequate stimulation being provided to each. Since the frequency of stimulation and duration of recovery periods differ for each, it is necessary to plan them individually and conduct distinct microcycles and macrocycles depending upon the respective developmental objectives. These considerations necessitate extensive time periods for training. Most team games have individual and team skill factors that are more important for competition outcomes and the development of those skills should not be reduced because of misdirected emphasis on 'conditioning'. One should not place undue emphasis on attempting to improve performances by training 'harder': skills are learned.

The physiological status of the body must be such that learning will occur under the best of conditions. Any form of fatigue or stress interferes with learning. A large part of team game practice should be devoted to learning and providing the appropriate environment (both internal and external to the learner) for it to occur. Training for physical capacities must occur after the technical and tactical skill aspects of team game performances have been accommodated. Several physical capacities can be stimulated during the practice of learned activities under simulated game conditions. Interval skill drills appear to be one of the most effective forms of achieving this outcome. Other physical capacities may have to be stimulated outside all individual and team skill-learning situations.

The programming of multi-capacity training is not easy. A knowledge of the training parameters of each is essential. Their development according to ideal frequencies of work and recovery is crucial. It is no longer acceptable to have physical training occur on, for example, three separate occasions per week where each capacity is 'trained'. That form of programming may lead to overstimulation of some capacities (e.g., muscular endurance), understimulation of others (e.g., cardio-respiratory endurance and flexibility), while others may be accommodated adequately (e.g., strength and speed). To refine the energizing capacities of a multi-capacity sports player, each capacity has to be trained to the level that is appropriate for the sport and the person. The programming of the training needs careful planning and close adherence to sound principles.

VI
Training Plans

18

Planning Training Sessions, Microcycles, and Macrocycles

A macrocycle constitutes a number of microcycles which aim to achieve certain fitness training objectives. Since performance consists of a number of fitness components, the structuring of macrocycles is not an easy task. Consideration of what is to be contained in a macrocycle requires careful deliberation about how training sessions and microcycles are planned. This chapter looks at these two training structures as building blocks for the sane development of macrocycles.

The Importance of Skill Learning

This text focuses on the development of fitness components without pretending to assert that fitness is the most important feature of an athlete's development. Training session plans need to consider where technical and tactical skill training should occur to supplement fitness training so that the best learning will be produced.

The skill learning capacity of an individual is moderated by the state of fitness. For the most efficient learning to occur, the fitness elements that are required for the performance of a skill need to exist in a sufficiently trained state to allow the skill to be performed adequately. For example, it would be difficult for a swimmer to attempt an 'elbows-up' position early in the crawl stroke technique, if he or she did not have sufficient body strength to be able to maintain a stable upper body position that only permitted rotation about the longitudinal axis. The correct execution of the finer technique point is dependent upon having the postural strength to establish a solid foundation for the peripheral movements. As another example, it would not be advisable for an archer to contemplate very fine technique points if there were not a sufficient level of fitness to be able to maintain a consistent stature for the duration of the longest competition. If fatigue were to occur, it would interact with the skill precision and either cause performance deterioration or establish a need for a technique alteration. Both reactions are not characteristics of desirable high-level performance features. Thus, the most efficient development of technique will occur only when appropriate levels of fitness to support the technique have been attained.

The rate of skill learning is moderated by a considerable number of factors. These determine what is included in a training session, how learning opportunities are distributed in a microcycle, and what the learning objectives of a macrocycle are. Even though this text focuses on fitness components, their planning needs to be considered in light of other factors, a brief description of some of the more important moderators of which are:

□ Age of the Learner

Skill-learning capacity varies with chronological and maturational age. Infants, teenagers, and the aged all have different potential capacities for learning. Two people with the same chronological age, but different maturational ages, learn at different rates. The amount of practice time allocated to learning will depend upon the interaction of both ages.

□ Degree or Stage of Training

Strength, endurance, and precision skills are affected by training. The more training that has occurred, the better skill learning is likely to be, given certain restrictions. In a group of athletes, with different amounts of exposure to training in the same season, each individual should train on a program that is appropriate for his or her stage. A single program for a group assumes that all individuals are equal, but that assumption is not appropriate for efficient and productive coaching (see Chapter 7, The Principle of Individuality). The state of fitness development will influence the level of skill precision that can be attained.

□ History of Training

The longer the history of participation in sports, the greater is likely to be the number of skill elements that could be transferred to the early stages of the learning of a new skill. The richness of the history determines the level and initial speed of learning when new skills are attempted. The directions and activities used in coaching should be geared to each person's sporting background so that initial skill-learning experiences will be efficient.

☐ Skill Level

The skill of a person governs the potential rate of improvement. For example, it is much easier to improve from 8 to 12 meters in the shot-put than it is to improve from 20 to 24 meters, although the absolute distance changes are the same. Improvements of a specified magnitude will be more difficult to attain for more advanced athletes: the expectations for activity development will be determined by the skill level of the athlete. More training time for skill improvement will need to be provided for highly skilled athletes to achieve noticeable performance changes.

☐ Nature of the Skill

The more difficult or complex the skill, the greater will be the time required to reach specific proficiency levels. For programming training sessions, complicated skills and tactics should be allocated more time than simple activities. The concept of variable programming, that is, assigning learning time opportunities that fit the requirements of the skill learning experiences, needs to be introduced into planning training content.

☐ Reinforcers Derived from the Activity

Strong reinforcers derived from learning experiences produce faster rates of skill acquisition than do weak reinforcers. The reinforcers and incentives which exist in the training environment should be personalized and maximized.

☐ Reasons for Participation

When an individual likes an activity, faster skill learning results than when an activity is not liked. A coach will have to be skilled in establishing the need and desirability for skill change/development (see Chapter 10, Social and Psychological Factors).

☐ Stimulus Variation

The more constant the learning environment, the faster is the rate of skill acquisition. Training environments should provide consistent coaching situations, particularly for early stages of learning. Distraction reduces the rate of learning, particularly in the early stages of skill acquisition. Distractions should be eliminated through self-preoccupied instructional techniques. The cues for instruction and directions need to be as clear as possible.

These features indicate the need to avoid group instruction sessions when coaching skills. Because group instruction methods have been perpetuated and are easier to administer than individual instructional procedures, this does not mean they are the best for learning to occur. Individualized training programs may seem more difficult, but they have to be followed to produce the best training responses in athletes.

There is another feature that must be considered when planning skill development and its inclusion in a training session. It is that *fatigue impedes learning*. Skills and tactical elements are learned faster and retained better when learning occurs in non-fatigued states. This means that all learning should precede any occurrence of fatigue in a training session. To some coaches, this principle may be contradictory to their understanding of the use of the principle of specificity. It is commonly asserted that if skills are to be performed when an athlete is tired, then learning those skills while experiencing the level of fatigue that will occur in the sporting event is the best procedure. However, it has been shown that techniques and tactics learned in non-fatigued states produce better performances in fatigued states than do skills which have been learned in the presence of fatigue (Williams, McEwan, Watkins, Gillespie, and Boyd 1979). The physiology of learning supports this finding. The formation of neuromuscular patterns is inhibited by increases in the acidity of the supporting physiological environment. Thus, when lactic acid accrues as a result of fatigue, the potential for learning is reduced.

The structural changes which occur with fatigue also reduce the efficiency of learning. In fatigued states, the recruitment of extra muscle fibers, to support or replace those which are fatigued, produces a different neural organization from that required for an efficient performance. The nature of specific fiber recruitment has not been studied very intensively, but it does appear that patterns of recruitment are situation-dependent. The fibers that are recruited depend upon the circumstances which exist at a particular time. Hence, the pattern of movement in fatigue will vary from experience to experience. This response variation does not increase performance efficiency. Thus it does not make sense to attempt any skill learning when athletes are in fatigued states. Attempts at learning should occur after adequate recovery from previous training-session fatigue and should precede increases in accrued fatigue in the training session. Attempts to learn skills and tactics at other times will produce less than efficient, and often undesirable, outcomes. All learning experiences should be planned for the initial stages of a training session.

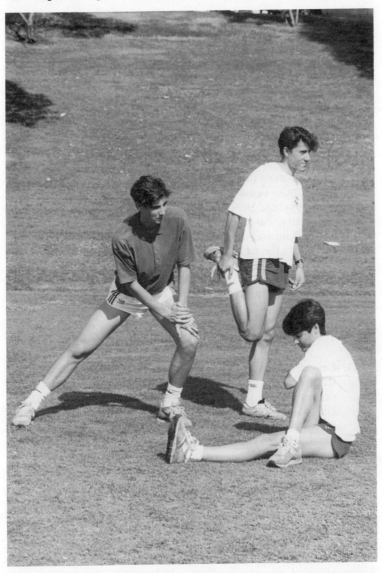

A warm-up should initiate every training session, and should include general exercises to warm the muscles, followed by specific flexibility exercises to increase the range of joint motion

Structuring a Training Session

The energizing forces of training are the fitness components that are stimulated. Because each component makes different physiological and neurological demands on the body, how those components are presented in a training session should occur in a particular order, intensity, and volume. The duration of a training session will depend upon the tasks that are presented as training stimuli, the activity forms in these tasks, the athlete's level of physical preparation for each fitness component, and the general training load.

Fatigue is the most important phenomenon that must be considered in the conduct of a training session. It has been explained at length that psychological and fatigue states affect the learning of skills and tactics. Fatigue also inhibits the development of speed and coordination, and these performance components should only be trained when the muscles are rested. A particular hierarchy for training fitness components exists, indicating that some training items must occur before others for desirable training outcomes to be produced. Not to adhere to the hierarchy is to diminish the potential value of a training session. The hierarchy of training session activities is:

1. *General warm-up.* A general warm-up should initiate every training session. The activities should involve all body components with a view to increasing the temperature of the large and deep muscles. Once an adequate temperature increase is achieved, usually indicated by a light sweat, flexibility activities that involve the major joints, and those joints of particular importance to the sport, should be undertaken. This order is often different from what is commonly seen during warm-ups. Flexibility should follow activity which makes muscles warm, because warm muscles and joint structures are more flexible than cold ones.
2. *Learn techniques and tactics.* If learning occurs in non-fatigued states, sufficient time should be allocated to ensure that it takes place by producing desirable patterns of response. Hurried learning sessions could result in the development of more errors than desirable outcomes.
3. *Perfect techniques and tactics.* Previous learning should be practiced at medium and maximum intensities. Goals for execution precision should be established. Adequate recovery times between repetitions should be provided so that no performance deterioration occurs due to fatigue.

4. *Develop speed.* Training stimuli that attempt to improve speed should next be planned. These should be of short duration. Complete recovery between each trial should be permitted. Any fatigue that exists at the start of a trial will reduce the specific nature of any training effect.

5. *Develop power.* Activities which require speed and strength (power) should next be considered. The rest period between each repetition will depend upon the importance of the speed factor. Interval training, which requires total recovery between repeats, is the preferred training format for this fitness component. Since the application of power is skill-dependent, obvious incursions of harmful fatigue should be avoided.

6. *Develop specific strength.* Within a training session, specific strength is best developed through a few maximum efforts (low repetitions with high resistance) with almost complete recovery between trials. It is not advisable to attempt supplementary training (e.g., weights, pulleys, etc.) during a training session. Supplementary training is best scheduled after or outside of training sessions, not before training as it is commonly practiced.

7. *Develop muscular endurance.* Muscular endurance should be presented in two stages. The first bout of repetitions should comprise a moderate amount of repetitions with moderate resistance. The volume then should be increased to a higher number of repetitions with moderate resistance. The repetitions and resistances will depend upon the fitness component requirements for the sport and the individual.

8. *Develop aerobic endurance.* The first level of aerobic endurance work should be the hardest.

9. *Develop aerobic endurance.* The remaining endurance work should be of a moderate intensity to initiate the winding-down of the training session.

10. *Recovery routine.* A training session should employ a recovery or cool-down routine. The work intensity is reduced and the specific nature of activity may also be reduced. This training segment should allow athletes to leave the practice environment partly recovered and with a positive disposition to promote interest in and enhance motivation for the next training session.

The sequence that has been described above indicates an initial learning emphasis, an intensity peak in the middle, and an endurance dominance at the end (Bompa 1986). It should be realized that not all the activity emphases which have been described will occur in each training session. Training segments, once they are selected, should be ordered according to this scheme.

In its simplest form, a training session may consist of only one segment, such as when a distance runner goes for a 12-kilometer fartlek run. The planning of what components are to be stimulated in a session depends on the requirements of the individual athlete, the sport, the microcycle, and the macrocycle in which the session occurs.

The organization of specific training items during a session should consider the following (Bompa 1986):

1. Exercises should be alternated between each training objective and segment to allow within session recovery/regeneration. Thus a decathlete would consider cycling through weight events in a training session rather than dedicating one part purely and totally to discus throwing, then the next to the shot, and the final part to javelin. Those events would be ordered: javelin (greatest speed requirement), discus (speed and strength), and then shot (strength and speed). Some javelin training would be done. As soon as performance or technique started to deteriorate, discus training would commence. This would allow some recovery to occur for javelin throwing. As soon as the discus work began to decline in quality, the shot activity would commence. This would allow even more recovery for the javelin, while recovery for the discus commenced. Then, as the performance features of the shot began to deteriorate, javelin would be once again reintroduced. Cycling activities in this manner may be difficult to organize, but will yield a greater volume of better quality training responses in each training session. This, in turn, would promote faster rates of fitness component improvement. Activity alternation, within the same fitness component, will allow some amount of within session recovery and regeneration.

2. The greater the training intensity, the less will be the volume of training in a standard time-period. Recovery needs increase as the intensity of training elements increase. The use of recovery periods for instruction in other domains, such as the development of psychological skills and the performance of managerial activities, should be considered to introduce increased productivity in training-time utilization.

3. The duration of a training session is inversely proportional to the intensity of the training stimulus. Low-intensity sessions can be more time-consuming because of the large amounts of fuel stores that can be accessed and the ability

of the organism to maintain activity levels without incurring debilitating fatigue.

4. The more intense and stressful a training session, the simpler should be its organization. That organization will be enhanced if the content of the session is posted before it commences. Athletes will better be able to appropriate their capacities to the training segments when they know what will occur.

5. The heavier and more intense the overall load of one training session, the lighter should be the next session. Thus the alternation in training sessions of volume and intensity would be a sound planning principle.

The final coaching determinant of training session content is employed during the actual session. When an athlete fatigues during a session, techniques deteriorate and performances become less consistent. When that performance diminution occurs, it could reach a stage where any continued participation would serve no productive purpose, and with extreme fatigue, the consequences may even be counter-productive. Since no planning procedure for sports training is precise, coaches will have to exercise their judgment as to when a training segment should be interrupted or altered because of performance deterioration. There seems to be an irrational principle in coaching lore, to the effect that once an athlete commences a training segment, or attempts to achieve a training item goal, activity is not terminated until either or both have been achieved. This is done despite the possible futility of the experience and detrimental effects that such a procedure might have on an athlete. The 'hell-week' of swimming and rowing is a good example of the abuse of sound coaching principles. It is better to subject athletes to a few good quality experiences than it is to subject them to a few good and a large number of poor experiences. The counter-productivity of excessive and damaging work has not been investigated fully, probably because of the ethics involved in deliberately subjecting athletes to such harmful experiences. However, such considerations do not seem to concern some sport coaches, when they should. As a general rule of thumb for coaching, the advice that was given many years ago by the great Australian swimming coach-scientist, Forbes Carlile, is most appropriate here: 'It is better to undertrain than to overtrain'.

Structuring Session Microcycles

To develop a training effect, a training stimulus needs to be repeated at least two or three times and followed by a short unloading session in a microcycle. The basic structure of a microcycle for a fitness component has been described in Chapter 3, Generalized Responses to Training. It is convenient that most microcycles can be accommodated in one calendar week.

Since the overload factor for a microcycle is constant, progressions between microcycles are step-like. This contrasts with a common procedure of making each training session gradually more demanding. The step-like versus continual-gradual overloading presents a contrast of training philosophies. The step-like progression focuses on recovery as the primary determinant of training benefits (sometimes called the 'East-European' approach). The continual-gradual progression focuses on workload assignments as being the major determinants of training benefits, and is sometimes called the 'Western' approach to training. It is our proposal that coaches draw back from emphasizing increases of workload as being the major focus for planning training, and instead present training stimuli in accordance with the recovery capacities of athletes. Thus progression in training states is determined by recovery features in athletes, not their capacities to handle ever-increasing training loads. The distinction between these two orientations is important for applying modern training principles.

The discussion of microcycles so far has centred on the training stimulus of one training segment. However, training sessions contain several training stimuli which often attempt to develop different fitness and learning capacities. This complicates the design picture of training programs for it introduces training microcycles as being a period of time in which segment microcycles are coordinated. Fitness components develop and recover at different rates. Thus the timing of successive exposures to training stimuli within a segment microcycle will depend upon the fitness component, and intensity and volume of the stimulus. If one were to apportion the same amount of time and frequency of presentation to each fitness component, then an unbalanced preparation would result. Some capacities would peak and then overtrain, while others would still be adapting, destroying the harmonious development of an athlete with a resulting decrease in performance potential. *For maximum performances to be achieved, all fitness components that are to be trained must be coordinated to achieve their peak adaptation levels at the same time.* Figure 18.1 illustrates the concept of independent planning of fitness component microcycles within a training microcycle.

The independent planning of fitness component microcycles within a weekly training microcycle requires some explanation. The illustrated structure is purely hypothetical. The power/speed microcycle segments are presented four times to develop a training effect, on 2 evenings and 2 mornings. An unloading stimulus occurs at Saturday morning's training session. The muscular endurance stimuli occur on 3 successive evenings with two 24-hour recovery periods. Then a 36-hour recovery period precedes the occurrence of a stimulus at the Friday morning training session, with the unloading stimulus occurring on Friday evening. Three days are then allowed for full recovery. Flexibility is stimulated in moderate amounts on each of 6 mornings. The unloading cycle occurs under the athlete's self-monitoring on Sunday morning.

Figure 18.1 Hypothetical Integration of Fitness Component Microcycles into a Week-long Training Microcycle

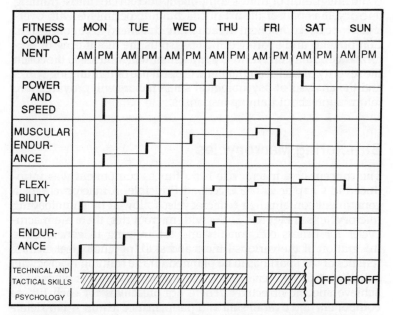

Each component is presented a number of times and followed by an unloading cycle. Mid-week recovery is facilitated by there being no fitness training on Thursday evening. Saturday morning to Monday morning is a period of no training that serves as the opportunity for regeneration to occur.

Flexibility development requires frequent stimulation, and this program has attempted to provide opportunities. Endurance training is mainly stimulated at the morning sessions. There are 5 exposures in the endurance microcycle with the unloading stimulus occurring on Saturday morning. Thus it can be seen that the components are stimulated according to the different schedules involved in each component's microcycle, which are coordinated into the overall training microcycle. Thursday evening has no scheduled fitness training to allow for extra recovery, although the following morning has all components stimulated. The training of these fitness components occurs along with technical and tactical skill training and psychological development. No skill/psychological training occurs on Friday morning, since that session is heavily loaded with fitness segments. Saturday evening and all day Sunday are rest days to facilitate the development of training effects. Only the isolated flexibility unloading stimulus occurs during these regeneration days.

The integration of fitness component microcycles into a training microcycle is part of the art of coaching. Experiments with overloads for each component in each individual need to be conducted. Component- and sport-specific tests, plus the monitoring of performance quality and recovery capacities, will indicate to the coach the severity of each training item. Careful use of training log books and the analysis of psychological stress factors will provide more information about training responses.

Structuring Macrocycles

The concept of a macrocycle for a fitness component was introduced in Chapter 4, The Overload Principle. A macrocycle for a component contains 5 or 6 microcycles followed by an unloading microcycle (see Figure 4.1). As with microcycles, there are macrocycles for fitness components and for training in general. The integration of the various fitness and skill/psychological characteristics of the sport has to be planned for the training macrocycle.

A distinguishing feature of a macrocycle is that it is planned to achieve specific objectives. There are objectives for each fitness component and overall skill and performance features. The determination of whether or not those objectives are achieved at the completion of a macrocycle is important, for it governs the content of subsequent macrocycles.

Objectives should be established for each fitness component as well as other performance features. The assessment of these objectives is to be through component testing (see Chapter 12). Initial tests of each fitness component should be conducted before the macrocycle is started. Periodically throughout the macrocycle, tests should be repeated to give indications of developmental progress or maintenance. A final testing should be conducted to indicate the resultant component state and degree of training objective fulfillment. The use of physiological testing in this manner has to become an integral feature of any modern training program. It serves both diagnostic and motivational purposes.

The objectives of component macrocycles change once desirable or maximum development levels are attained, the focus then shifting to maintaining attained fitness levels. Maintenance training will require an alteration of the frequency of training stimuli in the microcycles within the macrocycle.

To plan a macrocycle, weekly microcycles should be designed so that coordinated improvement in all fitness components occurs. Similar decision criteria to those for formulating microcycles are used. The only difference is that macrocycles are considered on a grander scale. Increases in training stimuli should occur as an athlete's capacities increase. These increases are best provided in steps, each step containing a number of exposures to component overload followed by an unloading cycle for regeneration and the attainment of training effects.

The most important stage of a macrocycle is at the end when evaluations of component states are performed. If a training factor has been found not to develop at a predicted rate, the initial emphasis of training in the next macrocycle should be shifted to correcting that weakness. Recovery programs should be monitored more frequently than those which occur with normal development. Coaches should always be aware of the possibility of the plateau stage and not misinterpret no-change observations. Thus the end of a macrocycle is the stage where important decisions are made about the continuation of a training plan. If corrective steps are necessary, they should be implemented immediately so that performance improvement will not be hindered.

To serve as a summary for this section, Bompa (1986) has highlighted the following features:

1. Any competitions should be scheduled for the end of the macrocycle.
2. For the preparatory phase of training, macrocycles are usually longer than in other stages of training plans.
3. Macrocycles have as their objectives: to improve competitive performances, to improve test scores, and to develop training/fitness factors.
4. The attainment of objectives should be analyzed at the end of a macrocycle.
5. Macrocycles are the major building block of any training program progression.
6. The last microcycle of a macrocycle is a regeneration/unloading one.

7. For sports which involve a great amount of skill learning, microcycles should be of uniform intensity within a macrocycle.

Planning Training Programs

☐ Training Sessions

Figure 18.2 illustrates one possible format for use when planning a training session. Those training factors which are not appropriate for the sport in question should be eliminated. The session number in the microcycle should be recorded along with the date and an estimate of the session training load. The training factors are ordered in the appropriate sequence for their occurrence in a training session. Some indication of acceptable performance levels should be indicated in the objectives column. The alternation of exercises to allow more in-session recovery should also be indicated. The recovery factor should list the activities to be undertaken at training to assist in recovery from session fatigue. Some general indication of the projected intensity, such as heavy, medium, or light, of each training stimulus should be included under the 'Intensity' column heading.

☐ Microcycles

Figure 18.3 illustrates one possible microcycle planning sheet format. Those factors which are not appropriate for the sport should be eliminated. Daily activities should be indicated for each training factor including rest and recovery opportunities. The time when an unloading session occurs for each factor should also be indicated. This category of testing has been introduced so that it can be planned in a consistent manner that is in concert with the aims of the training phase.

☐ Macrocycles

Figure 18.4 illustrates a possible planning sheet for developing macrocycles. The phase of training that the macrocycle is planned for should be recorded at the top of the page. The major items recorded are the progressions in training stimuli across the macrocycle. The macrocycle objectives for each training factor should also be planned. The decisions made concerning the macrocycle, testing results, and the attainment of objectives will determine the content of the subsequent macrocycle. Competition experiences and an unloading microcycle should be included in this plan.

Figure 18.2 A Training Session Planning Sheet that Lists the Correct Order of Session Activities

TRAINING SESSION PLANNING SHEET

Microcycle session . . . .   Training session severity:

Date . . . .   Heavy___ medium___ light___

Training Factor	Activities and Coaching Points	Intensity	Objectives
1. Warm-up			
2. Technique learning			
3. Tactical learning			
4. Technique practice			
5. Tactical practice			
6. Speed			
7. Power			
8. Strength			
10. Aerobic (H) endurance			
11. Aerobic (L) endurance			
12. Recovery			

Figure 18.3 A Suggested Format for Planning Microcycles

MICROCYCLE PLANNING SHEET

Microcycle session ___ of ___   Inclusive dates: .... to ....

Training Factor	Activities and Coaching Points							Objectives
	M	T	W	Th	F	S	Su	
1. Techniques								
2. Tactics								
3. Testing								
4. Technique practice								
5. Speed								
6. Power								
7. Strength								
8. Muscular endurance								
9. Aerobic (H) endurance								
10. Recovery								

The activities and training stimuli and objectives for each training factor are planned and recorded on the sheet.

Figure 18.4 Suggested Planning Sheet for Determining the Progressions Within a Macrocycle

MACROCYCLE PLANNING SHEET

Training phase _____   Inclusive dates: .... to ....

Training Factor	Microcycle/Activity Progressions							Objectives
	1	2	3	4	5	6	7	
1. Competitions								
2. Techniques								
3. Tactics								
4. Testing								
5. Speed								
6. Power								
7. Strength								
8. Muscular endurance								
9. Aerobic (H) endurance								
10. Recovery								

The maximum number of microcycles is seven. What is recorded in each box is an index of how the overload for each microcycle changes for each training factor.

19

Planning a Training Year

Not every sporting program can be accommodated by a calendar. Athletes who participate in more than one sport have to compromise some training elements for one or more of their sports. These days, for an ideal development of an athlete's capacities, dedication to one sport is necessary. This does not mean that multi-sport athletes are not possible. However, for an individual to have the chance to achieve performances that tax their potential to the fullest, it is necessary to have training experiences which allow appropriate developments to occur. If an athlete is not able, or is not prepared to train for a sport in the best manner possible, then he or she cannot perform to the level that is possible with full training.

For this chapter it is assumed that an athlete will be able to take part in a 12-month training program, and the features of an annual training plan will be discussed. If the training program cannot be accommodated as a full-year activity then the coach will have to reduce parts of the annual plan requirements with the understanding that an athlete's potential performances will be reduced by the degree of compromise that occurs.

There are five phases of an annual training plan:

1. Basic preparatory phase
2. Specific preparatory phase
3. Pre-competition phase
4. Competition phase
5. Transition phase

There is very little research that points to the ideal stages of an annual training plan. Conclusions about appropriate content are gathered by analyzing the philosophies and practices of successful sporting nations. The five-phase structure outlined above results from such an analysis. It mainly reflects the characteristics of Eastern bloc countries as well as some of the more advanced and (in sport) improving Western nations.

Annual training programs are planned. They should be based on scientific principles and experience. The habit of vague planning and then constructing the content of training sessions as they occur is no longer adequate. Plans need to be developed and structured according to specific features. This text so far has provided most of the tools for determining the features of sport fitness training. It now remains for coaches and athletes to plan the way the principles and characteristics of training given can be used in a year-round training program, one that is built on known principles of training and which should not be altered in any drastic manner once it is implemented. Alterations should be guided by test and performance results, as well as by careful athlete-involved discussions. A commitment must be made not to panic in an attempt to change a training program by suddenly altering the loadings of volume or training intensities. Sudden shifts in training regimens are stressful for athletes, and these stresses, plus the obvious inconsistency that develops from sudden changes, may be more harmful to an athlete's development, outweighing the benefits that can be gained from change.

Establishing Objectives

Before any detailed training plan is structured, objectives need to be established for the overall year and for each training phase. There are six categories that should be considered for the total and phase objectives. They are:

1. performance levels and characteristics
2. fitness capacity measures
3. the biomechanical features and performance characteristics of technical elements
4. the nature and features of tactical elements
5. behaviors and psychological factors
6. items and knowledge about the sport and its technical bases

Objectives that are formulated should be conceptualized and worded in such a way that they can be observed and measured. Statements such as 'improving tenacity', 'increasing aerobic power', etc. are useless. Each objective should state what quantities and qualities of behaviors are to be developed. For example, increasing aerobic power should be defined in terms of ultimate test scores and/or performance features. All objectives should be able to be directly interpreted by athletes and should be decided on jointly by the coach and athlete.

The time when training plans should be altered is when the attainment or non-attainment of training phase objectives is determined. With such alterations it is better to be too conservative than too radical. All alterations should be made jointly by the coach and athlete.

Testing Programs

The monitoring of fitness developments is a necessary feature of planning and implementing annual training plans. The tests that are selected should have direct utility and be meaningful for both coach and athlete. It is a good idea to have a mix of laboratory and field tests for each of the fitness capacities that are essential to the sport. Within macrocycles, some periodic testing should occur. At the end of each macrocycle, there should be extensive testing. At the end of each training phase there should be full testing.

Testing in an annual plan should be used to establish the following:

1. progress in the development of fitness capacities
2. the level of fitness that has been attained
3. the degree to which objectives have been achieved
4. program modifications for successive macrocycles

The types of tests that are selected will be influenced by available resources, facilities, and testing opportunities. Those tests which are finally decided upon should be scheduled and coordinated with the testing agencies, if necessary. As sport testing is no longer an unusual occurrence, the demand on existing facilities is starting to extend these facilities to near their maximum capacities. It is a good feature of planning to organize the times and locations of testing that will occur well before they are needed.

General Planning Considerations

□ Training Emphases

The dominant physical capacities that have been determined for the sport need to be considered when planning training volumes and intensities. Coordinating the development of these capacities and the length of time in change-training and maintenance-training stages should be decided. The shift from change to maintenance will release time for more concentrated development of other objectives. Some objectives, particularly technical, tactical, and psychological ones, cannot be fully attempted until fitness capacities attain certain levels.

□ Fitness Foundation

The degree of fitness in the capacities essential to a sport, as already emphasized, is the foundation upon which other aspects of training occur. The maintenance of that foundation is essential for adequate performance. There are two factors that govern this: the degree of general fitness, which includes both specific and non-specific fitness, and the degree of specialized fitness, that which can be directly used in a sport's activities. In developing the fitness foundation, there will be a constant push and pull between the need to maintain general fitness and the need to develop specific fitness. Too much general fitness may interfere with performance precision. Too much specific fitness training may lead to over-trained states which also interfere with performance.

□ Basic Training

The ultimate level of performance that can be attained in a year will largely be determined by the volume of basic training that is performed. Programs that emphasize the development of essential fitness capacities as well as those capacities that may be used sparingly in a performance constitute the basic preparatory phase for fitness. Training groundwork affects performance level and the length or number of times that level can be performed.

□ Emphasis Shifts

The annual plan should exhibit a shift in emphasis from an initial provision of general activities to final specialized training. The length of time that is allocated to each extreme of training is determined by the complexity of the activity. Generally, the more complicated a sport, that is, the more fitness components and the difficulty of the technical features, the earlier the shift into specialized training will occur. On the other hand, with particularly specialized activities such as power-lifting, the specialized nature of training will occur after a much greater base of general training. Determining when the change from general to specific training occurs is one of the responsibilities of a coach.

□ Overloading Stimuli

The progression of macrocycles which are planned for a year should follow similar guidelines to those which determine their own structure. The overall training loads of the macrocycles should change in a step-like fashion, with a noticeably different load/form of work between them. There should be an obvious increase in workload between change-training macrocycles up to the point of maximum adaptation. From then on, the number of exposures to training stimuli within a maintenance-training macrocycle will decrease although the intensity is maintained. At various stages in the annual plan, for example, the macrocycle preceding the period of serious competitions, there should be reductions in load for physical and psychological regeneration. One of the valuable features of step-like training load developments is that a plateau will become evident to indicate that full adaptation in fitness has occurred. If training loads were changing constantly it would not be possible for adaptation to be obvious because the body would be in either a state of adaptation or overtraining.

Across the annual plan, the training emphasis should shift from one of volume in the preparatory phase to intensity/quality in the competition phase. Within that shifting emphasis, there always should be an awareness of, and opportunity for, physical and psychological regeneration. The latter is particularly important in long-term programs. At various stages in annual plans, perhaps after each two macrocycles, there should be an unloading, short macrocycle that allows an athlete to recover enthusiasm for training and commitment to the sport. This is necessary because the psychological state of the athlete will mediate the quality and response to training (see Chapter 10). Bompa (1986) suggested the following options for producing an unloading macrocycle:

1. reduction in training volume
2. reduction in training intensity
3. reduction in training frequency
4. reduction in outside-of-sport stressors

These four factors will depend on the developed capacities that are to be retained, and the balance of training reduction with training stimulation. Unloading macrocycles generally should take no longer than two weeks.

Basic Preparatory Phase

The basic preparatory phase of training is characterized by the following features:

1. a dominant emphasis on volumes of physical activity rather than intensity
2. programming of related and remotely related activities

3. a length that is dictated by the needs/complexity of the sport
4. the establishment of training habits and commitment

The longer and more substantial is this basic form of training, the better and longer an athlete will be able to hold a peak performance capability when serious competitions occur. The corollary to this statement is: an athlete's ability to hold a peak performance status is directly proportional to the amount of base (preparatory or background) training that is done. The substantiation of this principle occurred when the sport of swimming underwent a radical change in training regimens in the late 1950s and early 1960s from 6 months to 12 months. Rushall (1967: 209–11) noted:

> . . . when one refers to the 1964 Olympic Games, and the swimming events where America and Australia took all but one of the Gold Medals, the American . . . swimmers were mostly representative of an all-year training and competitive program . . . Most of these people had been nurtured in the great increase in tempo of training and competition of the AAU age-group swimming program, started after the 1956 Olympic Games. Then eight years later, the greatest swim team ever was formed of individuals who were generally able to endure a year-round intensive program of very hard training and competition . . . They were so well adapted, that most competitors were able to produce and better their own personal, and in some cases world, best times in heats, semi-finals, and finals at the Games. The Australian Gold Medalists, Windle, Fraser, and Berry, and to a lesser extent O'Brien, all displayed similar training histories to those of the Americans, although Dawn Fraser had one more of years rather than intensity. They too displayed the ability to withstand great amounts of training and to produce great performances relatively on top of each other.
>
> The main feature being stressed here is that these swimmers had endured all-year programs in their development, and were able to produce 100 percent efforts on top of each other without their performances dropping off.
>
> Now contrasted to these all-enduring athletes of the USA . . . were the European swimmers [who had training histories of a half-year in the water, and a half-year out]. They contained among them world-record holders, Caron, Gottvales, McGregor, Kok, plus several others who were the fastest in the world at that time . . . Most European swimmers produced very good times in the qualifying heats; but as the semi-finals went on they were unable to improve as much as the Americans and Australians, and in some cases fell away in their performances. It was as if their adaptation capacities were more strained by one event than were the others. This is suggestive of the Europeans being good for only one top-class performance within such a short space of time as demanded by the Olympic program. This contrasted to the Americans and Australians who were able to produce world-class performances continually.

Harre (1971) reported a study that showed athletes who emphasized the general physical component in the preparatory training phase, as opposed to those who specialized, had their best results occur later but at superior levels and with more consistency. This can be interpreted as meaning that specialized training effects *were added to* a very substantial fitness base. Bompa (1986: 36) has stated that what is being discussed here is a principle that justifies the emphasis on a general physical preparation: 'The higher the athlete's working potential (obtained through preparatory training), the easier it is to adapt to the physical and psychological demands of [specialized] training'.

The basic preparatory phase can include activities drawn from sports which are related to the athlete's own sport. For example, a squash player may participate in table-tennis (for speed and agility), and tennis (for endurance) to supplement other forms of squash-related training. These activities usually contribute to some basic physical capacity that is required in the sport. This phase of training would also include the greatest amount of auxiliary training (medicine ball work, free-standing exercises, specific remedial resistance work, etc.). However, because such activities are beneficial for establishing a physiological base, this does not mean that they are just as beneficial when highly specialized training is employed. At that time they have the potential to disrupt refined neuromuscular patterns associated with skill.

The basic preparatory phase of training is characterized by the following:

1. There is improvement in the general fitness of the athlete.
2. There is heightened improvement in the capacities that are essential for the sport.
3. The development of *basic techniques* is the only major emphasis associated with the sport, that is, physical training is general, technique training is sport-specific.
4. Volume of vigorous activity is the predominant emphasis of the training program. Overtraining is avoided because the variety of activities allows various physical capacities to regenerate, even though activity persists, and the neuromuscular patterns remain understressed because of the variety of activities pursued.
5. It is the longest phase of training (possibly two macrocycles).
6. There are no competitions.
7. An attempt is made to improve an athlete's weaknesses in physical capacities.

8. It is similar for young athletes no matter what their sport. That similarity gradually disappears the more experienced and older the athlete becomes.
9. Testing usually occurs after the first two weeks of training, so that the tests themselves will not be too stressful. It also occurs at the end of the phase.

Specific Preparatory Phase

This phase represents a progression to more specialized training. At least half the training that is done should be directly related to the sport. The remainder still involves volume-oriented, remotely related work. Since technique was principally basic or general in nature in the basic preparatory phase, fitness training now has to become more specific so that finer points of technique, which probably rely on the existence of particular fitness levels, can be trained. Auxiliary training also becomes more specialized.

The length of time in this phase is usually one macrocycle. Care should be taken not to introduce specific work too quickly. If that were done, the intensity of the training stimuli might be too high, possibly leading to an early occurrence of overtraining. Untimely overtrained states usually disrupt training at the most crucial times, such as when leading up to competition preparation. It is prudent to avoid overemphasizing specific training too early.

The volume of training still remains relatively high but drops slightly when compared with the previous training phase. Some of the remotely related activities of the basic preparatory phase are replaced by greater attention to technique and tactical instruction, and a slightly increased volume of specific fitness training.

The amount of time spent training each week is no less, and possibly slightly more, than that spent in the previous training phase. This phase marks the start of 'committed' training and a serious attitude.

Tests should be conducted before, during, and after the phase. The objectives of improvement should be considered in relation to the year's plan. One should take care not to overemphasize too rapid an improvement at this stage. The reader is referred back to Figure 4.4, which highlights the benefits of moderate training loads as opposed to heavy loads, on ultimate performance achievements.

The volume of work done, in terms of caloric output, should peak at the end of this training phase. The concentration on training volume that has endured for about twelve weeks should produce a substantial capacity to perform large amounts of low to moderate intensity work.

The theme of this specific, but preparatory, training phase should be one of improving technical and fitness competencies according to some defined plan. Established objectives should be met but not exceeded.

Pre-competition Phase

The pre-competition phase of training marks the stage where specialized training dominates the content. Fitness capacities should achieve their maximum developmental levels. In terms of training load, this phase is the most demanding of all. Work intensity is increased and displaces volume as the primary emphasis. The heaviest loading should occur in the next-to-last microcycle, which is followed by an unloading microcycle which concludes the phase.

The pre-competition phase is the most critical part of an annual training plan. It is likely that most problems associated with fitness training could occur in this phase. Coaches will have to be very cautious and objective in their assessments of the training responses of athletes. Since this text concentrates on fitness development, it downplays the attention that should be given to technique development. Coaches have to decide whether the training fatigue that is developed during this stage hinders more important technique development. If it does, then opportunities for recovery should be increased so that harmful fatigue can be dissipated. The severity of training stimuli will be governed by the coaching decision of how much fatigue can be tolerated with each training stimulus and the effect of that fatigue on skills.

From the completion of the previous specific preparatory phase to the onset of the next phase should be a period of about 6–8 weeks — two relatively stressful macrocycles. Fitness capacities should be fully developed by the end of this training period. This will allow athletes to move into maintenance-training programs in the subsequent training phases. The intensity of the overall training load will be governed by when competitions will occur. The activities of this training phase should gradually approximate and model the intensities and forms of movement that will occur in competitions.

Thus this training phase emphasizes, from a fitness viewpoint, the final development to maximum levels of those specific fitness capacities that govern the performance of the sport. Remotely related activities are almost non-existent in the latter microcycles. The only purposes for their inclusion would be to assist in recovery and regeneration and, for psychological reasons, training program variety. Auxiliary training activities should cease by the end of this phase.

Testing should continue. The specificity of the tests and their relationship to critical features of the sport should be emphasized. Previous tests which have less than a relevant and direct implication for competition performances should cease. The results of these tests should be used to indicate progress to athletes or the achievement of maximum fitness states. The frequency of fitness testing should be at its highest during this stage. During the final intense training bouts, testing and monitoring should be increased to note at the earliest possible time the attainment of development plateaus or any onset of overtraining.

General non-specific activities are beneficial in the early stages of an annual training plan, but are potentially harmful in the latter stages of training. The reason for this reversal in benefit is that the nervous system is particularly fragile. Technique training emphasizes the development of specific neuromuscular patterns. Non-specific activities have the potential to confuse or disrupt the development of those fine-technique structures. If irrelevant patterns become dominant over desired movement patterns, the state of 'erroneous specialization' occurs. Examples of these errors were discussed in Chapter 6, The Principle of Specificity. As the competition period approaches, potentially incorrect patterns of movement should be removed from the training content so that those which remain are competition-specific. This also has direct relevance to how much training is done in debilitating fatigue states in training sessions. With each occurrence of fatigue, imprecise patterns of movement are enacted. The volume of these patterns should never come to exceed those of precise patterns (another form of 'erroneous specialization'). If that were to occur, the body would be dominated by incorrect repetitions of movement. In competition fatigue, it is likely that these incorrect movements would be evoked since they had been strengthened ('conditioned') through large amounts of training repetition. Coaches should constantly weigh the value of the volume of poor-quality technique work with that of good-quality work. Training efforts should cease as soon as the poorer work approaches the good work volume. The techniques to be used in competitions should achieve their highest levels of precision by the end of this phase.

The success of the pre-competition phase is dependent upon the volume of training achieved in the previous two phases; the introduction of judicious amounts of intense training; the achievement of peak fitness levels in all critical capacities; the performance of skills under competition-like circumstances; and the final refinement of skills.

Competition Phase

Competitive performances are built on a foundation of training. The training which precedes the competition phase should demonstrate a gradual improvement in the amount of specific training that has occurred. *Prior to entering this phase, all physical capacities and technical elements should have reached their highest levels of development.* The competitive phase involves the implementation of the benefits of previous training. The focus of athlete development in this phase is psychological and tactical.

The amount of fitness work that is done in this stage should be that which is appropriate for maintenance training. Each competition should be preceded by an unloading microcycle, the primary function of which is to allow for adequate resources to be applied to the other stresses which surround competitions (travel, competition hype, media, etc.).

The normal Western-orientation to competition-phase training is to start with a period of reduced work called the 'taper'. A taper is necessary if an athlete is unduly fatigued and recovery is required. With this suggested annual plan, the unloading cycle at the end of the pre-competition phase allows for regeneration. Thus the competition phase is not confounded by the anxiety associated with trying to time a 'taper' to allow maximum regeneration to occur in concert with the competition. The maintenance training associated with this phase should not allow athletes to be fatigued to any unnecessary degree. They should be able to proceed with competition-specific training. This marks a major difference from the excessive work ethic training of the West and the Eastern judicious rest form of training. The latter, as has been emphasized throughout this text, is supported by scientific research findings and principles.

Some training sessions should model the psychological atmosphere of competitions, and athletes should perform their competition routines in these simulated conditions. Such simulations will reduce the stress of competition (Rushall 1979c, 1986, 1987c). The degree to which simulations do mimic the actual organization, atmosphere, and expectations of competition will govern the success of the preparatory experience.

Usually, it is too late to attempt technique changes in this stage of training. There will be insufficient practice trials to allow newer technique features to be conditioned to sufficient strength to supersede previously established movement patterns. There is a psychological principle that indicates that the more stressful a situation, the more primitive will be the responses. This means that the more important is competition, the further back in training an athlete will regress with regard to the movement patterns used. Performance consists of the most frequently used movement patterns in that athlete's recent history of training. It is for this reason that the pre-competition phase stresses the final attainment of competition-level technical features. During the competition phase, athletes should condition those elements to an even stronger degree. No attempts to alter them should occur. The stress of late (panic) learning should be avoided so that competition performances can be attempted with confident techniques.

The training stimuli of the competition phase should be the most specific of any training phase. The major emphasis is on training intensity, which should, in major part, be the same as parts of the competition performance. The various forms of training that have been discussed in earlier chapters describe how specific training can be attempted without covering the actual competition in its entirety. Non-specific activities are done purely as active-recovery pursuits.

Within this phase there still is a transition. Right throughout the annual plan, the transition from one phase to the next should be subtle and hardly, if at all, noticeable to the athletes. The early stage of the competition phase should include practice and low-level competitions that are interspersed with stimulating, maintenance-training sessions. These early competitions should be used as testing grounds for the tactical, technical, and psychological features which have been developed. The latter part of the phase should be the period of serious competitions, and by this time, all elements of the sport should have been developed. Only alterations in the emphasis or sequence of already established performance elements should be new features. From a fitness viewpoint, maintenance training should continue to provide the energy base for superior performance. The nature and amount of that training will depend upon what training has occurred in previous phases. The latter stages of this phase should concentrate on providing positive and enjoyable training sessions, only involving activities that have been demonstrated at earlier training sessions or in competitions.

The nature of the competitions and their scheduling will determine what occurs in this training phase. Ideally, it would be best to have a period of serious training, perhaps two microcycles, and then an unloading microcycle at the end of which is the competition. After each competition, there should be a brief unloading microcycle to allow the athlete to recover from the other-than-physical stresses of competitions. Unfortunately, most high-level competitions and sporting agendas do not allow these ideal conditions to occur. An important coaching decision will be whether or not to permit alternations of training and competition micro-cycles.

The schedule of competitions will affect coaching decisions. The greater the number of competitions, the more stressed athletes will become. In the absence of stimulating training, stresses on frequent competitors tend to accumulate, placing them in a detraining spiral. This is the problem that occurs with professional or enter-tainment sports, such as baseball and basketball in the United States, and cricket in British Commonwealth nations. The stimuli that result from participation do not occur with sufficient volume or frequency to generate a training overload. Thus the benefits that have been gained from a final intense training phase are lost. Consequently, an athlete can detrain while being engaged in com-petitions. The occurrence of other competitive disruptions and consequences, such as unexpected travel, rescheduled compe-titions, injuries, etc., all produce lessened occurrences of training stimuli.

Close attention should be paid to the activities of the athlete outside the sporting environment. A conscious attempt should be made to minimize the stress of other features of his or her life-style.

If an annual training plan has been completed successfully, the competition phase will replace the taper procedure of older forms of training. The competition phase should be one of enjoying the fruits of training completed beforehand. It should allow ideal physiological and psychological states to be achieved for imple-mentation in serious and important competitions.

Transition Phase

The transition phase occurs between annual plans. The major task of this phase is to maintain an acceptable level of fitness. Passive rest periods, or periods between seasons where no structured activities occur, usually result in a loss of the trained states which have been achieved. *It makes no sense to allow an athlete to detrain*, since if detraining occurs, a period of time is required purely to attain previous levels of training. If fitness and other sporting features are maintained between annual plans, then further im-provements in performance could occur early in the next annual plan. Attained fitness is easier to maintain than it is to regain. Athletes should not detrain once they have achieved a high level of fitness.

The purpose of the transition phase is not to maintain the highest levels of performance potential possible. Rather, it should be to avoid detraining. This means that some reduction in fitness poten-tial can occur. The amount of activity in this period should be reduced gradually after the final competition. There should be no sudden cessation of activity. A post-competition unloading phase should occur first. This should develop into activity of a diverse nature which allows psychological regeneration without allowing physical degeneration. The reduction should reach an acceptable level of training frequency and stimulation to maintain a good proportion of what was attained through the previous year's efforts. Many of the characteristics of the basic preparatory phase are included in the program. Varied activities of both a specific and a general nature should occur. Training volume once again becomes the predominant emphasis. The degree of training that is maintained in the transition phase will determine the nature of the initial microcycle of the basic preparatory phase in the next annual plan.

Peaking

Peaking concerns the development of an athlete to the point where he or she is capable of performing his or her best. It is a feature that is influenced more critically by psychological factors than by either fitness or skill. Psychological factors mediate the peaking response. The annual plan that is proposed here asserts that both fitness and skill factors should be fully developed before peaking is attempted.

Where possible, competitions should be planned for the end of macrocycles. This time period facilitates adequate development and unloading to occur before the competition. Peak performances generally occur after maximum fitness and skill states have been attained — one of the reasons for attempting to attain those states at the end of the pre-competition phase. Peak performances cannot be accelerated by sudden increases in training loads or the introduction of new technique items. The maximum training response will only occur when the stimulation is optimum for an individual. Unexpected distractions and stresses detract from the peaking response, reducing the quantity of resources that can be applied to the competitive performance. The success of a peaking program rests with timing the competitive performance with the final over-compensation. This means that peaking occurs at different times and in different ways when it is attempted in change training, maintenance training, and recovery from overtraining. Peaking in a maintenance fitness state is the least complicated procedure. Consistent fitness states will yield consistent performances.

Peaking under the plan that has been described here will be new in concept and implementation when compared to traditional Western training procedures. Indications of performance capacities occur well before the competition, and fitness and skill levels will have been attained. Their maintenance will allow other performance factors to be stressed. This means that gradually, as the competition approaches, athletes should feel good about their fitness and skill precision, and be encouraged by the greater emphasis on factors that are purely related to the competition (e.g., tactics, psychology). This will occur as a refreshing change in the training regimen and will do much to promote high levels of self-efficacy in athletes. This contrasts with the 'normal' peaking procedure (tapering) where recovery, skill refinement, tactical development, and psychological focusing all appear to occur simultaneously. The problem with this simultaneity is that a coach or athlete cannot tell which area is progressing well and which is not: it deteriorates into a hit-or-miss process. Such a situation does not need to arise if training plans have been formulated properly and implemented as described above.

Other Training Plans

Not all sports accommodate annual training plans. There are many variations, each of which must sacrifice some of the benefits that can be gained from a single-focus annual training program.

□ Two-peak Annual Plan

The partitions of the training program that have been outlined for the annual plan are maintained, but in abbreviated form, when there are two major competition periods in a year. The alterations that are needed are:

1. Assuming the first competition allows a full six months of training, all phases are programmed.
2. In the second part of the plan, the transition phase and the basic preparatory phase are disregarded. An unloading microcycle occurs after the competition and then the athlete enters the next specific preparatory phase. All other stages of planning remain the same in intent, but diminished in extent.

Sports which have more than two, but distinct, periods of competition, should have the competitive phases linked by unloading and specific preparatory phases.

□ Excessive Competitions Plan

For sports where weekly or even more frequent competitions occur, it is generally not possible to maintain peak performances. As has been explained above, there are not enough meaningful training stimuli that occur frequently enough to produce a maintenance training form of program. Fitness states deteriorate over the period of competitions. Psychological fatigue ('loss of form', 'in a slump') is quite prominent at various stages throughout an excessively long competition period. Training intensities, when they occur, diminish as the season of competition wears on.

The best alternative for this form of competition is to schedule non-competition periods 2–3 weeks in length after about 6 weeks of competition. These periods can be used for healing injuries, recovery from psychological fatigue, and retraining of fitness capacities. Such an alternative is rarely, if ever, used, but it remains a viable option.

Unloading microcycles should be planned for athletes who have qualified for play-offs prior to the commencement of the final competitions. These microcycles should be used to stimulate fitness while allowing psychological regeneration.

□ Scholastic Sports

Scholastic sports in Western nations used to be the training grounds for athlete development. However, they no longer provide adequate training for satisfactory improvement. They are limited in two ways. First, they do not allow adequate training to occur prior to the first competition. In most situations, sport seasons commence and athletes are expected to perform within the first month of the season. This means that they become used to competing in a less-than-adequately-prepared state. Second, after the competitive program has commenced, further frequent competitions interfere with the quality of ensuing training. This means that programs of this nature have two major deficiencies.

1. They expose athletes to competitive circumstances with inadequate training. Legislating maximum periods of training may be good for the organizers, but is not beneficial for the athletes. As a reaction to this restriction, athletes attend outside-of-school competitions and train elsewhere to gain extra experience and fitness conditioning. However, these haphazard experiences are less than adequate, for they do not provide a soundly-based coordinated program of development.
2. Because athletes receive less than optimum stimulation for training their sporting development will be retarded.

The existence of scholastic sports organizations that inhibit the development of sound training programs may be the single most important factor that has added to the decline in international sporting prowess of nations such as the United States, Australia, and Britain.

It is not possible to achieve one's maximum potential without adequate stimulation from a sound training program. Any decision made about the content of training should consider all the principles and factors that underlie sound planning rather than isolating a single item or a few. Sound planning, year-round training, and decisions based on known principles of human performance are the major ingredients required for successful sporting programs. The diminution of any of these factors will degrade a sporting experience.

Planning

Figure 19.1 illustrates a planning sheet for determining the general content of a training phase. The major decisions concern how many macrocycles will be included, and the number of microcycles in each macrocycle. The objectives of the training phase covering all facets of the sport should be described. The types and frequency of both skill and fitness testing should also be indicated. A requirement that is included is the determination of competitions that will be entered and an indication of the relative importance of each. This facet is supposed to produce a commitment and understanding as to the nature of the competitions that will occur and their relationship to the various training stages and content of the phase. The final feature highlights the importance of considering unloading microcycles in the training phase plan. This emphasis is in keeping with the major philosophy of this text: rest is as important as work in the development of sports fitness.

Figure 19.2 depicts a general decision-making sheet for establishing the content of an annual plan. It focuses on the general objectives of the year's experience, the types of competitions and their importance, and the training phases and their dates. Figure 19.3 is another form of a decision-making sheet for an annual plan. The use of this item was illustrated in Chapter 17.

Figure 19.1 Suggested Planning Sheet for Determining the Phases of Training

---

TRAINING PHASE PLANNING SHEET

Phase Type ....   Dates: .... to ....

1. Number of microcycles for   Macrocycle 1 ___   Macrocycle 2___

                                              Macrocycle 3 ___   Macrocycle 4___

2. Objectives: 1._____
   Technical,
   Tactical, and   2._____
   Psychological
                      3._____

                      4._____

                      5._____

3. Objectives: 1._____
   fitness
                      2._____

                      3._____

                      4._____

                      5._____

4. Tests and   1._____
   frequency:
                      2._____

                      3._____

                      4._____

                      5._____

5. Competitions and ratings of their importance:

       1._____   2._____

       3._____   4._____

       5._____   6._____

6. Dates of   1._____   2._____
   unloading
   microcycles: 3._____   4._____

Figure 19.2 Suggested Decision-making Sheet for Planning Year-long Activities

---

ANNUAL PLAN DECISION SHEET

Dates: .... to ....

A. GENERAL DEVELOPMENTAL OBJECTIVES

1. Fitness Components: _____

_____

2. Technical Components: _____

_____

3. Tactical Components: _____

_____

4. Psychological Skills:_____

_____

B. COMPETITION TYPES AND IMPORTANCE (Dates and ratings)

_____

_____

_____

_____

C. TRAINING PHASES AND DATES

1._____   2._____

3._____   4._____

5._____   6._____

7._____   8._____

9._____   10._____

Figure 19.3 Alternative Decision-making Sheet for Planning Annual Activities

MONTHS												
COMPETITIONS												
PERIODIZATION												
MACROCYCLES												
ENDURANCE												
STRENGTH												
FLEXIBILITY												
SPEED												
TECHNIQUE (SKILL)												
TACTICS (TEAM PLAYS)												
PSYCHOLOGY												
% TRAINING TIME	CONDITIONING											
	SKILL											
	TACTICAL											
	100%											
TRAINING LOAD	80%											
	60%											
KEY												

The reader will notice that the planning forms and sheets which have been illustrated have been presented in the reverse order of their use. As well, the content has been loosely defined for demonstrative purposes. Each sporting situation will have its own requirements and important considerations that need to be heeded. Thus it is very likely that planning forms will be designed that best meet the needs and circumstances of a particular coaching environment. The guideline forms included in this and the previous chapter aim to help in the construction of suitable decision-making guides. This approach is different from other texts, in which one form is usually recommended. That form includes information on all stages of at least an annual plan. But determining exact information early in the planning process would seem to be counterproductive. The exact content of microcycles and training sessions should not be determined until the end of a previous macrocycle. The progress of an athlete through a training program will, in large part, determine the future training experiences that will be provided. It is believed that the forms and planning process presented in this text will assist a coach to focus on the concepts of training, while still remaining flexible in specific programming. This flexibility should provide for the individual needs of athletes as they progress through a year's training, and the planning process advocated should allow the coach to be consistent throughout the year with regard to training decisions while tuning these experiences to the needs of athletes for obtaining specific and general objectives.

20

Planning a Sporting Career

The greatest extent of planning possible for athlete development is that which encompasses a total career of participation, with the ultimate objective being to develop the highest possible caliber of performance. This chapter considers some general factors underlying the decisions needed to develop the fitness aspects of long-term sports participation. These aspects cannot be contemplated without some consideration of growth, skill, and psychological development.

Sporting career planning can only involve the consideration of general principles. These develop a training philosophy in the coach. The reason that one should not attempt to be exact in prescribing the activities that can be followed over a period of many years is that sound training plans react to, and are altered by, the performances of athletes as they undergo training experiences.

The prediction of the nature of developments in young athletes is still in the realm of a guessing game. The state of current sports science is such that it is not possible to estimate how individuals will react to long histories of sporting participation. Thus, for determining extended programs of involvement, it is economical to consider only a general framework of principles when planning sporting careers. The details of such plans would be filled in as athletes' reactions to training, and the assessments of goal achievements, are revealed throughout the years of involvement. With very long-term planning, a coach should consider only a general set of principles. It makes no sense to be overly specific.

An ideal sporting career would start at a young age and continue through a considerable number of years of participation as a mature athlete. With this span in mind, there are a number of principles which can be followed that will assist understanding as to why career programs should be developed in the manner that is recommended.

Growth and Development

The capacity to improve in physical fitness functions increases during the growth period. Once physical maturity has been achieved, further improvements in already maximally-trained fitness capacities are not possible. Figure 20.1 illustrates this principle. During successive training seasons that occur during the growth period, the potential for performance able to be affected by fitness features continually improves. There are no studies to date which indicate the nature of this improvement. It is not known whether the amount of improvement steadily diminishes or remains constant. It has been shown that many features of the physiology of an individual change with age during growth (Astrand 1960); once growth stops, however, it is no longer possible to increase the potential of physiological capacities. Thus, during growth, performance improvements can be attributed partly to 'growing' physiological capacities. Once maturity has been achieved, performance improvements will have to come from increases in either or both skill and psychological factors.

This simple picture of growth as being a limiting factor in fitness development is confused slightly by the observed developments in fitness capacities of mature individuals who undergo training programs. There is no doubt that an untrained mature person improves in physical capacity when training is commenced. Figure 20.2 illustrates the $\dot{V}O_2$ max responses of both élite athlete and normal subject responses to intensive training over a number of years. The three élite skiers did not display any change in maximum oxygen uptake although there are fluctuations between sets of test data. The untrained individuals did improve over the first one- to two-year period. From then on, the $\dot{V}O_2$ max remained relatively stable. If one were to generalize on the basis of the first two or three observations on the untrained subjects, it would be incorrectly concluded that physical capacities increased as a consequence of training. However, the more accurate interpretation would be that training produces a reorganization of existing capacities. This reorganization produces increased physiological measurements until the finite capacity that has been established by growth at the age of maturity is fully taxed. From that stage on, further improvements in physiological potential are not possible.

Figure 20.1 Long-term Physiological Training Responses of Mature and Growing Athletes

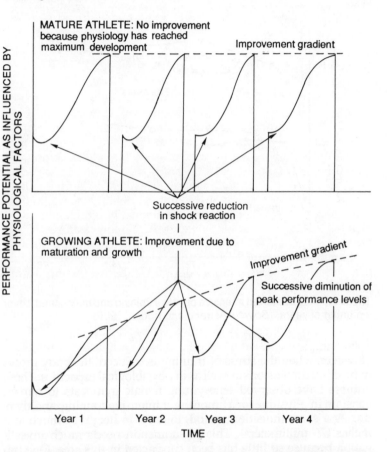

During the period of growth, changes in physiological performance capacities are dependent upon cycles of training and unloading. An athlete who trains very hard may exhibit no growth at all. The demands of training could consume all the physical resources of the individual. When this occurs, training could produce a level of fitness component development that seems not to change any further while training demands remain high. During an extended unloading phase or transition period, when training demands are greatly reduced, some energies and capacities of the body can be diverted to bodily growth. It is not uncommon to observe that no growth in stature occurs during training in young athletes who are being subjected to a highly intensive and demanding regime.

Figure 20.2 An Adaptation of Data on Maximal Oxygen Uptake of Three Internationally Successful Cross-country Skiers and Two 'Normal' Subjects

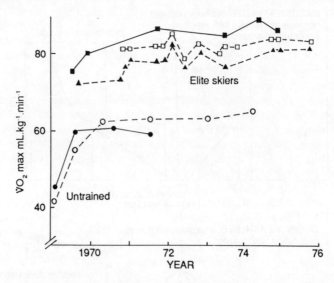

These athletes all started intensive physical training and maintained it over a number of years. (*Source:* Astrand and Rodahl 1986)

However, when the stress of training is reduced, the body grows in physical dimensions as well as in physiological capacities. These authors have observed élite young female gymnasts to remain constant in physique for 11 months of intensive training, and then, during a short transition period, to grow in height as much as 3 inches (76 millimeters). This phenomenon needs much investigation because so little has been conducted in this area. One can hypothesize that long durations of intense training that *do not adhere to the principle of periodization* may actually retard the development of physiological capacities. What affect such practices may have on the health of the athlete in later life is also unknown. It can be imagined that alternating work and rest in a sensible fashion throughout a whole career will allow the natural development of physiological capacities under the stimulation of exercise. These capacities would improve to their inherent maximum potential. On the other hand, if growth is suppressed because of excessive training loads it may be possible that it will be retarded and physiological capacities may never achieve their full potential. This is purely conjecture at this stage but it is a possibility that seems plausible. It means that too much intensive training in young people not only could be counter-productive in the short-term, as has already been discussed, it may also be counter-productive in the long term as well. It is our opinion that physical training should be used to stimulate growth to achieve maximum physiological potential. Using it to suppress growth is ill-advised and probably unethical. Thus sports which try to suppress growth in participants (e.g., gymnastics, weight-lifting, wrestling, boxing, etc.) need to rethink their philosophies and ethics.

The stage of growth also should be considered when determining the type of activities to be performed. The tendency to introduce weight training at an early age is inadvisable (*Coaching Review* 1985). Free-standing exercises and games that can produce enjoyable and beneficial training effects should be extensively used before the highly specialized and probably overrated (in effectiveness) forms of weight and resistance training. It has been advocated that weight training not start until the post-pubertal stage of growth.

To summarize: training during the period of growth, which constitutes the early years of a sporting career, *should be provided in sufficient amounts to produce the maximum stimulation of all physiological capacities*. When growth stops, fitness training should be followed with a view to training the athlete to maximum capacity and then improving performance through refinements in skill and psychology.

Prediction of Sport Specialization

The pursuit of talent identification programs that should allow one to select youngsters for particular sport participations at an early age has to date been a futile pursuit. There are stories of programs of exact selection occurring in countries behind the Iron Curtain, but these stories are more fiction than fact. The reason that many Eastern bloc nations are becoming superior to Western nations in sports is more attributable to their sound developmental programs than any selection process. Given the state of sport science as it is today, there should be no attempt to specialize young athletes too early. There is really no telling what potential for activity excellence exists in a young person. The appeal to specific cases of champions starting at an early age as evidence to support early specialization is a spurious procedure. There are just as many examples of late starters achieving world-standard sporting excellence as there are early starters.

It is the nature of early participation, however, that is important for developing athletes. No athlete should be denied the opportunity to participate in a sport if he or she shows interest in it. An individual's interest is just as good a predictor of athletic success as is any currently available physical test. This supports the notion of natural selection in sports participation as being the best talent identification process currently available. Individuals will gravitate towards activities which provide the most rewarding experiences and indications of self-improvement.

Skill Development

The single most influential principle of sports participation is that the first emphasis of training in a sporting career should be on skill development. Stegemann (1981: 264) highlighted this principle as being one of the major responsibilities of a coach:

> The coach or physical education teacher thus has a special responsibility because he brings the first movement pattern of a complicated type of sport to the student. If a false, ineffective technique of the arm-pull was learned in the breast stroke, then a movement stereotype would be formed. If the student then wished to become a competitive swimmer, he would find that relearning would be more difficult than learning from scratch. It is also possible that under the stress of competition, the old stereotype would take effect once more. In the case of such technically difficult types of sports as skiing, lessons should be taken from the beginning. A self-taught, false movement pattern can be a great hindrance on the way to perfection.

When young athletes are placed in competitive circumstances, those with superior strength and size usually dominate, and the attitude is developed that performance success comes to those who are the strongest and biggest. Thus physical attributes are seen as the secrets of success. Smaller and weaker children will have to resort to skill and guile, it is thought, to compensate for their physiological deficiencies. Initial training programs for youngsters typically aim at developing work-ethic attitudes to a sport. While sporting successes may be obtained at first from physiological training emphases, these are short-sighted. Once growth limits have been achieved, sporting successes will be determined by skill and psychology. Hence, if an athlete has been deprived of adequate skill development in the formative years, the bad technical patterns that have been established will serve as a hindrance to later improvements. The conditioned strength of neuromuscular patterns that have been ingrained over many years cannot be weakened over a short time. There comes the time in an athlete's career when attempts to change technique faults which have been practiced for a very long time will be counter-productive. When these technique faults are basic, for example, performance posture, gross-timing factors such as the number of turns in the circle in a discus throw, and positional play, attempts to change them will never yield benefits that supersede the value of their tolerance. The reasons for the counter-productivity are several. First, when an established technique is altered, performance deteriorates until the new technique element becomes more highly conditioned than the element being replaced. Second, the length of time to achieve new levels of conditioned strength for element substitution to occur may not be possible. In this case, performance is harmfully affected by the attempted change and remains in a state of reduced functioning for the remainder of the athlete's participation. Third, experienced athletes who practice incorrect technique elements minimize the effects of these. Thus, even with a basic technique flaw, an athlete may be performing at the highest level of proficiency possible given the limitations of the erroneous element. If changes are attempted, the resultant performance reduction may be of sufficient severity not to warrant its attempt. If this is the case, even though training is followed to produce development of a new element, the altered skill may never reach the level of proficiency of the previous erroneous one.

This highlights the need for the development of skill proficiencies in athletes early in their sporting careers. The younger the athlete, the simpler should be the technique that is instructed, because more complex and finer elements of skill may be dependent upon physiological capacities which have not been developed. No attempt should be made to teach youngsters technical features which are beyond their current capacities even though these may be displayed by older athletes. In work-oriented programs, it is the underdeveloped individual who participates most. The requirement to compensate for a size/strength deficiency through the employment of superior skill and tactics will serve them better once their growth has been fully attained. As a consequence, the initially strong and dominant athlete will be ill-served by the use of strength and size as a means of generating early competitive successes. In later years, when the initially smaller and weaker athletes have grown fully, they will have a similar physical potential plus established good technique and tactical skills that further influence performance. The superior early-age performer will not have the technique/tactical skill grounding or development to assist them in later participation years. Thus athletes who experience initial sporting success because of accelerated physical maturation capacities will suffer as a consequence in later years of participation

in the sport. This deficiency can be removed by providing programs where skill factors are emphasized to a high degree no
matter what the physical maturation of the athlete.

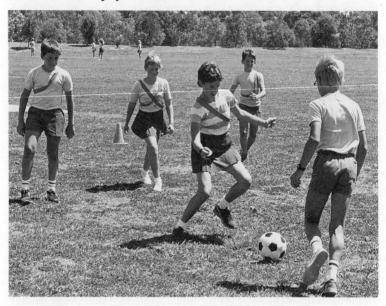

Rather than concentrate on fitness work and highly specialized techniques,
young children should be encouraged to learn a variety of basic movement
skills that they can refine as they mature during adolescence

Perhaps the most striking feature of the philosophies of many
currently successful sporting nations is the philosophy of minimizing competitive opportunities before adequate skill levels have
been developed. The development of skill competencies before
subjecting athletes to intense training and serious competitive
experiences is a sound tenet.

The General Basis of Development

There is a strong tendency in the Western world for sport programs
to initiate specific training and participation at early ages. Such
specialized emphases have, however, been discarded by Eastern
bloc nations. Mizerski (*Coaching Review* 1985) reported that nations
which specialized athletes too early produced quick results but
little improvement thereafter. He cited Russia and East Germany
as having this philosophy in the early days of their entry onto the

international sporting scene. When this approach to developing athletic talent was replaced by a thorough and well-balanced base of youth sports and physical education, national performances and world statuses ultimately exceeded previous levels in these nations.

With regard to fitness, there is sound support for the contention that non-specialized activities form the best basis for later specialization. Sports which rely heavily on fitness as a determinant for success need to have certain attributes developed to support the specialized nature of the sport. For example, in swimming it is essential to have good overall body strength to maintain a firm posture as the basis for arm–shoulder and leg actions. Postural strength and integrity can be adequately developed by participating in a variety of activities that stimulate the development of the musculature of the trunk (e.g., games which require dynamic adjustments of stance, such as soccer, football, wrestling; activities which require body control, such as dance, gymnastics, canoeing). Shoulder girdle strength can be developed by a selection of appropriate activities. Thus, for swimming there are activities that can occur very early in a sporting career that develop a general basis upon which later specialized movement patterns can be superimposed. This approach contrasts with the current emphasis of attempting to teach specialized techniques to young people *who have not developed the appropriate general physical basis to support these techniques*. As a consequence of experiencing development on an inadequate physical basis, compromises in technique are made. For reasons stated above, these compromised elements tend to perpetuate themselves throughout a sporting career. Consequently when an athlete with physical potential for a particular sport enters a standard of competition where even slight inefficiencies in movement cost dearly, he or she is hindered by the originally developed techniques.

A general program of non-specialized activity in the early years should ensure the general all-round development of physical capacities. When the stimulation for development is coupled with the maturation process, an individual is prompted to grow in a balanced fashion. This means that should a young person have a capacity to perform in a sport, but that capacity is not realized until later in the athlete's young life, when the physiological basis for good fitness training will have been established.

What has to be determined are the benefits of this approach over early specialization. If a child were to specialize early, only to find later that the specialization was wrong for his or her 'real capacities' which are better suited to another sport, then the lack of development of the requirements for good fitness and technique training in a new sport means that full potential in it cannot be achieved.

General growth and training stimulation from a variety of different sporting activities serve individuals, and a population in general, in a better fashion than does early specialization. More on this topic will be presented later in this chapter.

Sporting Career Programs

Sporting careers should change gradually, from a general basic form of participation (multilateral activity) to specialization. The length of time spent in specialization should be longer than that spent in multilateral activity. This book primarily emphasizes the decision criteria and structure of programs that should be provided for athletes in the specialization phase of their sporting careers. To balance that emphasis, a number of features that should be included in the early stages of a career are presented below.

☐ Multilateral Physical Development

Multilateral development refers to the enhancement of all the physical capacities of the body. Experiences and programs to develop strength, speed, flexibility, endurance, and coordination should be the focus of youth-sport training programs. The stimulated development of these capacities provides a fitness basis for acquiring the necessary skill fundamentals of a variety of sports before specialization is determined. This means that children will be able to participate with physical competence in developmental programs in a variety of sports. This will serve as a better system of talent identification than that which is currently favored, early specialization. When coaching programs are devised for young children it is better to err on the side of providing too much multilateral-development training, than to attempt too much specialization.

The desirable length of time spent in multilateral development cannot be exactly defined. There is little research that indicates an appropriate time period. It does seem that multilateral work should be continued throughout an athlete's growth period, although the emphasis would diminish during the latter stages. It would be better to consider that multilateral development should never stop while an athlete is growing. However, coaches must determine the balance between multilaterality and specialization. One should never underemphasize multilaterality to achieve the short-term benefits of early specialization, because of the long-term deficiencies which result. Young athletes who participate in many sports and activities as well as being instructed in basic techniques will improve in their performances because of their general fitness capacities and the emphasis placed on technique development.

Multilateral development consists of two emphases. The first is that young athletes are exposed to activities which develop all their fitness capacities. One capacity should not be emphasized over another. The second is that these exposures contain a large variety of exercises. Thus, it would be wrong to develop endurance in young children purely by running. A mix of swimming, running, cycling, and even long-distance walking (e.g., challenging hikes) would be more appropriate. Alternating different activities which stimulate different capacities means that the interests of young people will be maintained in sport training as well as providing the opportunity to recover between exposures to the specific stresses developed by particular exercises.

☐ The Acquisition of Simple Skills from Related Sports

The programming of skill development is the most important feature in the early career of an athlete. However, as with fitness capacities, the skills that are learned early in a career should not be overly specialized. Participation in cricket, field hockey, baseball, and tennis would seem to be appropriate activities for developing a ball-awareness capacity in a budding cricketer. It is participation in a variety of activities such as these that serves as the establishment of good skill bases that will later become the foundation for more advanced techniques. Such a general orientation is very different to the approach of many swimming coaches who prohibit young swimmers from participating in water-polo and swimming in the surf because of a supposed 'interference' of these activities with the specialized techniques of speed swimming.

The individualization of simple skills should also be considered early in career development. The accommodation of technique features to best suit the attributes of a youngster (his or her particular 'style') will mean that learning experiences will be easier and more pleasant than those which arise from athletes being forced to attempt movement patterns that are not suited to their capacities.

☐ Diverse Competitive Experiences

Competitions should be experienced by young athletes. However, their importance should be minimized while the diversity across sports and activities is maximized. The intent of scheduling competitions should be to develop an approach response to competing because of associated positive experiences. The introduction to competitions is very important for formulating attitudes towards competing. As long as young athletes can feel competent in their initial competitive efforts, they will enjoy competitions. The problem that will face many coaches is that entrenched competitive programs force children to compete when they are not competently skilled or adequately trained (see the previous chapter).

□ Training Discipline and Commitment

The election to participate in sports in a serious manner requires certain character features to be developed. To achieve this, coaches of young athletes need to be more of a psychologist than physiologist or biomechanician. The gradual shaping of behaviors which indicate training discipline and sport commitment should be part of the program of multilateral development.

Multilateral development is the basis of an athlete's sporting career. When training is started, the younger the athlete, the more diverse and simple should be the tasks and activities required for sport participation.

Progression Factors in Sporting Career Programs

□ Amounts of Training

The greater the degree of training adaptation, the better will be the performance potential. Thus, performances can only be as good as the amount of training that has preceded them. This means that high levels of performance have to be based on large amounts of training experience. The volume of training that serves to influence performances covers the volume that has occurred in the sporting career of the athlete. In every year of training, whether in multilateral or specialized phases, the volume of training should be increased. The imposition of volume should always be moderated by considerations of periodization and avoidance of states of overtraining.

When planning programs, conscious efforts should be made to avoid detrained states. This text has indicated that modern training theory calls for the maintenance of adapted states. 'Rests' from specific sport training are accommodated within the transition phase. With the introduction of such phases, athletes should remain competent and physically fit, and detraining should not occur. The major negative experiences that are associated with retraining, symptoms of the alarm reaction phase and the loss of potentially productive time, will be avoided.

□ Types of Training

Contrary to popular opinion, young athletes tolerate volume/endurance training better than intensity/strength activities. However, many sporting programs for young people only provide opportunities to participate in wrong forms of physical activity. For example, age-group swimming and running programs feature competitions over short distances. Strong and big youngsters have a definite advantage over lesser-developed individuals, although neither is helped in any great way by such events. It is interesting to contemplate why programs which are ill-adapted for their target participants are conceived. One possible explanation is that adults wrongly transfer their perceptions of activity difficulty to youngsters. For adults, it is endurance events that are perceived as being harder than strength events. Consequently, when youth competitive programs are formulated adults think that short sprint events are best for young children for they are easier for adults. Short competitive events may seem to be easiest for adults but they are not appropriate for the physical capacities of young children.

As a further consequence, since competitive programs are inappropriate, the training programs that are devised for them are also inappropriate. This results in a less-than-desirable starting phase for a competitive career. In the majority of sports, a reorientation of youth sports is warranted. This should be more in tune with what is known in sports science rather than what has been traditionally done in a sport.

☐ Variety in Training

Variety is an important factor in motivation. It is also a good safety valve for training programs to retard or defend against overtraining. Young children need programs that contain much variety *and* rest as well as the opportunities to follow other pursuits. No matter how rapid the development of young children, multilateral development and variety cannot be compromised. The short-term gains that result from early specialization and excessive workloads will always be a strong attraction for coaches and parents but will not be sufficient to compensate for the long-term losses that also result.

☐ Progression in Emphases

The age at which an athlete should change from a multilateral development to a specialized one will depend on the sport and the degree of multilateral exposure that has occurred. The introduction of specialized training should be in concert with growth/development and psychological factors. There should be no hesitancy in programming a possible return to a multilateral emphasis for young children if specialization has occurred too early.

Too often an absence from training, or a reduction in training load, is interpreted as a critical event that will produce irreparable harm to an athlete's ultimate sporting development. It is now known that isolated and brief training reductions or fluctuations have no effect on the long-term productivity of a sporting career. In fact, the science of training is still crude enough to be able to say that as long as the work gets done, performance will improve. To support this latter statement, Overend, Paterson, Cunningham, and Taylor (1985) and Bhambhani and Singh (1985) found that completely different training programs produced similar training results. The failure to detect differences was not so much a matter of any form of training always producing a training effect but rather that athletes require training programs that best suit their particular individual needs. Herb Elliott (1961) presented the athlete's point of view:

> The more I speak to athletes, the more convinced I become that the method of training is relatively unimportant. There are many ways to the top, and the training method you choose is just the one that suits you best.

Having just implored the reader to not specialize athletes too early in their sporting careers, it is realized that such training is the main element that is required to obtain sporting success. Specialized training is, as discussed, most effective when it has as its base an extensive exposure to volumes of multilateral development.

Some general areas that should be assessed when determining progression throughout an athlete's sporting career are:

1. *Objectively evaluate performances.* Since the precision of performance types and standards for young people is not great, it is often not possible to accurately consider their developmental progress in sports. Even though accurate performance and physical capacity measures are possible, whether these are appropriate for the maturation stage or inherent potential of the young athlete usually remains a mystery. Consequently a lot of coaches turn to subjective measures for assessing further potential and current progress. There is a strong tendency to rely on such assessments of psychological factors, as evidenced by statements such as 'having the right attitude', 'not being committed enough to training', 'having a negative influence on other performers', and so on, as being the determinants of adequate career progress. These vague measures are often a result of the type of sporting experience that has been provided for the athlete. Boring programs, specialization that has occurred too early, excessive overloading, insufficient rest opportunities, and inappropriate exercises for the age of development, are examples of programming errors that cause psychological

problems which, in turn, are used as reasons for removing or demotivating 'problem' athletes.

Better coaching will be achieved if objective measures are taken of the physiological, psychological, and biomechanical developments of athletes. Problems which are located should be initially interpreted as being a result of the exercise programs provided for the athletes. Alterations in these programs should be attempted to remove problem causes. Only when such attempts have been made should the coach start to look at the inner athlete as a potential cause.

2. *Assess the positive and negative aspects of performance.* The preoccupation of many coaches with concentrating on error detection when determining training progressions often leads to the neglect of desirable features of training. If a change in training is promoted as a means for correcting a deficiency, before that change is implemented its potential effect on good performance should also be considered. Another factor that is rarely considered is what would occur if no corrective action were taken at all. The consideration of these three alternatives before instituting training changes is called the 'full-picture concept'. It requires coaching decisions to be made on the basis of sound, fully-contemplated reasons and data, rather than hastily-conceived impulsive hunches.

Another important consideration when changes are to be made is the impact of changes on the positive nature of the sporting experience. Changes often are stressful and could result in reduced performance efficiency. Participants often cannot see the benefits to be derived from training changes which contain more negative than positive aspects. Usually, the more drastic the alteration in a training experience, the greater is the negative potential of a change. Once the negative features of a sporting situation exceed the positive, a real problem has occurred for an athlete. Progressions in a career should be considered in terms of their impact on the positive aspects of the experience for the performer, and should be moderated if negativism appears to threaten an acceptably positive level in the sport.

3. *Construct changes to improve performance and performance capacities.* Program phases and activities should be aimed at improvements. Not all improvements will immediately translate into performance enhancements. For example, the development of basic capacities in multilateral training experiences may not be immediately reflected in specialized performances, although the capacity base which has been

developed will affect such performances at a much later date when that kind of training has been instituted. The value of testing such capacities, with the feedback derived, serves a motivational function. Thus the performance factors against which training alterations are measured should be both performance improvements and improvements in capacity measures. Those evaluations are the measures against which training effectiveness should be judged.

Sporting Career Plans

The foundations of long-term training rest on a coordinated plan that reacts to specific objective assessments of performance and performance capacities in the areas of physiological adaptation, psychological capacities, and biomechanical efficiencies. Programs that carry individuals from very young ages through to extensive participation as mature athletes, perhaps over a period of some 20–25 years, need to be formulated on a basic progression concept for the development of physical capacities. That progression is:

1. an initial program that overwhelmingly emphasizes multilateral development through diverse activities, exercises, and competitive experiences
2. a period of assessment to determine tendencies of potential for certain types of activities (hints of specialized abilities)
3. a foundation of specialized training that is mixed with continued multilateral development, but to a lesser degree than at the start of the career
4. a final stage of highly specialized training that still looks at some general multilateral training as being part of the preparatory phase of an annual training plan

Within these gradual changes of emphases there are further qualifiers for programming (Bompa 1986):

1. Increase the number of training sessions and hours each year.
2. Increase the number and frequency of competitive experiences.
3. Increase training volume each year with the types of capacities that are stimulated being appropriate for the maturation stage of the athlete.
4. Increase the intensity of training each year, but not at the expense of achieving a substantial performance base derived from volume training.

5. Gradually introduce performance and physical capacity objectives as being the objective measures of improvement.

The definition of more exact principles and concepts is not possible at this time. There just has not been the research conducted to indicate specific functions. In fact, it is possible that there will never be exact specifications.

Within the general framework that is described in this and the previous two chapters, progressions in and content of training are determined by performances and measures that are taken as the athlete proceeds through macrocycle stages. The prescription of training content should be based on objective measurements taken at these stages. These prescriptions are easier to make with fully adapted high-level athletes, where capacities are more consistent and growth has ceased. It is in the early stages of an athlete's career that coaching judgments will have to be made based more on beliefs and philosophies than hard and fast data. With very young people, the coach's preoccupation should be with general physical and skill development and experience in a variety of activities. Any signs of special preferences or capacities should be noted. Indications of special talents and interests should be used to explore the reactions of young athletes to slightly more specialized training while still maintaining an overall emphasis on multilateral development. As a career progresses, more and more testing of greater volumes of experiences in specialized exposures should be conducted. This procedure will result in the determination of the special activity that best suits the talents and interests of each athlete. At this stage, the considerations and features that have been outlined in this text will be appropriate.

21
Coaching Implications

This text has described the general principles and guidelines that underlie the development of maximum physical conditioning for sports. These principles have been demonstrated across a number of activities. A coach is advised to take this information and apply it to the sport and athletes for which he or she has responsibility — a task that may be daunting to some. There has always been a tendency for coaches to require precise training prescriptions for developing the physiological state of athletes. It is not uncommon to hear questions such as 'How many repetitions are best?', 'How often should we train?', and 'When is the best time to start a taper?' It should be clear, however, that very little is exact when coaching athletes in any sport. Individual differences, biophysical, social, and psychological modifiers, and the demands of each sporting task must be considered, and coaches should expect great variation in the training formulae for the members of a team. It is the responsibility of the coach to adapt to the individual specifications of sound training programs rather than succumb to the erroneous assumption that all athletes should train in the same way. More athletes will be poorly served by group-oriented training programs and philosophies than will be benefited. This is a reality of modern coaching and it makes the task more difficult and time-consuming than many are willing to admit.

When superior performances are sought, the level of excellence that is achieved will be dependent upon the level of coaching decisions that are made. Occasionally, élite athletes will be developed despite poor coaching. However, these occurrences are becoming more rare as world standards continue to progress at a

366

remarkable rate. Superior athletes will have to be coached by individuals who make superior decisions and who run superior programs. This text has attempted to illustrate the parameters of decision-making that surround the development of the highest level of fitness in athletes.

This chapter attempts to tie together the themes of this book. These are:

1. The definitions of the physical requirements of each sporting role and the physical capabilities and training status of each athlete, something provided by research and testing.
2. The determination of the objectives and general structure of a total training plan, requiring an understanding and recognition of those long-term factors which are associated with sporting excellence while also allowing some programming flexibility depending upon the short-term progress of the athlete.
3. The specific definitions of the training stimuli, recovery periods, and microcycle and macrocycle structures. These will be determined by the training history and life-style of the athlete, the nature and schedule of competitive performances, and the supporting environment.

Research and Testing

☐ Determine Exact Sporting Requirements

There is still much to be learned in describing the nature of sporting activities, their physiological demands, and the appropriate training activities to produce maximized conditioning. One needs to know the precise requirements for each of the physiological capacities for each role and event in a sport. Such exact knowledge is not yet available although there are many opinions on it. Without this knowledge coaching decisions will cause athletes to emphasize some forms of training at the expense of others in a manner that will not encourage maximal adaptation or development in a sport. Training programs must have sound bases and objectives.

Participation in unproductive and/or excessive training activities, which consume training time, produce fatigue, and alter motivation, could be eliminated if training prescriptions were based on verified knowledge. It is assumed that determinations of the physical requirements of the sport would also accurately specify the activities that need to be undertaken to provide a capacity to meet unusual physical demands, particularly those in multi-skilled and body-contact sports. Since some of this information is not yet known, it is sorely needed. National and international sport governing bodies need to embark upon research programs to specify the maximum physiological demands of the various events and participant roles in their sports. Without that knowledge, athletes cannot engage in the most efficient forms of training to allow them to achieve their maximum potentials in their sports. Participation is discouraged when performance improvements do not result from the demands of extensive training. On the other hand, if the demands cover functional activities that directly produce performance benefits, then participation would be encouraged.

The capacities that need to be trained and the level for each role in each sport need to be determined by the sport and sport-science communities.

☐ Determine the Physical Capacities of Athletes

The effectiveness of training programs needs to be monitored. This has not always been done well. If the performance itself is used as the criterion for improvement, it is not possible to accurately attribute performance changes to any specific aspect of training. When a number of capacities are being developed at the same time, performance improvements could be due to one, or even a subset, of those capacities, while others are inconsequential. This confusing picture can lead the coach to retain ineffective training methods that in turn will detract from the benefits of more effective ones. To solve this problem, frequent physiological capacity testing needs to be conducted under controlled conditions in both laboratory and field settings.

The determination of what valid tests are, how they can be administered in an objective and reliable fashion, and how they can be made freely available need to be examined. Thus the provision of testing centers and facilities is an important ingredient for successful modern coaching programs. In some Western and Eastern bloc countries, these have been established for élite athletes. In Australia and Canada, for example, there have been attempts to establish geographically distributed sport-science testing centres that should reach a greater number and variety of athletes. The value and use of these facilities is not yet optimal. They have been restricted because of variations in understanding of the best tests for use in each role in each sport. Testing must be standardized and subjected to stringent quality control. Athletes need to be tested with assessment procedures that will exactly evaluate the training effects and physiological statuses that have been achieved. *It may be best not to conduct any testing if testing is not valid for or sensitive to the training aspects that are to be measured.* Testing for testing's sake usually does not yield information that can benefit coaching decisions and training prescriptions.

Physiological testing needs to provide evaluations of the effects of training that are appropriate for the sport performance. This information will indicate the capacities that have changed and contributed to performance improvements or changes. This is important, for it will tell where adjustments in the training program have to be made so that optimal training effects are achieved in all performance-relevant capacities. Without such knowledge, training cannot be optimized.

Sport physiologists and coaches need to develop specific sport-role tests for all physiological capacities. The determination of the training status and the provision of the resultant information should be frequent so that developmental programs can be adjusted and refined on an ongoing basis. Unless coaches know the physiological capabilities and statuses of athletes, training effects cannot be maximized.

The sporting world is not yet fully serviced with testing capabilities. Sport scientists could embark on a very beneficial program of test development, evaluation, and service provision that would provide results which would allow coaches to make better and more informed decisions. Research programs aimed at the construction and standardized administration of tests and various forms of sport analysis are needed if performances are to benefit.

Planning

The quality of program planning is dependent upon the consideration of all the finite factors that affect performance in a specific activity. Planning is governed by the physical requirements for the sport and the athlete capacities that exist. Since neither of these can be provided exactly, a large number of coaching decisions will have to be based on existing knowledge. 'Experts' in the various fields of sport science should be incorporated into the coaching decision process, particularly when the coach feels inadequate in the scientific area. Thus, the provision of coaching decisions should be supported by the best and most extensive advice and knowledge that is available. The structuring of sport-science support staffs for sports is part of the 'team-coaching' concept. The combined wisdom of a group of experts, when added to that of a very knowledgeable coach, will produce a higher level of decision-making than that which can be provided by the coach alone. With the deficiencies that currently exist in sport testing and knowledge, a stop-gap measure to partly make up for that inadequacy would be to conduct valid and reliable testing on some aspects of performance and to employ 'experts' to provide sound and reasoned advice. The personal dynamics or 'chemistry' of such a group is the largest stumbling block to the success of this form of coaching team.

After obtaining knowledge of the physical requirements and athlete capacities for performance, the coach still has to establish reference points for program development. The establishment of goals and objectives are these reference points.

First, the most general goals of training should be structured and then followed by greater degrees of specification. More remote objectives serve as the ultimate reference points for a program even though they are usually the most vague in terms of performance. This means that coaches should have an understanding of what it takes to train athletes in a sporting career so that the end product will be the best performances of which they are capable.

The general planning process largely involves the determination of objectives, major competitions, developmental emphases, and training volumes. Such decisions usually encompass the planning of careers, four-year programs, annual plans, and training phases. Chapters 18 and 19 include some forms that will assist the coach in making those plans. It makes no sense to plan in detail too far ahead because programming flexibility and adaptability to the needs of athletes must be maintained. The unpredictable rate of capacity improvement and intrusion of uncontrolled events, such as injury and selection to representative teams, interfere with even the best-laid plans.

It is advisable that coaches only plan specific details for a training phase, and in particular for the current macrocycle. It has been proposed that physiological testing be employed as a standard feature of the training plan. It is important to test not only during but particularly at the end of a macrocycle to determine which training objectives have been accomplished. The content of the next macrocycle will be determined partly by these test results. Failures and successes will determine the planning of the next macrocycle.

Thus the planning of training should be balanced between meeting general objectives that guide specific content, and specifying exact training stimuli. The success of the program in achieving training and testing objectives will determine the coaching decisions that are made: these decisions should be made only after the appropriate information and results have been achieved. *This means that a coach should constantly evaluate training effects and specific program content against specific and general objective assessments.* This activity is completely opposite to the common coaching behaviors of copying others' training programs, or developing a session's training content without careful consideration and the thematic direction that is afforded by long-term objectives.

The principle of specificity has been promoted as being essential for sporting success. However, it is not proposed that the only training conducted should be specific. It has been advocated that one-sport athletes who train throughout the year should:

1. keep a considerable level of fitness all year, particularly in the transition phase
2. train initially in a more general way that establishes a broad base for withstanding the stresses of life and the overall sporting experience
3. gradually develop more specific sport-appropriate training that is primarily a fine-tuning of physiological capacities, neuromuscular (skill) efficiency, and the competitive strategies (tactics) of the sport.

When athletes undertake too much general training, the failure to fully develop specific capabilities will result in achievements that are below potential. When athletes attempt to participate seriously in more than one sport, the compromises that result will detract from achieving maximized states in any of them. When athletes engage in too much specialized training, their performances improve quickly at first, but fail to reach performance levels that are possible through a program that establishes a performance base through general preparatory work followed by specific work to refine the athlete's state for serious competitions.

Coaches have to be prepared to alter a planned program based on knowledge of an athlete's progress and forms of response. For many coaches this will be a difficult behavior to adopt. Coaches often justify 'their' method or program of training as being the 'only' way to train. Indeed, it may be the only way that they know but it is hoped that this text will have contained sufficient information to offer coaches new information, procedures, and perspectives that will allow them to function more efficiently when training the physical capacities of athletes.

A central theme of this text is that coaching has to be an adaptive process, where coaching programs can be adjusted according to performance and test results. It is a 'control system' that develops athletes by responding to uncontrolled factors, such as stressors outside sport and social pressures, that alter the response capacities and characteristics of an athlete.

Specific Coaching Factors

A large portion of this text has attempted to provide guidelines for structuring programs of physical training. It is not possible to recount all of these in this concluding chapter. However, there are some main points that are central to the approach to training that is proposed in this work:

1. Recovery is as important as work. The amount of recovery that is required is that which will facilitate the occurrence of training effects. The current focus on doing 'as much work as possible' without providing for recovery is short-sighted and foolish.

2. It is pointless to continue a training activity when both performance and technique deteriorate. When these two behavioral characteristics occur, adaptation to the specific training stimulus has ceased and the athlete mobilizes a variety of resources to combat the general fatigue that is experienced. The end result of this excessive fatigue is a non-specific coping response that in no way benefits performance improvement. Coaches have to learn when to stop exposing athletes to excessive and sometimes harmful amounts of training stimuli.

3. The way in which workloads are increased is in a step-like fashion. This approach differs from the traditional approach of increasing workloads on a daily basis. The step-like progression allows the body to adapt through a variety of repeated exposures to a particular level of training stress. It allows the body time to develop the familiarity and adaptation that results from repeated exposure to a constant stimulus. Daily exposures to constantly changing workloads do not allow for that familiarity and response refinement to develop. A further change in the training response that occurs with the step-like progression is that the first exposure to the stimulus is the most fatiguing. As the microcycle (usually a week of training) progresses, training should become easier. This contrasts with the single-incremental training progression where Thursday's and Friday's sessions are usually deemed to be the hardest of all and usually warrant more than one-and-a-half days of rest over the weekend. Thus a valuable index of whether the loading in a microcycle is correct is the perception of the athletes that the sessions in the microcycle are gradually becoming easier.

4. Each physical capacity should be planned and trained according to its own program. The frequency, loadings, and number of training sessions are usually particular to each capacity. Thus coaches should not attempt to train all capacities at each practice session.

5. Physiological capacities of mature athletes have finite levels that can be attained but not exceeded. Performances can still improve due to biomechanical and psychological skill developments. Once a finite level in a capacity is achieved, programming for maintenance training should be instituted. A reduction in the quantity of training without decreasing quality is sufficient to maintain peak physical adaptation for an extended period of time. This principle contravenes the approach of many coaches that extra and harder training will somehow develop extra physical capacities. This is just not true. It is an unwise procedure that almost guarantees the occurrence of overtrained states.

6. Exceptional levels of performance cannot be achieved without the correct amount of specialized training. Early competitions when athletes are in basic or specific-preparatory training phases are not the times to expect exceptional performances. There is a distinct difference between what one would like or hope to do and what one is capable of doing. This reality should be recognized.

7. The greatest responsiveness of an athlete is determined by how much of his or her finite physical resources can be applied to training. The influence of distracting or detracting stresses will diminish that capacity and, consequently, the potential training effects that can be achieved. This means that ideal training environments should be established to develop athletes to their greatest physical potential.

8. Training sessions should be structured according to a particular sequence. Fatigue is the most influential factor thwarting the occurrence of training effects. The existence of lactic acid inhibits the development of neuromuscular patterns. Consequently, all learning and physical capacities that are dependent upon the neuromuscular reorganization of existing capacities have to be completed before activities which generate lactic acid are attempted in a training session.

These general factors are the major implications for training physical capacities. There are many minor principles that have not been recounted but should be considered when developing specific capacities and plans.

This text maintains that the principle of specificity is the single most pervading factor that influences the improvement of performance from a physiological perspective. Training effects are, in the main, so specific that even minor departures from movement forms, velocities, and intensities result in undesirable training effects. This means that incorrectly designed training activities, *no matter how well intentioned*, will have no carry-over value for a particular movement form, and may even have the potential to negatively influence activities. The adherence to the principle of specificity will govern the rapidity of performance improvements. When performances do not change, the commonest possible faults are the unrelated nature of training activities, excessive fatigue, and an unpreparedness to seek improvements from biomechanical or psychological sources.

It is hoped that reading this text has inspired coaches to approach the training of physiological factors in athletes in a beneficial way so that their responses can be maximized.

A

Daily Analyses of Life Demands for Athletes Material

How To Use This Book

This set of questions asks you to make some decisions about how you feel at a particular time. You are asked to compare your present feelings with your normal feelings. It is important for you to answer as truthfully and accurately as possible. The information that you provide will be used to determine your immediate training programs so it is important for you to answer each question conscientiously and honestly. Your coach will indicate to you how often you should fill in the answer sheets which are provided. If this is not done, then complete the analysis every other day.

This appendix contains a single set of questions, an answer sheet, and two graphs which are called Data Logs. You should familiarize yourself with the questions. Read them carefully and understand them. If you have any problems ask your coach to clarify your difficulties. The explanations and directions before each question set should help your understanding further.

In the early stages of completing the log book you will have to refer to the questions quite often. In time, you will come to memorize them. So that you will not have to keep turning back and forth to the questions, the answer sheets have key words printed alongside each set of question responses. Consequently, you will only have to turn to an answer sheet when you become familiar with the questions.

What to Put on the Answer Sheet

Fill in all information. Make sure you record the correct date. Answer every question. Remember that an 'a' response indicates worse than usual, a 'b' response indicates normal, and a 'c' response means better than usual. After you finish each part, total the responses for each category and enter them in the spaces provided. In this way, you know the number of items which are worse than usual, normal, and better than usual.

How to Use the Data Logs

There are two summary sheets called Data Logs. These are used to graph the total number of response categories for each part of each day.

When you complete the answer sheet, totaling the number of responses for the 'a', 'b', and 'c' categories is important. This is what you do:

1. Turn to the Data Log for Part A.
2. Write the date of the day's testing below a vertical line at the very bottom. Start at the left.
3. Mark a very small dot or 'x' on the vertical line for the number of responses to 'a', 'b', and 'c' on the appropriate graph.
4. Turn to the Data Log for Part B. Repeat the process, entering the information for Part B in the same way as you did for Part A.

Part A

In the various things that you do throughout your daily living, events happen which may cause you worry, upset you, cause you to work harder than usual, or even make you tired. Happenings of that nature are commonly termed 'stressful'. On the other hand, there are events which make life seem to be very easy and enjoyable. You may seem to have no worries or upsets and whatever you do seems satisfying. In such cases life seems 'less stressful' than it normally is. The purpose of this set of questions is to get you to decide whether certain aspects of your everyday living are more or less stressful than usual.

Nine areas of your life are described below. You are to indicate whether each is (a) 'more stressful' than usual, (b) 'about normal', or (c) 'less stressful' than usual. For example, one of the items is sleep. If you have not been sleeping well then you would answer 'more stressful' than usual. For the item concerning friends, if you are very happy with your relationship with all your friends, have had no upsets or arguments, you would probably answer 'less stressful'. Alternatively, if things were going normally with your friends, maybe an occasional argument or feeling that some people do not like you, you probably would answer 'about normal'.

You are asked to picture what is *normal* for you. Then consider each item *as it is at the time of completing the answer sheet*. Make a careful judgment before you respond to each of the items described. Answer on the answer sheet and plot the results on the Data Logs, as described.

Definitions for Part A

1. *Diet.* Consider whether you are eating regularly and in adequate amounts. Are you missing meals? Do you like your meals?

  (a) more stressful   (b) normal   (c) less stressful

2. *Home life.* Have you had any arguments with your parents, brothers, or sisters? Are you being asked to do too much around the house? How is your relationship with your wife/husband? Have there been any unusual happenings at home concerning your family?

  (a) more stressful   (b) normal   (c) less stressful

3. *School/college/work.* Consider the amount of work that you are doing there. Are you required to do more or less at home or in your own time? How are your grades or evaluations? Think of how you are interacting with administrators, teachers, or bosses.

  (a) more stressful   (b) normal   (c) less stressful

4. *Friends.* Have you lost or gained any friends? Have there been any arguments or problems with your friends? Are they complimenting you more or less? Do you spend more or less time with them?

  (a) more stressful   (b) normal   (c) less stressful

5. *Training and exercise.* How much and how often are you training? Are the levels of effort that are required easy or hard? Are you able to recover adequately between efforts? Are you enjoying your sport?

  (a) more stressful   (b) normal   (c) less stressful

6. *Climate.* Is it too hot, cold, wet, or dry?

  (a) more stressful   (b) normal   (c) less stressful

7. *Sleep.* Are you getting enough sleep? Are you getting too much? Can you sleep when you want to?

  (a) more stressful   (b) normal   (c) less stressful

Data Log Part A

Number of Responses to 'a' Alternative (note any increases)

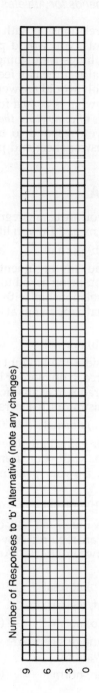

Number of Responses to 'b' Alternative (note any changes)

Number of Responses to 'c' Alternative (note any decreases)

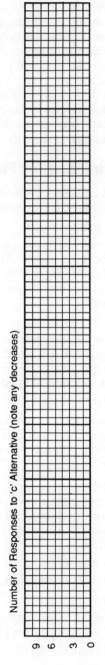

ENTER THE DATE FOR EVERY RECORDING

Data Log Part B

Number of Responses to 'a' Alternative (note any increases)

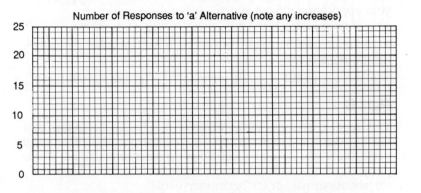

Number of Responses to 'b' Alternative (note any changes)

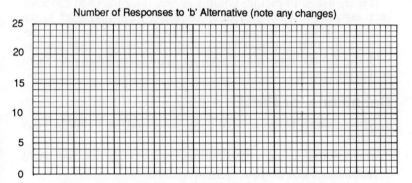

Number of Responses to 'c' Alternative (note any decreases)

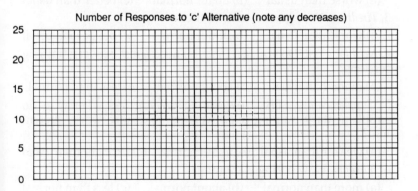

ENTER THE DATE FOR EVERY RECORDING

8. *Recreation.* Consider the activities that you do outside of your sport. Are they taking up too much time? Do they compete with your application to your sport?

    (a) more stressful   (b) normal   (c) less stressful

9. *Health.* Do you have any infections, a cold, or other temporary health problems?

    (a) more stressful   (b) normal   (c) less stressful

Part B

This section asks questions about a number of behaviors and feelings that could occur in athletes. You are to read each item and decide how you normally feel. Then consider how you are at this particular time and decide whether you are (a) 'worse than usual', (b) 'about normal', or (c) 'better than usual'.

You are asked to picture what is *normal* for you. Then consider each item *as you feel at the time of completing the answer sheet*. Make a careful judgment before you respond to each of the items described. If any of the questions do not apply to you then answer with the '(b) about normal' response. Answer on the answer sheet that is provided.

Definitions for Part B

1. *Muscle pains.* Do you have sore joints and/or pains in your muscles?

    (a) worse than usual   (b) about normal   (c) better than usual

2. *Techniques.* How do your techniques feel?

    (a) worse than usual   (b) about normal   (c) better than usual

3. *Tiredness.* Your general state of tiredness is:

    (a) worse than usual   (b) about normal   (c) better than usual

4. *Need for a rest.* Do you feel that you need a rest between training sessions?

    (a) more than usual   (b) about normal   (c) less than normal

5. *Supplementary work.* How strong do you feel when you do supplementary training (e.g., weights, resistance work, stretching)?

    (a) weaker than usual   (b) about normal   (c) stronger than usual

6. *Boredom.* How boring is training?

    (a) more than normal   (b) about normal   (c) less than normal

7. *Recovery time.* Do the recovery times between each training effort need to be longer?

    (a) longer than usual   (b) about normal   (c) shorter than usual

8. *Irritability.* Are you irritable? Do things get on your nerves?

(a) more than usual   (b) about normal   (c) less than usual

9. *Weight.* How is your weight?

(a) lighter than usual (b) about normal (c) heavier than usual

10. *Throat.* Have you noticed your throat being sore or irritated?

(a) worse than usual   (b) about normal   (c) no troubles felt

11. *Internal.* How do you feel internally? Have you had constipation, upset stomachs, etc.?

(a) worse than usual   (b) about normal   (c) better than usual

12. *Unexplained aches.* Do you have any unexplained aches or pains?

(a) more than usual   (b) about normal   (c) less than usual

13. *Technique strength.* How strong do your techniques feel?

(a) worse than usual   (b) about normal   (c) better than usual

14. *Enough sleep.* Are you getting enough sleep?

(a) less than necessary (b) about normal (c) more than normal

15. *Between-sessions recovery.* Are you tired before you start your second training session of the day?

(a) more than usual   (b) about normal   (c) less than usual

16. *General weakness.* Do you feel weak all over?

(a) worse than usual   (b) about normal   (c) better than usual

17. *Interest.* Do you feel that you are maintaining your interest in your sport?

(a) worse than usual   (b) about normal   (c) better than usual

18. *Arguments.* Are you having squabbles and arguments with people?

(a) more than usual   (b) about normal   (c) less than usual

19. *Skin rashes.* Do you have any unexplained skin rashes or irritations?

(a) more than usual   (b) about normal   (c) less than usual

20. *Congestion.* Are you experiencing congestion in the nose and/or sinuses?

(a) worse than usual   (b) about normal   (c) better than usual

21. *Training effort.* Do you feel that you can give your best effort at training?

(a) less than usual   (b) about normal   (c) more than usual

22. *Temper.* Do you lose your temper?

(a) quicker than normal (b) about normal (c) less than normal

23. *Swellings.* Do you have any lymph gland swellings under your arms, below your ears, in your groin, etc.?

(a) more than normal   (b) about normal   (c) less than normal

24. *Likability.* Do people seem to like you?

(a) less than usual   (b) about normal   (c) more than usual

25. *Running nose.* Do you have a running nose?

(a) worse than usual   (b) about normal   (c) better than usual

Answer Sheet

ANSWER SHEET

Name: ....   Date: ....

RESPOND BY CIRCLING the appropriate response alongside each item.

a = worse than normal   b = normal   c = better than normal

PART A

1. a	b	c	Diet
2. a	b	c	Home life
3. a	b	c	School/college/work
4. a	b	c	Friends
5. a	b	c	Sport training
6. a	b	c	Climate
7. a	b	c	Sleep
8. a	b	c	Recreation
9. a	b	c	Health

Total 'a' responses   ....
Total 'b' responses   ....
Total 'c' responses   ....

Record these values and the day's data on the Data Log Part A

8. a	b	c	Irritability
9. a	b	c	Weight
10. a	b	c	Throat
11. a	b	c	Internal
12. a	b	c	Unexplained aches
13. a	b	c	Technique strength
14. a	b	c	Enough sleep
15. a	b	c	Between sessions recovery
16. a	b	c	General weakness
17. a	b	c	Interest
18. a	b	c	Arguments
19. a	b	c	Skin rashes
20. a	b	c	Congestion
21. a	b	c	Training effort
22. a	b	c	Temper
23. a	b	c	Swellings
24. a	b	c	Likability
25. a	b	c	Running nose

Total 'a' responses   ....
Total 'b' responses   ....
Total 'c' responses   ....

Record these values and the day's data on the Data Log Part B

PART B

1. a	b	c	Muscle pains
2. a	b	c	Techniques
3. a	b	c	Tiredness
4. a	b	c	Need for a rest
5. a	b	c	Supplementary work
6. a	b	c	Boredom
7. a	b	c	Recovery time

B

Monitoring Training Responses Using Ergometer Scores and Recovery Heart Rates

This section explains, in greater detail, the compilation of and monitoring of the relationship between performance and recovery heart rate measures. For convenience, Figure 8.8 is repeated as Figure B.1.

Steps in Developing a Performance Monitoring Graph

1. Decide upon what measure of physiological response will be used. In this example, it is the total of three 10-second pulse counts taken immediately, 30 seconds, and 60 seconds after the completion of the performance. It is to be expected that the total value will vary depending upon the intensity of the effort, the level of performance, and/or the state of training fitness. It is helpful if a maximum recovery heart rate is known.
2. Decide upon the physical performance that will be the standardized testing task. This activity should be repeated for each assessment under the same conditions of pre-test diet, rest, and time of day. In this example, the task was the completion of a 2,500-meter row on a Concept II ergometer under USRA national team testing conditions (small sprocket, flywheel cover).
3. Construct the graph axes that will cover all ranges of heart rate totals and performance possibilities. In Figure B.1 the heart rate range is from 40 to 100 bpm and the performance time range is 7 minutes 45 seconds to 9 minutes. It is helpful

383

Figure B.1 Graph of Recovery Heart Rate Totals and Concept II Rowing Ergometer Performances for a Male Varsity Rower

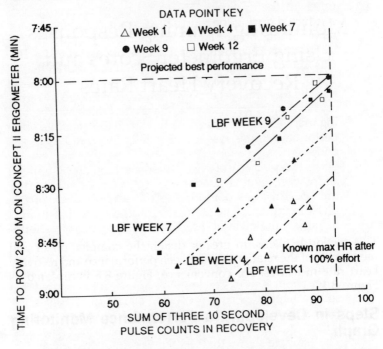

to have this graph constructed on graph paper so that the preprinted lines can be used to record data points accurately.

4. Early in the specific preparatory training phase collect data from at least 5 performance efforts. In this example, an effort was done each weekday and on Saturday after completing a standard warm-up. Those points should be plotted on the graph and a 'line of best fit (LBF)' entered. The LBF is the central tendency of all the data points. *It is important to vary the percentage of effort between the tasks so that a wide distribution of points is obtained.* If all efforts were done near maximum, then the points would be clustered and no LBF could be constructed that would serve any valuable purpose. Assuming that the maximum recovery heart rate total is known, the LBF can be extended to that maximum value. The point where the two lines intersect can then be aligned with the performance time axis. The value of that alignment is the 'predicted best performance time' given the current state of fitness/technique of the athlete. In Figure B.1, that predicted value is in the region of 8 minutes 30 seconds.

5. As training progresses, fitness should improve. To evaluate this another bout of standardized testing should be instituted. In the example, the second series of testings was conducted during the fourth week of the specific preparatory training phase. Four data points were plotted after standardized warm-up and assessment conditions. A LBF was drawn to best represent the data. It can be seen that all 4 points had moved to the left of the Week 1 LBF. This meant that the physical cost of performance, as reflected by recovery heart rates, was lessening, that is, the athlete was becoming more efficient or fitter. At this stage the 'predicted best performance time' was in the vicinity of 8 minutes 17 seconds.

6. Since the purpose of this procedure is to track training adaptation, another standardized set of tests should be conducted. This was done during the seventh week of this phase of training. The exampled data points had continued to move to the left indicating that the energy cost of performance was still improving. The first near-maximum heart rates were recorded during this period. The 'predicted best performance time' was near 8 minutes 5 seconds.

7. After about 8 weeks of serious training, it is possible that some athletes will be approaching maximum fitness states. At that time, the frequency of testing increases so that the critical overtraining state is at least located in its early stages. The example shows that testing was conducted again during the ninth week. Performance improvement was still being evidenced but the amount of improvement was reduced when compared to that which occurred between weeks 4 and 7. This suggests that the returns from challenging overloads may be starting to diminish. The 'predicted best performance time' during this time was 8 minutes 1 second.

8. Further testing was conducted during week 12. Four of 5 data points had moved back slightly to the right of the week 9 LBF. One point was in the range of the best performance recorded. This regression indicates that peak fitness has been obtained. Since top-quality performances were not exhibited for the week, several of them dropping below those standards exhibited in week 7, these data also suggest that quality performances cannot be maintained over an extended period. The regression and performance deterioration within week 12 suggest that the athlete was beginning to deteriorate in performance potential and that his restorative/regeneration capacity was degrading. These signs

indicate that at least one unloading microcycle is warranted as is a cessation of overload increases. The athlete would seem to have entered the early states of overtraining.

General Comments

As an athlete improves in fitness, the LBFs and data points move to the left. Once peak fitness is attained, that migration ceases. When overtrained states begin, the points move back to the right. Once that regression occurs, and if a LBF were drawn, it might be noticed that the slope of the line also becomes steeper. This increase is because the cost of work at lower effort levels increases in overtrained states.

To use this measurement technique, it will be necessary to do some experimenting to learn the recording and graphing principles as well as interpreting the data and trends. It is best to educate athletes to do this in a self-monitoring mode so that the coach will not be overburdened with the task.

The assessment of performances and physiological measures provides a means of predicting performance. These predictions serve a strong motivational function and allow testing to be related directly to training.

A Final Concern

The value of using performances to indicate the state of training is dependent upon the only factor affecting performance being that state. A coach should make every effort to standardize testing conditions. The athlete's preparation (e.g., diet, fluid intake, amount of rest, warm-up) and the environmental conditions (e.g., temperature, clothing, number of spectators) need to be as similar as possible for all testing sessions. This consideration requires the development of testing protocols by the coach and rituals by the athletes. If these factors are not controlled then performances will be caused by other variables as well as the state of training. The confounding effect of uncontrolled variables will increase the variability of performances and obscure the sensitivity of this method of monitoring an athlete's training progress.

Physiological Fitness Test Standards

1. Endurance Tests

Typical Values for Maximal Oxygen Consumption (V̇O₂ max) in Highly Trained Young Adult Athletes (various sources)

☐ Running Sports   Treadmill (mL.kg⁻¹.mm⁻¹)

		Mean	Usual Range
Distance Runners	Male	75	70–80
	Female	65	60–75
Soccer Players	Male	60	55–65
	Female	50	45–55
Field Hockey Players	Male	60	55–65
	Female	50	45–55
Basketball Players	Male	55	50–60
	Female	45	40–55
Australian Football Players	Male	60	55–65

☐ Rowing   Rowing Ergometer (L.min⁻¹)

	Mean	Usual Range
Heavyweight Male	5·5	5·0–6·2
Heavyweight Female	3·8	3·3–4·4

☐ Cycling   Cycling Ergometer (L.min⁻¹)

		Mean	Usual Range
Track	Male	5·3	4·5–6·0
	Female	3·3	2·6–4·0
Road	Male	5·4	4·5–6·1
	Female	3·5	3·0–4·0
Road (mL.kg⁻¹.min⁻¹)	Male	75	6·5–8·0
	Female	65	5·5–7·0

☐ Kayaking   Kayak Ergometer (L.min^{-1})

Sprint	Male	4·8	4·4–5·2
	Female	3·1	2·8–3·4
Distance	Male	4·6	4·0–5·2
	Female	3·1	2·8–3·4

☐ Standards for PWC-170 Test: Cycle Ergometer
(kgm.kg^{-1}.min^{-1})

	Male	Female
Very Good	> 20·0	> 18·0
Good	18·5–20·0	16·7–18·0
Average	17·0–18·4	15·3–16·6
Fair	15·5–16·9	14·0–15·2
Poor	< 15·5	< 14·0

☐ Standards for Tri-level Aerobic Power Index: Cycle Ergometer
(W.kg^{-1})
From Telford *et al.* 1987

	Male	Female
Elite	> 3·4	> 3·1
Very Good	2·9–3·4	2·7–3·1
Good	2·4–2·8	2·2–2·6
Average	1·8–2·3	1·6–2·1
Fair	1·1–1·7	1·0–1·5
Poor	< 1·1	< 1·0

☐ Standards for 15-minute Run for Team Game Players (m)

	Male	Female
Very Good	> 4200	> 3800
Good	3900–4200	3500-3800
Average	3600–3899	3250–3499
Fair	3300–3599	3000–3249
Poor	< 3300	< 3000

2. Anaerobic Power and Speed Tests

☐ Standards for Tri-level Alactic Power Index: Cycle Ergometer
(Peak power in 10 s (W.kg^{-1})
From Telford *et al.* 1987

	Male	Female
Elite	> 19·5	> 16·6
Very Good	17·0–19·5	14·3–16·6
Good	14·4–16·9	11·9–14·2
Average	11·8–14·3	9·5–11·8

| Fair | 9·2–11·7 | 7·1–9·4 |
| Poor | < 9·2 | < 7·1 |

☐ Vertical Jump (cm)

	Male	Female
Very Good	> 67	> 57
Good	60–67	50–56
Average	52–59	43–49
Fair	44–51	36–42
Poor	< 44	< 36

☐ 35 Meter Dash (s)

	Male	Female
Very Good	< 4·80	< 5·30
Good	4·80–5·09	5·30–5·59
Average	5·10–5·29	5·60–5·89
Fair	5·30–5·60	5·90–6·20
Poor	> 5·60	> 6·20

☐ 5-0-5 TEST* (s)

	Male	Female
Very Good	< 2·20	< 2·40
Good	2·20–2·39	2·40–2·54
Average	2·30–2·49	2·55–2·74
Fair	2·50–2·60	2·75–2·90
Poor	> 2·60	> 2·90

*this test involves running 5 meters to and from an end line, from a moving start

3. Anaerobic Endurance Tests

☐ Tri-level Anaerobic Work Capacity Index: Cycle Ergometer
(Work done in 30 s ($J.kg^{-1}$))
From Telford *et al.* 1987

	Male	Female
Elite	> 366	> 325
Very Good	324–366	278–325
Good	284–323	244–277
Average	244–283	214–243
Fair	204–243	179–213
Poor	< 204	< 179

□ 400 Meter Run (s)

	Male	Female
Very Good	< 53·0	< 59·0
Good	53·0–55·9	59·0–61·9
Average	56·0–58·9	62·0–64·9
Fair	59·0–62·0	65·0–68·0
Poor	> 62·0	> 68·0

4. Other Tests

□ Sit and Reach Test (cm)

	Male	Female
Very Good	> 13·0	> 15·0
Good	10·1–13·0	12·1–15·0
Average	6·1–10·0	8·1–12·0
Fair	1·0–6·0	3·0–8·0
Poor	< 1·0	< 3·0

□ Skinfold Thickness (mm)

		Mean	Range
Basketball	Male*	67	40–89
	Female**	84	54–133
Cycling (Track)	Male	48	33–79
	Female	75	56–104
Gymnastics	Male	39	29–57
	Female	45	34–55
Field Hockey	Male	49	34–68
	Female	71	55–92
Rowing	Male	55	36–76
	Female	94	55–133
Swimming	Male	50	38–75
	Female	66	47–90
Track and Field			
Sprinting	Male	42	32–69
	Female	67	39–97
Middle-distance Running	Male	38	32–44
	Female	63	31–90
Throwing	Male	107	45–224
	Female	135	103–220

*Males: sum of eight skinfolds.
**Females: sum of seven skinfolds.

From Telford *et al.*
'Skinfold measures and weight control in élite athletes',
Excel 5 (2) 1988: 21–6

Bibliography

Aggis, R. (1985) '15-minute run v 5-minute run', *Sports Coach* 9 (2): 55–6.

Akerstedt, T. (1977) 'Inversion of the sleep–wakefulness pattern: Effects on circadian variations in psychophysiological activation', *Ergonomics* 20: 459–74.

Andrisani, P. J., and Nestel, G. (1976) 'Internal–external control as contributor to and outcome of work experience', *Journal of Applied Physiology* 61: 156–65.

Arakelyan, E. E., Raitsin, L. M., Manzhuev, C. H., and Brazhnik, I. I. (1985) 'Specialized sprint exercises on a training aid with lightened loading', *Soviet Sports Review* 20: 45–7.

Asfour, S. S., Ayoub, M. M., and Mital, A. (1984) 'Effects of an endurance and strength training programme on lifting capability of males', *Ergonomics* 27: 435–42.

Ashy, M. H., Landin, D. K., and Lee, A. M. (1988) 'Relationship of practice using correct technique to achievement in a motor skill', *Journal of Teaching in Physical Education* 7: 115–20.

Asmussen, E., and Boje, O. (1945) 'Body temperature and capacity for work', *Acta Physiologica Scandinavica* 10: 1–22.

Asmussen, E., and Bonde-Petersen, F. (1974) 'Storage of elastic energy in skeletal muscles in man', *Acta Physiologica Scandinavica* 91: 385–92.

Astrand, I. (1960) 'Aerobic work capacity in men and women with special reference to age', *Acta Physiologica Scandinavica* 49, Supplement 169.

Astrand, P-O., and Rodahl, K. (1986) *Textbook of Work Physiology*, New York, McGraw-Hill.

Atha, J. (1981) 'Strengthening muscle', *Exercise and Sport Science Review* 9: 1–73.

Athletic Performance Review (1986) (Rusko, H.) 'Analysis of physiological response to training and competition among Finnish endurance athletes' (abstract).

Bedi, J. F., Cresswell, A. G., Engel, T. J., and Nicol, S. M. (1987) 'Increase in jumping height associated with maximal effort vertical depth jumps', *Research Quarterly for Exercise and Sport* 58: 11–15.

Belcastro, A. N., and Bonen, A. (1975) 'Lactic acid removal rates during controlled and uncontrolled recovery exercise', *Journal of Applied Physiology* 39 (6): 932–6.

Berg, K., Miller, M., and Stephens, L. (1986) 'Determinants of 30-meter sprint time in pubescent males', *Journal of Sport Medicine and Physical Fitness* 26: 225–30.

Berger, R. (1962) 'Optimum repetitions for the development of strength', *Research Quarterly* 33: 334–8.

Bergstrom, J., Hermansen, L., Hultman, E., and Saltin, B. (1967) 'Diet, muscle glycogen, and physical performance', *Acta Physiologica Scandinavia* 71: 140–50.

Bhambhani, Y., and Singh, M. (1985) 'The effects of three training intensities on $\dot{V}O_2$ max and $\dot{V}E/\dot{V}O_2$ ratio', *Canadian Journal of Applied Sport Sciences* 10: 44–51.

Blattner, S. E., and Noble, L. (1979) 'Relative effects of isokinetic plyometric training on vertical jumping performance', *Research Quarterly* 50: 583–8.

Bleier, R., and O'Neil, T. (1975) *Fighting Back*, New York, Stein and Day.

Bobbert, M. F., Van Ingen Schenau, G. J., and Huising, P. A. (1985) 'Plantar flexion torques in jumping and isokinetic plantar flexion: A comparison' in S. M. Perren and E. Schneider (eds), *Biomechanics: Current Interdisciplinary Research*, Dordrecht, Netherlands, Martinus: 403–8.

Bompa, T. O. (1986) *Theory and Methodology of Training*, Dubuque, Iowa, Kendall/Hunt.

Bosco, C., and Komi, P. V. (1979) 'Potential of the mechanical behavior of the human skeletal muscle through prestretching', *Acta Physiologica Scandinavica* 106: 467–72.

——, Rusko, H., and Hirvonen, J. (1984) 'The effect of extra-load conditioning on muscle performance in athletes', *Medicine and Science in Sports and Exercise* 18: 415–19.

Brooke, J. D., and Knowles, J. E. (1974) 'A movement analysis of player behaviour in soccer match performance', in *Proceedings of the British Society of Sport Psychology Conference*, Salford, England.

Brouha, L. (1945) 'Specificite de l'entrainement au travail musculaire', *Review of Cardiac Biology* 4: 144.

Brown, M. E., Mayhew, J. L., and Boleach, l. W. (1986) 'Effect of plyometric training on vertical jump performance in high school basketball players', *Journal of Sports Medicine and Physical Fitness* 26: 1–4.

Burton, A. C., and Edholm, O. G. (1969) *Man in a Cold Environment*, New York, Hafner.

Campbell, C. J. (1979) *Information on Jet-lag*, Package 1, Item #3, Ottawa, Coaching Association of Canada.

Campbell, R. E. (1944) 'A study of factors affecting flexibility', Unpublished Master's thesis, University of Wisconsin.

Carlile, F. (1955) 'The athlete and adaptation to stress', Part I of an address delivered to the Symposium on Training, NSW Amateur Swimming Association, Sydney, Australia.

—— (1956) 'The effects of preliminary passive warming on swimming performance', *Research Quarterly* 27: 246–7.

—— (1964) *Forbes Carlile on Swimming*, London, Pelham.

—— (1981) 'Fifty years of swimming research', in *Proceedings of the Pacific Coaches' Conference,* Sydney, Australia, Australian Swimming Union.

—— and Carlile, U. (1961) 'Physiological studies of Australian Olympic swimmers in hard training', *Australian Journal of Physical Education,* October–November.

Chalip, L. (1980) 'Social learning theory and sport success: Evidence and implications', *Journal of Sport Behavior* 3: 76–85.

Chevrier, C. D. (1981) 'The short-term retention of flexibility in varsity ice hockey players', Unpublished Master's thesis, Lakehead University, Canada.

Chu, D. (1984) 'Plyometric exercise', *NSCA Journal,* January: 57–62.

Clarke, H. H. (1975) 'Joint and body range of movement', *Physical Fitness Research Digest* 5: 1–22.

Clarke, H. H. (1976) 'Exercise and the knee', *Physical Fitness Research Digest* 6: 1–17.

Clutch, D., Wilton, M., McGown, C., and Bryce, G. R. (1983) 'The effect of depth jumps and weight training on leg strength and vertical jump', *Research Quarterly for Exercise and Sport* 54: 5–10.

Coaching Review (1985) (Matt Mizerski) September–October: 9–13.

Cochrane, C., and Pyke, F. S. (1976) 'Physiological assessment of the Australian soccer squad', *Australian Journal of Health, Physical Education, and Recreation* 73: 21–5.

Colquhoun, D., and Chad, K. E. (1986) 'Physiological characteristics of Australian female soccer players after a competitive season', *Australian Journal of Science and Medicine in Sport* 18 (3): 9–12.

Conlee, R. K., McGown, C. M., Fisher, A. G., Dalsky, G. P., and Robinson, K. C. (1982) 'Physiological effects of power volleyball', *The Physician and Sportsmedicine* 10 (2): 93–7.

Costill, D. L. (1979) *A Scientific Approach to Distance Running,* Los Altos, Calif., Track and Field News.

—— (1986) *Inside Running: Basics of Sports Physiology,* Indianapolis, Benchmark Press.

——, Kammer, W. F., and Fisher, A. (1970) 'Fluid ingestion during distance running', *Archives of Environmental Health* 21: 520–5.

——, King, D. S., Thomas, R., and Hargreaves, M. (1985) 'Effects of reduced training on muscular power in swimmers', *The Physician and Sportsmedicine* 13: 94–101.

——, Sharp, R., and Troup, J. (1980) 'Muscle strength: contributions to sprint swimming', *Swimming World* 21: 29–34.

—— and Winrow, E. (1970) 'A comparison of two middle-aged ultramarathon runners', *Research Quarterly* 41 (2): 135–9.

Cureton, T. K. (1941) 'Flexibility as an aspect of physical fitness', *Research Quarterly,* Supp. 12: 381–90.

Davis, E. C., Logan, G. A., and McKinney, W. C. (1961) *Biophysical Values of Muscular Activity with Implications for Research.* Dubuque, Iowa, Wm C. Brown.

Dawson, B., and Pyke, F. S. (1988) 'I: Responses to wearing sweat clothing during exercise in cool conditions. II: Training in sweat clothing in cool conditions to improve heat tolerance', *Journal of Human Movement Studies* 15: 171–83.

Denk, G. M. (1971) 'The changes occurring in strength and flexibility during a competitive gymnastics season involving high school boys', Unpublished Master's thesis, University of Kansas.

Derbaba, L., and Petrov, V. (1984) 'Learn to jump', *Soviet Sports Review* 19: 17–21.

Derriman, P. (1989) 'Tuning the champions', *Good Weekend* (The *Sydney Morning Herald* Magazine), 20 May, 28–32.

de Vries, H. A. (1962) 'Evaluation of static stretching procedures for improvement of flexibility', *Research Quarterly* 32: 468–79.

—— (1974) *Physiology of Exercise*, Dubuque, Iowa, Wm C. Brown.

Dons, B., Bollerup, K., Bonde-Petersen, F., and Hancke, S. (1979) 'The effects of weight lifting exercise related to muscle fiber composition and muscle cross-sectional area in humans', *European Journal of Applied Physiology* 40: 95–106.

Draper, J. A., and Lancaster, M. G. (1985) 'The 505 test — A test for agility in the horizontal plane', *Australian Journal of Science and Medicine in Sport* 17 (1): 15–18.

Draper, J. A., and Pyke, F. S. (1988) 'Turning speed — A valuable asset in run-making', *Sports Coach* 11 (3): 30–1.

Dudley, G. A., Abraham, W. M., and Terjung, R. L. (1982) 'Influence of exercise intensity and duration on biochemical adaptation in skeletal muscle', *Journal of Applied Physiology* 53: 844–50.

Elliott, B. C., Champion, N., and Morrison, D. (1980) *Squash*, Adelaide, ACHPER Publications.

Elliott, H. (1961) *The Golden Mile*, London, Cassell and Co.

Ekblom, B. (1986) 'Applied physiology of soccer', *Journal of Sports Medicine* 3: 50–60.

Faulkner, J. A. (1964) 'Effects of cardiac conditioning on the anticipatory, exercise and recovery heart rates of young men', *The Journal of Sports Medicine and Physical Fitness* 4: 79–86.

Fleck, S. J., and Kraemer, W. J. (1987) *Designing Resistance Training Programs*, Champaign, Ill., Human Kinetics.

—— and Kraemer, W. J. (1988a) 'Resistance training: basic principles', Part 1 of 4, *The Physician and Sportsmedicine* 16 (3): 161–71.

—— and Kraemer, W. J. (1988b) 'Resistance training: physiological responses and adaptations', Part 2 of 4, *The Physician and Sportsmedicine* 16 (4): 109–24.

—— and Kraemer, W. J. (1988c) 'Resistance training: physiological responses and adaptations', Part 3 of 4, *The Physician and Sportsmedicine* 16 (5): 63–75.

Fleishman, E. A. (1964) *The Structure and Measurement of Physical Fitness*, Englewood Cliffs, NJ, Prentice-Hall.

Fox, E. L., Bartels, R. L., Klinzing, J., and Ragg, K. (1977) 'Metabolic responses to interval training program of high and low power output', *Medicine and Science in Sports* 9: 191–6.

—— and Costill, D. L. (1972) 'Estimated cardio-respiratory responses during marathon running', *Archives of Environmental Health* 24: 315–24.

Gettman, L. R., and Pollock, M. L. (1981) 'Circuit weight training: a critical review of its physiological benefits', *The Physician and Sportsmedicine* 9: 44–60.

Goodyear, M. D. (1973) 'Stress, adrenocortical activity and sleep habits', *Ergonomics* 16: 679–81.

Grabe, S. A., and Widule, C. J. (1988) 'Comparative biomechanics of the jerk in Olympic weightlifting', *Research Quarterly for Exercise and Sport* 59: 1–8.

Graves, J. E., Pollock, M. L., Leggett, S. H., Braith, R. W., Carpenter, D. M., and Bishop, L. E. (1988) 'Effect of reduced training frequency on muscular strength', *International Journal of Sports Medicine* 9: 316–19.

Gregory, L. W. (1979) 'The development of aerobic capacity. A comparison of continuous and interval training', *Research Quarterly* 50: 199–206.

Grobaker, M. R., and Stull, G. A. (1975) 'Thermal applications as a determiner of joint flexibility', *American Corrective Therapy Journal* 29: 3–8.

Harre, D. (1971) *Trainingslehre*, Berlin, Sportverlag.

Harris, M. L. (1969) 'A factor analytic study of flexibility', *Research Quarterly* 40: 62–70.

Hempel, L. S., and Wells, C. L. (1985) 'Cardio-respiratory cost of the Nautilus Express Circuit', *The Physician and Sportsmedicine* 13 (4): 82–97.

Hickson, R. C., Bomze, H. A., and Hollaszy, J. O. (1977) 'Linear increase in aerobic power induced by a strenuous programme of endurance exercise', *Journal of Applied Physiology* 42: 372–6.

——, Rosenkoetter, M. A., and Brown, M. M. (1980) 'Strength training effects on aerobic power and short-term endurance', *Medicine and Science in Sports and Exercise* 12: 336–9.

Holmer, I. (1972) 'Oxygen uptake during swimming in man', *Journal of Applied Physiology* 33: 502–9.

—— (1974) 'Physiology of swimming man', *Acta Physiologica Scandinavica*, Supp. 407.

Holt, L. E. (1973) *Scientific Stretching for Sport*, Halifax, Nova Scotia, Dalhousie University.

——, Travis, T. M., and Okita, T. (1970) 'Comparative study of three stretching techniques', *Perceptual and Motor Skills* 31: 611–16.

Houston, M. E., Bentzen, H., and Larson, H. (1979) 'Interrelationships between skeletal muscle adaptations and performance as studied by de-training and re-training', *Acta Physiologica Scandinavica* 105: 163–70.

Hurley, B., Seals, D., Ehsani, A., Carter, L., Dalskey, G., Hagberg, J., and Holloszy, J. (1983) 'Effects of high-intensity strength training on cardiovascular function', *Medicine and Science in Sports and Exercise* 18: 483–7.

Ikai, M., and Steinhaus, A. H. (1961) 'Some factors modifying the expression of human strength', *Journal of Applied Physiology* 16: 157–63.

Jackson, A., Jackson, T., Hnatek, J., and West, J. (1985) 'Strength development: using functional isometrics in an isotonic strength training program', *Research Quarterly for Exercise and Sport* 56: 234–7.

Jacobs, M. (1976) 'Neurophysiological implications of slow active stretching', *American Corrective Therapy Journal* 30: 151–4.

Kabat, H. (1952) 'Studies of neuromuscular dysfunction XV — the role of central facilitation in restoration of motor function in paralysis', *Archives of Physical Medicine and Rehabilitation* 33: 521–33.

Karlsson, J., Komi, P. U., and Viitasalo, J. H. (1979) 'Muscle strength and muscle characteristics in monozygous and dizygous twins', *Acta Physiologica Scandinavica* 106: 319–25.

Karvonen, J., Peltola, E., and Saarela, J. (1986) 'The effect of sprint training performed in a hypoxic environment on specific performance capacity', *Journal of Sports Medicine* 26: 219–24.

Kaufman, W. C. (1982) 'Cold weather comfort or heat conservation', *The Physician and Sportsmedicine* 10: 70–5.

Keatinge, W. R., and Sloan, R. E. (1972) 'Effect of swimming in cold water on body temperatures in children', *Journal of Physiology* 226: 55–6.

Klissouras, V. (1971) 'Heritability of adaptive variation', *Journal of Applied Physiology* 3: 338–44.

Komi, P. U., Klissouras, V., and Karvinen, E. (1973) 'Genetic variation in neuromuscular performance', *Int. Z. Angew. Physiol.* 31: 289–304.

Konstanty, P. G. (1989) 'Acquisition of strength for a specific task', Unpublished manuscript, San Diego State University, Department of Physical Education, San Diego.

Kraemer, W. J., and Fleck, S. J. (1988) 'Resistance training: exercise prescription', Part 4 of 4, *The Physician and Sportsmedicine* 16 (6): 69–81.

LaDou, J. (1979) 'Circadian rhythms and athletic performance', *The Physician and Sportsmedicine* 7: 87–93.

Le Rossignol, P. (1985) 'Short sharp training compared to a long hard slog', *Sports Coach* 8: 3–8.

Lindh, M. (1979) 'Increase in muscle strength from isometric quadriceps exercises at different knee angles', *Scandinavian Journal of Rehabilitation Medicine* 11: 33–6.

MacDougall, J. D., and Sale, D. G. (1981) 'Continuous vs. interval training: A review for the athlete and coach', *Canadian Journal of Applied Sport Sciences* 6: 93–7.

——, Sale, D. G., Moroz, J. R., Elder, G. C., Sutton, J. R., and Howard, H. (1979) 'Mitochondrial volume density in human skeletal muscle following heavy resistance training', *Medicine and Science in Sports* 11: 164–6.

——, Ward, G. R., Sale, D. J., and Sutton, J. R. (1977) 'Biochemical adaptation of human skeletal muscle to heavy resistance training and immobilization', *Journal of Applied Physiology* 43: 700–3.

——, Wenger, H. A., and Green, H. J. (1982) *Physiological Testing of the Elite Athlete*, Ottawa, Canadian Association of Sport Sciences.

Martindale, W. O., Robertson, D. G., Coutts, K. D., and McKenzie, D. C. (1982) 'Mechanical energy variations in rowing', Paper presented at the annual meeting of the Canadian Association of Sports Sciences, Victoria, British Columbia, Canada, October.

Mayhew, J. L., Schwegler, T. M., and Piper, F. C. (1986) 'Relationship of acceleration momentum to anaerobic power measurements', *Journal of Sports Medicine and Physical Fitness* 26: 209–13.

Mayhew, S. R., and Wenger, H. A. (1985) 'Time–motion analysis of professional soccer', *Journal of Human Movement Studies* 11: 49–52.

McCue, B. F. (1953) 'Flexibility of college women', *Research Quarterly* 24: 316–24.

McDonagh, M. J., and Davies, C. T. (1984) 'Adaptive response of mammalian skeletal muscle to exercise with high loads', *European Journal of Applied Physiology* 52 (2): 139–55.

McKenzie, T. L., and Rushall, B. S. (1974) 'Effects of self-recording contingencies on improving attendance and performance in a competitive swimming training environment', *Journal of Applied Behavior Analysis* 7: 199–206.

—— and Rushall, B. S. (1980) 'Experimental controls of inappropriate behaviors in a competitive swimming environment', *Education and Treatment of Children* 3: 205–16.

McKethan, J. F., and Mayhew, J. L. (1974) 'Effects of isometrics, isotonics, and combined isometrics-isotonics on quadriceps strength and vertical jump', *Journal of Sports Medicine* 14: 224–9.

McNair, D. M., Lorr, M., and Droppleman, L. F. (1971) *POMS Profile of Mood States*, EdiTS, San Diego.

McPherson, B., Marteniuk R., Tihanyi, J., and Clark, W. (1977) *An analysis of the System of Age Group Swimming in Ontario*, Toronto, Ontario Section, Canadian Amateur Swimming Association.

Meyers, E. J. (1971) 'Effects of selected exercise variables on ligament stability and flexibility of the knee', *Research Quarterly* 28: 357–63.

Michael, E. D., and Horvath, S. M. (1965) 'Psychological limits in athletic training' in F. Antonelli (ed.), *Psicologia dello sport*, Rome, Federazione Medico Sportavia Italiana.

Moffroid, M. T., and Whipple, R. H. (1970) 'Specificity of speed of exercise', *Physical Therapy* 50: 1692–1700.

Montpetit, R., Duvallet, A., Serveth, J. P., and Cazorla, G. (1981) 'Stability of VO_2 max during a 3-month intensive training period in élite swimmers', Paper presented at the Annual Meeting of the Canadian Association of Sport Sciences, Halifax.

Morgan, W. P. (1980) 'Psychological monitoring of athletic stress syndrome', Paper presented at the 27th Annual Meeting of the American College of Sports Medicine, Las Vegas, May.

Moritani, T., and de Vries, H. A. (1979) 'Neural factors vs hypertrophy in the time course of muscle strength gain', *American Journal of Physical Medicine* 58: 115–30.

Nadel, E. R., Holmer, I., Bergh, U., Astrand, P-O., and Stolwijk, J. A. (1974) 'Energy exchanges of swimming man', *Journal of Applied Physiology* 36: 465–71.

Noakes, T. (1986) *Lore of Running*, Cape Town, Oxford University Press.

O'Reilly, K. P., Warhol, M. J., Fielding, R. A., Frontera, W. R., Meredith, C. N., and Evans, W. J. (1987) 'Eccentric exercise-induced muscle damage impairs muscle glycogen repletion', *Journal of Applied Physiology* 63: 252–6.

Overend, T., Paterson, D., Cunningham, D., and Taylor, A. (1985) 'Interval and continuous training: A comparison of training effects', Paper presented at the Annual Meeting of the Canadian Association of Sport Sciences, Laval University, Quebec City, October.

Payne, W. R., and Lemon, P. W. R. (1982) 'Metabolic comparison of tethered and simulated swimming ergometer exercise', Paper presented at the Annual Meeting of the Canadian Association of Sports Sciences, Victoria, October.

Pechar, G. S., McArdle, W. D., Katch, F. I., Magel, J. R., and De Luca, J. (1974) 'Specificity of cardio-respiratory adaptation to bicycle and treadmill training', *Journal of Applied Physiology* 36: 753–6.

Peterson, S. R., Holding, M. V., Morrow, A. G., and Wenger, H. A. (1981) 'The specificity of aerobic endurance: the influence of mode of training on $\dot{V}O_2$ max and anaerobic threshold', Paper presented at the Annual Meeting of the Canadian Association of Sport Sciences, Halifax.

Pickard, R., and Pyke, F. S. (1981) 'Assessment of the strength and endurance of surf-ski paddlers', *Sports Coach* 5 (1): 23–6.

Pipes, T. V. (1978) 'Variable resistance vs constant resistance strength training in adult males', *European Journal of Applied Physiology* 39: 27–35.

Poliquin, C. (1985) '10 common mistakes in strength training', *Coaching Review*, September–October: 14–16.

Prokop, L. (1963) 'Adrenals and sport', *The Journal of Sports Medicine and Physical Fitness* 3: 115–21.

Pugh, L. G., and Edholm, O. G. (1955) 'The physiology of channel swimmers', *Lancet* 2: 761–8.

Pyke, F. S. (ed.) (1980) *Towards Better Coaching*, Canberra, Australian Government Publishing Service.

—— (1986) 'Physiological testing of athletes', *Sports Coach* 10 (3): 4–6.

——, Craig, N. P., and Norton, K. I. (1988) 'Physiological and psychological responses of sprint and pursuit track cyclists to a period of reduced training' in E. R. Burke and M. Newsom (eds), *Medicine and Science in Cycling*, Champaign, Ill., Human Kinetics.

——, Elliott, B. C., and Pyke, J. E. (1974) 'Performance testing of tennis and squash players', *British Journal of Sports Medicine* 8 (2): 80–6.

——, and Hahn, A. G. (1981) 'Body temperature regulation in summer football', *Sports Coach* 4 (3): 41–3.

——, Minikin, B. R., Woodman, L. R., Roberts, A. D., and Wright, T. G. (1979) 'Isokinetic strength and maximal oxygen uptake of training oarsmen', *Canadian Journal of Applied Sports Science* 4: 277–9.

——, Ridge B. R., and Roberts, A. D. (1976) 'Responses to kayak and cycle ergometer training', *Medicine and Science in Sports* 8: 18–22.

Rasch, P. J., and Morehouse, C. E. (1957) 'Effect of static and dynamic exercises on muscle strength and hypertrophy', *Journal of Applied Physiology* 11: 29–34.

Reilly, T., and Thomas, V. (1976) 'A motion analysis of work rate in different postural roles in professional football match play', *Journal of Human Movement Studies* 2: 87–97.

Reitter, S. (1982) 'Isolating the motivation factors of athletes who competed in the 1981 Canada Summer Games', Unpublished BPE thesis, Lakehead University, Canada.

Rejeski, W. J., and Ribisl, P. M. (1980) 'Expected task duration and perceived effort: An attributional analysis', *Journal of Sport Psychology* 2: 227–36.

Robinson, T., and Sucec, A. A. (1979) 'The relationship of training intensity and anaerobic threshold to endurance performance', *Medicine and Science in Sports* 11: 124.

Rushall, B. S. (1967) 'The scientific bases of circulo-respiratory endurance training', Unpublished Master's thesis, Indiana University.

—— (1970) 'The value and use of weight training', *Compete* 2: 1–2.

—— (1975a) 'Applied psychology in sports' in B. S. Rushall (ed.), *The Status of Psychomotor Learning and Sport Psychology Research*, Dartmouth, Nova Scotia, Sports Science Associates.

—— (1975b) 'Psychological aids for swimming coaches' in R. M. Ousley (ed.), *1975 American Swimming Coaches Association World Clinic Yearbook*, Fort Lauderdale, American Swimming Coaches Association.

—— (1977) 'The team approach to the coaching of athletes' in J. Taylor (ed.), *Proceedings of the Post-Olympic Coaching Symposium*, Ottawa, Coaching Association of Canada.

—— (1979a) 'Coaches and sport psychology', *International Journal of Sport Psychology* 10: 164–7.

—— (1979b) *The Swimmer's Race Preparation Checklists*, Sydney, The Forbes and Ursula Carlile Swimming Organization.

—— (1979c) *Psyching in Sport*, London, Pelham.

—— (1981a) 'A tool for measuring stress in élite athletes' in Y. Hanin (ed.), *Stress and Anxiety in Sport*, Moscow, Physical Culture and Sport Publishers.

—— (1981b) 'Daily analyses of life-demands for athletes' in T. Valeriote (ed.), *Level 3 National Coaching Certification Supplement*, Ottawa, Coaching Association of Canada.

—— (1981c) 'Coaching styles: a preliminary analysis', *Behavior Analysis of Motor Activity* 1: 3–19.

—— (1986) *The Psychology of Successful Cross-country Ski Racing*, Ottawa, Cross Country Canada.

—— (1987a) *Daily Analyses of Life Demands for Athletes*, Spring Valley, Calif., Sports Science Associates — Canada.

—— (1987b) 'Caracteristicas conductuales de los campeones' in G. Perez (ed.), *Proceedings of the Jornades Internacionals de Medicina I Esport*, Barcelona, Spain, INEF.

—— (1987c) *The Psychology of Successful Competing in Endurance Events*, Pretoria, South Africa, South African Association for Sport Science, Physical Education, and Recreation.

—— and Fry, D. (1980) 'Behavior variables in superior swimmers', *Canadian Journal of Applied Sport Sciences* 5: 177–82.

—— and Garvie, G. (1977) 'Psychological characteristics of Canadian Olympic and non-Olympic wrestlers', Paper presented at the Ninth Canadian Psychomotor Learning and Sport Psychology Symposium, Banff, October.

—— and Roaf, W. A. (1986) 'Physiological, sociological, and psychological responses of training-adapted talented age-group swimmers under three levels of training stress', Paper presented at the XXIII FIMS World Congress of Sports Medicine, Brisbane, Australia, September.

—— and Siedentop, D. (1972) *The Development and Control of Behavior in Sport and Physical Education*, Philadelphia, Lea and Febiger.

—— and Smith, K. C. (1979) 'The modification of the quality and quantity of behavior categories in a swimming coach', *Journal of Sport Psychology* 1: 138–50.

Rutherford, O. M., Greig, C. A., Sargeant, A. J., and Jones, D. A. (1986) 'Strength training and power output: Transference effects in the human quadriceps muscle', *Journal of Sports Sciences* 4: 101–7.

Sale, D. G. (1975) 'Limitations to strength, power and speed' in J. Taylor (ed.), *Science and the Athlete*, Ottawa, Coaching Association of Canada.

—— and MacDougall, J. D. (1981) 'Specificity in strength training: A review for the coach and athlete', *Canadian Journal of Applied Sport Sciences* 6: 87–92.

Saltin, B. (1973) 'Metabolic fundamentals in exercise', *Medicine and Science in Sports* 5 (3): 137–46.

——, Blomquist, G., Mitchell, J. H., Johnson, J. R., Wildenthal, K., and Chapman, C. B. (1968) 'Responses to submaximal and maximal exercise after bed rest and training', *Circulation* 38: Supplement 7.

——, Brown, S. L., Savage, P., and Bannister, E. W., (1981) 'Physiological and performance correlates of training in swimmers', Paper presented at the Annual Meeting of the Canadian Association of Sport Sciences, Halifax.

Scala, D., McMillan, J., Blessing, D., Rozenek, R., and Stone, M. (1987) 'Metabolic cost of a preparatory phase of training in weight lifting: A practical observation', *Journal of Applied Sport Science Research* 1: 48–52.

Scott, G. M., and French, E. (1959) *Measurement and Evaluation in Physical Education*, Dubuque, Iowa: Wm C. Brown.

Secher, N. H., Vaage, O., and Jackson, R. C. (1982) 'Rowing performance and maximal aerobic power of oarsmen', *Scandinavian Journal of Sports Sciences* 4: 9–11.

Selye, H. (1950) *Stress*, Montreal, Acta Inc.

Sharp, R. L., Troup, J. P., and Costill, D. L. (1982) 'Relationship between power and sprint freestyle swimming', *Medicine and Science of Sports and Exercise* 14 (1): 53–6.

Sherman, W. M. (1987) 'Carbohydrate, muscle glycogen, and improved performance', *The Physician and Sportsmedicine* 15: 157–64.

Skinner, B. F. (1968) *The Technology of Teaching*, New York, Appleton-Century-Crofts.

Song, T. M. K. (1979) 'Flexibility of ice hockey players and comparison with other groups' in J. Terauds and H. J. Gros (eds), *Science in Skiing, Skating and Hockey*, Del Mar, Academic Publishers.

Stamford, B. A., Cuddihee, R. W., Moffatt, R. J., and Rowland, R. (1978) 'Task specific changes in maximal oxygen uptake resulting from arm versus leg training', *Ergonomics* 21: 1–9.

Stegemann, J. (translated by J. S. Skinner) (1981) *Exercise Physiology*, Chicago, Year Book Medical Publishers.

Sports (1986) 'Regeneration alternatives in high performance sport', February.

—— (1986) 'Recovery: Part two — Overtraining', August.

Talyshev, F. (1977) 'Recovery', *Legkaya Atletika* 6: 25–9.

Tanigawa, M. C. (1972) 'Comparison of the hold-relax procedure and passive mobilization on increasing muscle length, *Physical Therapy* 52: 725–35.

Taylor, D. E. M. (1979) 'Human endurance — Mind or muscle?', *British Journal of Sports Medicine* 12: 179–84.

Telford, R. D., Minikin, B. R., Hooper, L. A., Hahn, A.G., and Tumilty, D. M. (1987) 'The Tri-level Fitness Profile', *Excel* 4 (1): 11–13.

Tharp, G. D., Johnson, G. O., and Thorland, W. G. (1984) 'Measurement of anaerobic power and capacity in élite young track athletes using the Wingate test', *Journal of Sports Medicine and Physical Fitness* 24: 100–5.

Thorstensson, A., and Karlsson, J. (1974) 'The effect of strength training on muscle enzymes related to high energy phosphate metabolism', *Acta Physiologica Scandinavia* 91 (3): 21a.

——, Hulten, B., von Doblen, W., and Karlsson, J. (1976) 'Effect of strength training on enzyme activities and fiber characteristics in human skeletal muscle', *Acta Physiologica Scandinavica* 96: 392–8.

Travers, P. (1973) 'A regular warmup is advisable', *Swimming Coach* 66: 12.

Turner, A. A. (1977) 'The effects of two methods of flexibility training on joint movements'. Unpublished Master's thesis, Lakehead University, Canada.

Vandervoot, A. A., Sale, D. G., and Moroz, J. (1984) 'Comparison of motor unit activation during unilateral and bilateral leg extension', *Journal of Applied Physiology: Respiratory, Environmental, and Exercise Physiology* 56: 46–51.

Viitasalo, J. T. (1988) 'Evaluation of explosive strength for young and adult athletes', *Research Quarterly for Exercise and Sport* 59: 9–13.

Wankel, L. M., and Kreisel, P. (1982) 'Methodological considerations in measuring sport motivation: A comparison of open-minded and structured appraisals' in L. M. Wankel and R. B. Wilberg (eds), *Psychology of Sport and Motor Behavior: Research and Practice*, Edmonton, University of Alberta.

Weber, S., and Kraus, H. (1949) 'Passive and active stretching of muscles', *The Physical Therapy Review* 29: 407–10.

Weitzman, E. D., Kripke, D. F., Goldmacher, D., McGregor, P., and Nogeire, C. (1970) 'Acute reversal of the sleep–waking cycle in man: Effect on sleep stage patterns', *Archives of Neurology* 22: 483–9.

Wenger, H. A., and Green, H. J. (1982) *Physiological Testing of the Elite Athlete*, Ottawa, Canadian Association of Sport Sciences.

Whitehead, N. (1975) *Conditioning for Sport*, Wakefield, UK, EP Publishing.

Whithers, R. T., Maricic, A., Wasilewski, S., and Kelly, L. (1982) 'Match analysis of Australian professional soccer players', *Journal of Human Movement Studies* 8: 159–66.

Wilmore, J. H. (1974) 'Alterations in strength, body composition, and anthropometric measurements consequent to a ten-week weight training program', *Medicine and Science in Sports* 6: 133–8.

Williams, L. R. T., McEwan, E. A. S., Watkins, C. D., Gillespie, L., and Boyd, H. 'Motor learning and performance and physical fatigue and the specificity principle', *Canadian Journal of Applied Sport Sciences* 4: 302–8.

Wilt, F. (1975) 'Plyometrics, what it is — how it works', *Athletic Journal* 76: 89–90.

Woodman, L. E., and Pyke, F. S. (1990) 'Physiology of football training and performance' in *Level 2 Coaching Manual*, Jolimont, Victoria, National Football League of Australia.

Worthington, A. J. (1975) 'Causes and prevention of hamstring injuries', *Track Technique* 61: 1950–1.

Yakimovich, D. (1986) 'Why does running speed drop?', *Soviet Sports Review* 21: 22–3.

Index